NEW TRENDS IN CANCER FOR THE 21ST CENTURY

ADVANCES IN EXPERIMENTAL MEDICINE AND BIOLOGY

A Continuation Order Plan is available for this series. A continuation order will bring delivery of each new volume immediately upon publication. Volumes are billed only upon actual shipment. For further information please contact the publisher.

NEW TRENDS IN CANCER FOR THE 21ST CENTURY

Edited by

Antonio Llombart-Bosch

University of Valencia
Valencia, Spain

and

Vicente Felipo

Valencian Foundation for Biomedical Research
Valencia, Spain

Springer Science+Business Media, LLC

Library of Congress Cataloging-in-Publication Data

International Symposium on Cancer "New Trends in Cancer for the 21st Century" (2002:
Valencia, Spain)
    New trends in cancer for the 21st century/edited by Antonio Llombart-Bosch and
Vicente Felipo.
        p.   ; cm. — (Advances in experimental medicine and biology; v. 532)
    Includes bibliographical references and index.
    ISBN 978-1-4613-4914-3   ISBN 978-1-4615-0081-0 (eBook)
    DOI 10.1007/978-1-4615-0081-0
        1. Cancer—Treatment—Congresses.   2. Cancer—Molecular aspects—Congresses.   I.
Llombart Bosch, Antonio.   II. Felipo, Vicente.   III. Title.   IV. Series.
        [DNLM: 1. Neoplasms—immunology—Congresses.   2. Neoplasms—therapy—Congresses.
3. Angiogenesis Factor—therapeutic use—Congresses.   4. Antineoplastic
Agents—therapeutic use—Congresses.   QZ 266 1609n 2003]
    RC270.8.I5286 2003
    616.99'406—dc21

                                                                        2003047451

Proceedings of the International Symposium on Cancer: New Trends in Cancer for the 21st Century, held
November 10–13, 2002, in Valencia, Spain

ISBN 978-1-4613-4914-3

©2003 Springer Science+Business Media New York
Originally published by Kluwer Academic/Plenum Publishers, New York in 2003
Softcover reprint of the hardcover 1st edition 2003

http://www.wkap.nl/

10   9   8   7   6   5   4   3   2   1

A C.I.P. record for this book is available from the Library of Congress

Permissions for books published in Europe: *permissions@wkap.nl*
Permissions for books published in the United States of America: *permissions@wkap.com*

In Memoriam of Ms. Ana Viñes Rubert

PREFACE

This volume contains the majority of the conferences presented at the International Symposium on Cancer "New Trends in Cancer for the 21st Century", held in Valencia, Spain, November 10-13, 2002. This Simposium was one of the activities of the Cátedra Santiago Grisolía and of the Fundación Museu de les Ciències "Píncipe Felipe" of Valencia.

It is estimated that every year nearly 3 million Europeans develop cancer, leading to 750.000 deaths per year. This represents a tremendous burden that cannot be ignored by politicians and citizens, taking into account that these deaths occur not only in an ageing population but also in children and in adults in the most active period of their lives. The probability of cure for cancer patients, considering all types of cancer, within the different states of the European Union (EU), ranges from between one fourth and one half, and the survival rates in different European populations varies widely being low in western Europe. Everybody is conscious that cancer in Europe is without doubt a major health problem. Therefore greater effort is needed to achieve better results in decreasing both the incidence and the mortality.

In this sense, the European Parliament under the auspices of the European Commission Research Directorate-General has expressed the need for a more active policy in order to develop new strategies in prevention, cancer care and research. The following needs have been identified: a) developing evidence-based guidelines for early detection, diagnosis, treatment and after-care for the most common types of cancer; b) cancer research should be oriented towards a more interdisciplinary approach and should receive more financial support; c) more research on courses of treatment, introducing independent clinical assays on a higher number of patients; d) comparative research on the cost-effectiveness of various detection and treatment methods in order to increase efficiency and reduce costs in the health care system; e) development of European modules for continued training in research and of clinical specialists in the various fields; and f) to ensure that the existing networks can continue their successful activity in the future and that new ones will be created.

The main objective of the Symposium *"New Trends in Cancer for the 21st Century"* was to join outstanding scientists from over the world who develop their activities in different areas of the fight against cancer, giving them the opportunity to improve their knowledge in other areas and exchange ideas and information.

The causes of cancer and the many factors which influence its emergence are very complex and heterogeneous. The malignant transformed cell contains signals that stimulate or inhibit the disease and arise from the stepwise accumulation of genetic changes that confer the mutated cell the properties of unlimited growth and resistance to homeostatic regulatory mechanisms.

One of the main targets in cancer is the cell cycle machinery which is controlled by a number of extrinsic signals and tumour suppressor proteins that decide whether the cell should remain quiescent or enter into active growth and division. This decision is mainly taken at the restriction point at the middle of the G1 phase, but there are certain checkpoints that ensure the correct transition of each phase through the cell cycle. Several animal models have been developed with the aim of understanding the role played by the different elements integrating these cell cycle checkpoints. These animal models may be a valuable tool to design and validate new therapeutic strategies against tumor development.

From the pathological point of view, the diagnosis and clinical classification of tumours is based mainly upon the recognition of the microscopical tumoral pattern with the support of immunophenotyping and some other emerging molecular techniques that help to distinguish several tumor subtypes and grades and correlate them with the clinical stage and response to treatment. However, the molecular heterogeneity of cancer cells and of their supporting stroma and vascularization, produces numerous biological variations, within morphologically similar malignancies, that currently escape the current possibilities of diagnosis and prognosis and therefore to a rational therapeutic approach. The development of a novel and sophisticated technology for the study of tumour profiling, both at the genetic level (genetics and epigenetics) and at protein expression profiles (proteomics), is opening doors to what is considered the *new molecular pathology*. This represents an exceptional opportunity for histopathology since with the expansion of a large number of assayable markers, it is now possible to gather a better molecular portrait of tumors.

Most tumors acquire the capacity of invasion and metastasis and escape the barriers of the host's immune system. One of the main focuses of attention in this sense is the study of the phenomenon of angiogenesis: structural bases and main molecular players, as well as the therapeutic possibilities that exist to abrogate this process in tumors. On the other hand, stimulation of the host immune system by means of newly developed anti-tumoral vaccines has opened one of the most exciting fields in the fight against cancer.

The search for and development of new therapeutic drugs directed against specific targets such as inhibitors of tyrosin kinase receptors or monoclonal antibodies which down-regulate the hyperactive function of some oncogenes, has considerably improved the outcome for several patients (Phase II and III studies) which on the contrary would have approached to the outcome.

Special mention in the fight against cancer has to be made of organizations such as the EORTC (European Organization for Research and Treatment of Cancer), the OECI (Organization of European Cancer Institutes) and the comprehensive cancer centers that promote and co-ordinate high-quality laboratory research and clinical trials and also provide central facilities with scientific expertise and administrative support for this network of scientists and clinical investigators.

This book provides, therefore, an update on the knowledge on certain crucial aspects regarding the latest aspects on research in the field of cancer, such as basic diagnostic and therapeutic research.

We would like to express our gratitude to all the participants for their written contributions and for their enlightened and fruitful discussion.

We also acknowledge with deep gratitude the Gomez Mata family who take the initiative and provided financial support to organize this Symposium to honour the memory of Ms Ana Viñes Rubert who died of cancer. This represents an exceptional example of the society's feelings about this disease.

We also thank the Department of Pathology of the University of Valencia, the Fundación Instituto Valenciano de Oncología, the Oficina de Ciencia y Tecnología de la Generalitat Valenciana, the Catedra Santiago Grisolía and the Museo Principe Felipe of the Ciudad de las Artes y las Ciencias of Valencia, which provided the personnel and the facilities to organize both the Symposium and the sessions.

Antonio Llombart-Bosch
Vicente Felipo

CONTENTS

DRIVING THE CELL CYCLE TO CANCER

Marcos Malumbres[1], Sarah L. Hunt, Rocío Sotillo, Javier Martín, Jun Odajima, Alberto Martín, Pierre Dubus*, Sagrario Ortega and Mariano Barbacid

Molecular Oncology Progamme, Centro Nacional de Investigaciones Oncológicas Madrid, Spain and *University of Bourdeaux, Bourdeaux, France

ABSTRACT

Cell cycle progression requires the co-ordinated activation of several kinases, some of which are activated upon the binding of a cyclin subunit. At least four of these so-called cyclin-dependent kinases, namely Cdk4, Cdk6, Cdk2 and Cdk1, have specific roles at particular stages of the cell cycle, including passage through the various cell cycle transitions and the response to specific checkpoints. Not surprisingly, most human tumors carry mutations that deregulate at least one of these kinases. To analyze their specific role in vivo, we are generating strains of gene-targeted mice carrying either activated or defective alleles of these Cdks. As an example, Cdk4 expression appears to be expendable in most cell types since mice lacking Cdk4 are viable. Yet, Cdk4 mutant mice are smaller in size and infertile (only partial infertility in males). In addition, Cdk4 defective mice develop insulin dependent diabetes early in life. However, the importance of these Cdks in tumor cell cycles is underscored by the phenotype of knock in mice where the normal Cdk4 gene has been replaced by a Cdk4 R24C (insensitive to INK inhibitors) mutant. These animals develop a wide spectrum of spontaneous tumors and are highly susceptible to specific carcinogenic treatments. These models are being used now to understand how deregulation of these Cdks leads to cancer development and will be a valuable tool to design and validate new therapeutic strategies against tumour development.

---

[1] Correspondence: Marcos Malumbres (marcos.malumbres@cnio.es), Centro Nacional de Investigaciones Oncológicas, C/ Melchor Fernández Almagro 3, E-28029, Madrid

New Trends in Cancer for the 21ˢᵗ Century, edited by
Llombart-Bosch and Felipo, Kluwer Academic/Plenum Publishers, 2003

CANCER AS A CELL CYCLE DISEASE

Tumours are the consequence of a process of clonal selection in which multiple alterations, such as oncogene activation or the loss of tumour suppressers, are accumulated and give selective advantage to the cells that carry them. The outcome is the generation of a cellular clone with aberrant growth, and, in some cases, even metastatic properties. However, it is not clear yet how many different regulatory pathways must be altered in order to generate tumour cells and whether these pathways are the same in all the different types of cancer. Hanahan and Weinberg[1] have suggested that all cancer phenotypes are the manifestation of six essential physiological alterations shared by most, and perhaps all, types of human tumour. Self-sufficiency in growth signals, insensitivity to growth inhibitory signals and evasion of programmed cell death are alterations that uncouple the growth program of the cell from environmental signals. On the other hand, tumours frequently acquire new capabilities that bypass the normal anticancer defence mechanisms. These include the evasion of internal controls that regulate and limit replicative potential, the ability to form new blood vessels and properties such invasion and metastasis.

Although breaching of these physiological barriers seems to be necessary for most tumours to achieve full malignancy, cancer is increasingly viewed as a cell cycle disease. This view reflects the evidence that the vast majority of the tumours have suffered defects that derail the cell cycle machinery, leading to increased cell proliferation. Such defects can target either components of the cell cycle itself or elements of upstream signalling cascades that ultimately converge to trigger cell cycle events. Whilst consideration of cancer as a disease of the cell cycle implies that every tumour is defective in one or more aspect of cell cycle control, it clearly does not infer that oncogenesis targets only the cell division machinery. It simply regards cell cycle deregulation as an essential step in the process of tumorigenesis.

REGULATION OF CELL CYCLE ENTRY AND G1/S TRANSITION

Most cell cycle components so far implicated as targets of tumorigenic aberrations directly or indirectly control G1 progression and the G1/S transition. More specifically, these molecules regulate the Restriction point in the mid-to-late G1 phase and the onset of DNA replication. Why do defects of this transition, rather than S, G2 or M phases, provide such a growth advantage to tumour cells? Although speculative at present, the reason for this selectivity may reflect the decisive role of G1/S events in the commitment of differentiated cells to cell division. DNA replication, that takes place in S-phase, is extremely costly in terms of energy. Therefore not surprising that at this stage cells are already committed to continue the cell cycle unless catastrophic problems impair progression in subsequent phases. If such catastrophes do occur, cell cycle progression will be halted by the appropriate checkpoints. Before starting S phase, however, cells have to ensure that environmental conditions are appropriate for cell division. This decision is taken in response to a number of regulatory pathways that receive and integrate mitogenic signals and regulate the passage through the Restriction point[2-4]. Beyond this point, cells –at least those in tissue culture– are committed to complete a round of cellular division, independently of the stimulation by growth factors. Relaxed constraints on G1/S control therefore provide a direct and selective growth advantage. In the S phase, there is a branching in the proliferation pathway due to the activation of a large spectrum of transcription target. This very divergence in the signalling cascade makes it most unlikely that defects in the S/G2/M phase regulators would lead to a complete program of cell division. Any attempt to trigger incomplete cell cycles would either activate checkpoints to arrest or eliminate such defective cells, or would cause gross chromosomal changes mostly incompatible with cell proliferation[5-6].

Progression through the G1/S phases of the cell cycle is controlled mostly by three cyclin-dependent kinases (Cdk4, Cdk6 and Cdk2) and their substrates (Figure 1)[2, 4]. These Cdks phosphorylate and inactivate the retinoblastoma family of proteins (pRb, p107 and p130). The pRb proteins function in the repression of transcription through the binding and inactivation of transcription factors, such as E2F members (E2F1-5), and the binding to histone deacetylases (HDAC) and chromatin remodelling complexes[7, 8]. The initial phosphorylation of pRb induced by Cdk4 and Cdk6 partially inactivates pRb, resulting in the release of HDAC and the induction of the transcription of some genes including the E-type cyclins[8, 9]. These cyclins bind to and activate Cdk2, a kinase that is able to further phosphorylate pRb as well as other substrates[2]. Complete inactivation of pRb liberates the E2F transcription factors, activating the transcription of many genes needed for DNA replication, mitosis or the control of cell cycle progression beyond the R point. Consequently, the A-type cyclins, that are also partners of Cdk2, are now induced and participate in the phosphorylation of new Cdk2 substrates during S phase.

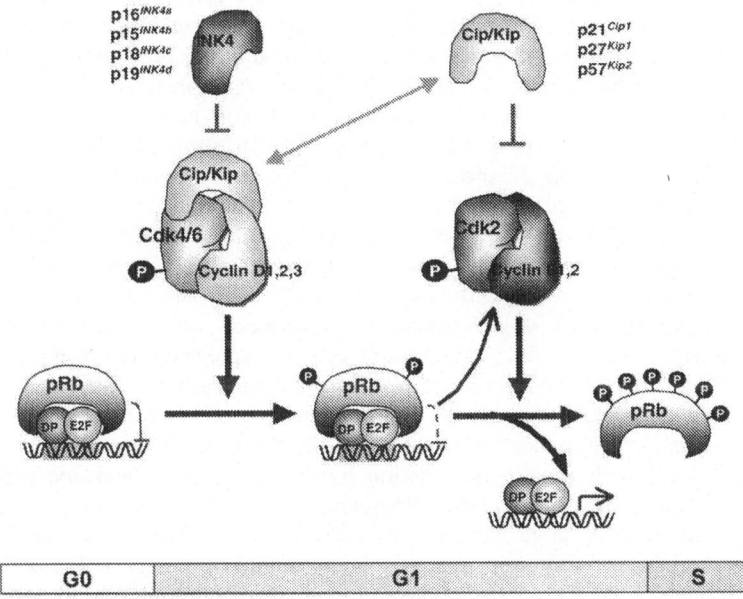

Figure 1. Control of G1 progression and the G1/S transition by the Cdk4/6 and Cdk2 kinases. Most molecules shown here are either oncogenes or tumor suppressors.

Regulation of these cell cycle kinases is therefore tightly controlled at different levels including interaction with positive and negative partners, regulation by phosphorylation, and subcellular localisation[2, 4, 10-11]. As previously discussed, the Cdks are activated by binding to specific cyclin subunits which provide residues for substrate recognition and induce changes in the Cdk conformation that allow kinase activity.

Cdk4 and Cdk6 are activated by the D-type cyclins (cyclin D1, D2 and D3) in G1 phase, Cdk2, by the E-type cyclins (E1 and E2) in mid G1, and A-type cyclins (A1 and A2) in late G1/S phase. Two families of Cdk inhibitors have been described: the INK4 family (p16^{INK4a}, p15^{INK4b}, p18^{INK4c} and p19^{INK4d}), and the Cip/Kip family (p21^{Cip1}, p27^{Kip1} and p57^{Kip2}). INK4 proteins specifically bind to and inhibit Cdk4 and Cdk6[2, 11, 12]. Cip/Kip proteins, on the other hand, are able to bind all Cdks. Whilst their interaction which Cdk2 complexes clearly blocks kinase activity, their role in Cdk4/6 inhibition is unclear. Indeed, Cdk4/6–cyclin D heterodimers can bind Cip/Kip inhibitors at stochiometric concentrations without losing their kinase activity[13-15]. It has been proposed that this interaction titrates these inhibitors away from Cdk2–cyclin E complexes facilitating the activation of the Cdk2 kinase[2]. These mechanisms are in agreement with results obtained with gene-targeted mice[16-18]. Gene replacement of cyclin D1 by cyclin E1 in the mouse restores most of the phenotypic defects of cyclin-D1-defective animals[16]. The most likely explanation is that one of the major roles of cyclin D1 in vivo is to activate Cdk2–cyclin E1 complexes. Likewise, loss of p27^{Kip1} in mice lacking cyclin D1 restores some of their phenotypic defects[17, 18].

CELL CYCLE DEREGULATION IN HUMAN CANCER

It has been shown that most, if not all tumours, lose control of the G1/S transition through alterations in the pRb pathway[3, 4, 19]. Most of these mutations occur in G1 regulators, thus underscoring the importance of maintaining proper control of cell cycle commitment to prevent human cancer. They include overexpression of cyclins (mainly D1 and E1) and Cdks (mainly Cdk4 and Cdk6) as well as loss of CKI expression (mainly p16^{INK4a}, p15^{INK4b} and p27^{Kip1}) and of pRb proteins. Tumour-associated changes in the expression of these regulators frequently result from chromosome alterations (amplification of cyclin D1 or Cdk4, translocation of Cdk6 and deletions of INK4 proteins or pRb) or epigenetic inactivation (methylation of INK4 or pRb promoters). Miscoding mutations in Cdk4 and Cdk6 resulting in loss of INK4 binding have also been identified, albeit with low frequency[20, 21].

Interestingly, although direct genetic or epigenetic alteration of Cdk2 or its regulators have rarely been described, loss of p27^{Kip1} expression and overexpression of cyclin E1 are among the most frequent events in human tumours. The levels of p27^{Kip1} protein dramatically decrease during tumour development and progression in some epithelial, lymphoid and endocrine tissues and this decrease occurs mainly at the post-translational level with protein degradation by the ubiquitin-proteasome pathway. In fact, these changes in the expression frequently correlate with poor prognosis in a variety of tumours. A large number of studies have characterised p27^{Kip1} as an independent prognostic factor in human cancers including breast, colon and prostate adenocarcinomas[22]. The involvement of p21^{Cip1} gene in human tumorigenesis however seems to be very sporadic since only a few tumour samples analysed show functional alteration in p21^{Cip1}. The third member of the family, p57^{Kip2}, is located on 11p15.5, a region implicated in both sporadic cancers and Beekwith-Wiedemann syndrome (BWS), a inherited syndrome that predisposes to tumour development. p57^{Kip2} inactivating mutations have been found in 10-20% of BWS patients.

How p27^{Kip1} and cyclin E1 expression is altered in tumour cells is not well understood yet. p27^{Kip1} degradation in tumours is mediated by the proteosome machinery. In fact, Skp2, a F-box protein involved in p27^{Kip1} degradation in G1, S and G2 phases[23], is altered in some tumour cells and has oncogenic properties[24, 25]. On the other hand, the F-box responsible for cyclin E1 degradation (hCdc4/Fbw7/Ago) is a putative tumour suppresser and is mutated and inactivated in some cancer cell lines[26, 27]. Alternatively, cancer-associated cyclin E overexpression could be explained in most tumours by the deregulated Cdk4/6 activity or pRb inactivation.

Within the pRb protein family, loss or inactivation of pRb is a rather frequent event in human tumours[19]. Children that inherit one defective autosomal allele have a high probability (>95%) of developing bilateral multifocal tumours of the retina (retinoblastoma) and are predisposed to other types of tumours later in life such as osteosarcomas, melanoma and brain tumours. Somatic alterations of the pRb locus have also been found in sporadic tumours such as lung, breast and bladder carcinomas (Table 1) and, in fact, the loss of pRb function in sporadic cancer is more frequent than in inherited eye tumours. In retinoblastoma, small cell lung carcinoma, bladder carcinoma and many sarcomas, pRb function is lost directly through mutations within the pRb gene. In many cases, tumours with wild-type pRb protein lose other tumour suppressers in the same pathway such as the cell cycle inhibitor p16[INK4a]. In addition to genetic and epigenetic (promoter hypermethylation) alterations in the pRb locus, pRb function can also be altered by the effect of several viral proteins, such as the human papillomavirus E7 oncoprotein, E1A, Large T antigen and the LNA viral oncoprotein from Kaposi's sarcoma-associated herpes virus[20]. Among the other members of the family, p130 is less frequently lost and p107 inactivation has not been reported[28]. These observations suggest that p107 and p130 may play a primary role in promoting differentiation rather than proliferation, a concept supported by results obtained with gene-targeted mice[29].

Table 1. Cell cycle regulatory elements altered in human neoplasia

Molecule	Alteration	Representative Tumor
Cdk4	Amplification, Mutation	Sarcomas, melanoma
Cdk6	Translocation, overexpression	Leukemia/lymphoma, gliomas, melanoma
Cdk2	Amplification	Hepatocellular carcinoma
Cyclin D1	Amplification, translocation, overexpression	Breast and prostate cancer, parathyroid adenoma, gastric and esophagic carcinoma, multiple myeloma
Cyclin D2	Overexpression	Germ-line tumors
Cyclin D3	Overexpression	Breast carcinoma, lymphoma, leukemia
Cyclin E1	Overexpression	Breast, ovary and gastric carcinoma
Cyclin A1	Overexpression	Hepatocellular carcinoma
p16INK4a	Deletion, Mutation, Methylation	Melanoma, lymphoma/leukemia, lung cancer, pancreatic carcinoma
p15INK4b	Deletion, Methylation	Leukemia/lymphoma
p27Kip1	Reduced protein levels/protein degradation	Colon, breast, prostate and other tumors
p57Kip2	Mutation	Beekwith-Wiedemann Syndrom
Cdc25A	Overexpression	Head and neck cancer, lung tumors
Cdc25B	Overexpression	Breast cancer, lymphomas, head and neck cancer, lung tumors
pRb	Deletion, mutation, methylation	Retinoblastoma, melanoma, lung tumors, sarcoma and bladder carcinoma
p130	Deletion, mutation	Breast, head and neck tumors and melanoma
Plk1	Overexpression, mutation	Lung tumors, melanoma, esophageal carcinoma, head and neck carcinoma
Aurora A & B	Overexpression	Breast, gastric and colorectal cancer
Cables	Deletion	Colon and head and neck tumors

As a direct consequence of the functional inactivation of pRb, E2Fs are liberated from pRb control and the progression of cells into late G1 and S becomes unconstrained. Consistent with a role for E2F activation in cancer development, several E2F family member genes have been shown to function as oncogenes in culture. Deregulated expression of E2F1, in co-operation with an activated Ras gene, can lead to oncogenic transformation of primary rat embryo cells. Cells transformed by E2F1 and Ras form foci, grow in soft agar, and form tumours when injected into nude mice. On its own, E2F1 confers anchorage-independent growth to immortalised murine cells. E2F2, E2F3, E2F4, and DP1 have each been shown to behave as an oncogene when tested in similar transformation assays. However, in spite of their central role in cell cycle regulation, deregulated E2F expression in human cancer has been rarely observed. Overexpression of E2F-1 has been reported in some human neoplasias such as lung tumours, although decreased expression has also been described in breast carcinomas[20].

Other proteins involved in the regulation of the G1/S kinases are also under investigation in cancer development although their causal role in human cancer is not clear yet. The Cdc25 phosphatases (Cdc25A, Cdc25B and Cdc25C) activate Cdks by removing inhibitory phosphates and are therefore candidate protooncogenes. In fact, Cdc25A or B but not C phosphatases accelerate G1/S transition leading to premature activation of Cdk2 and cooperate with both oncogenic Ras and loss of pRb in foci formation in rodent cells. Human Cdc25A maps to 3p21, a locus frequently involved in renal carcinomas, lung small cell carcinomas and benign tumours of the salivary gland. Cdc25A or Cdc25B are overexpressed in several tumour types such as head and neck cancer, gastric carcinomas, oesophageal squamous cell carcinomas, lung tumours, colorectal carcinoma, ovarian cancer, non-Hodgkin lymphomas and breast cancer [20].

Finally, some tumours display additional alterations in the proteins involved in the mitotic checkpoint. After all, chromosomal instability and aneuploidy, two events controlled during the M phase of the cycle, are hallmarks of cancer cells. Proper distribution of chromosomes among daughter cells is controlled by the spindle assembly checkpoint that separates metaphase from anaphase, two clearly defined stages within mitosis. Some molecules involved in controlling the spindle assembly checkpoint have been implicated in human cancer. They include Bub1, the polo-like kinase 1 (Plk1), two members of the Aurora family of protein kinases, Aurora-A and Aurora-B, and securin. In addition, Chfr1 –a ligase that ubiquitinates Plk1 and inhibits Cdk1 at the G2 to M transition– is also inactivated by hypermethylation in some lung tumours[4, 30].

GENETIC MODELS OF TUMOR DEVELOPMENT

Genetic analysis of cell cycle regulators has provided us with new insights on their roles in cell cycle control and the effect of their alteration in tumour development[21, 31]. Early gene targeting studies showed that pRb deficiency is lethal in mouse developing embryos, whereas pRb$^{+/-}$ mice develop tumours of endocrine origin (pituitary, thyroid and adrenal medulla). In contrast, deletion of the other pocket proteins, p107 or p130, has few or no effect on mouse embryonic development or tumour susceptibility[29]. Combined deficiency of pRb and p107, however, causes retinoblastoma in the mouse, showing that these proteins are partially overlapping in tumour suppression.

Genetic analysis of the function of cell cycle inhibitors has also resulted in several models of tumour development. Knockout mice for each of the INK4 proteins have been generated[21]. These mice develop normally to adulthood and are fertile, indicating that the individual INK4 proteins are not essential for development. However, p16^{INK4a}

deficiency results in a low susceptibility to spontaneous tumour development and increased tumour susceptibility under specific carcinogenic protocols. p15[INK4b] knock out mice develop lymphoproliferative disorders such as extramedullar hematopoiesis in the spleen and formation of secondary follicles in lymph nodes. Although lymphomas are rare (less than 1%), these animals develop other types of tumours, mostly hemangiosarcomas, albeit with low incidence (about 8%) and long latency. Mice lacking p18[INK4c] are larger than the wild-type littermates, although differences in size vary with their genetic background. These mutant mice develop pituitary hyperplasia that often progresses to form pituitary adenomas. They also display other types of neoplasias including testicular tumours, pheochromocytomas, hemangiosarcomas, lymphomas and renal cell carcinomas with limited incidence (5 to 20%). Finally, mice lacking p19[INK4d] are normal and fertile and do not develop tumours. Multiple mutants have also been derived from these strains [21, 31].

Ablation of p27[Kip1] in the mouse results in organomegaly and high penetrance of pituitary tumours. In addition, this protein is haplo-insufficient for tumour suppression, suggesting a functional effect for the decreased expression frequently observed in human tumours. p21[Cip1]-null mice also develop a variety of tumours (mainly sarcomas, B-cell lymphomas) although with long latency[21, 31].

CDK4 DEREGULATION: A CENTRAL MOTIF IN TUMOUR DEVELOPMENT

The functional characterisation of the Cyclin/Cdk4/INK4/pRb pathway in tumour development has been experimentally addressed in mouse models. Transgenic mice overexpressing D-type cyclins in various cell types or mice deficient in INK4 proteins or partially deficient in pRb develop spontaneous tumours and have been reviewed elsewhere[31, 32]. Cdk4 has also been expressed as a transgene in some particular tissues, such as the lens crystal or the epidermis, as well as in astrocytes. Although the sole overexpression of Cdk4 did not result in proliferation in terminally differentiated lens cells[33], expression of a transgenic human Cdk4 cDNA under K5 promoter resulted in hyperproliferation of the epidermis and mild hyperkeratosis[34]. This phenotype was also accompanied of changes in the dermis, such as dermal fibrosis and a decrease in the adipose tissue. Cdk4 overexpression in the epidermis also resulted in hypertrophy (detected by the presence of large nuclei) in addition to hyperplasia. Strikingly, these Cdk4 transgenics resulted in a stronger phenotype than transgenic mice carrying cyclin D1, D2 or D3 under the same promoter. The epidermis thickness of the K5-Cdk4 mice increased twofold whereas in the K5-D-type cyclin animals it increased an average of 1.25-fold[34-36]. These results were unexpected because Cdk4 was thought, from in vitro data, to be non-limiting whereas cyclin availability is usually limiting in several cultured cell types.

Recently, knock-in mice expressing the melanoma-associated mutated form of Cdk4 —Cdk4 R24C[37, 38]— have been developed and characterized[39-42]. Knock-in mice expressing normal levels of this mutant in the Cdk4 endogenous locus develop normally and are fertile[39]. However, they are slightly larger (about 10-20%) than their wild type littermates, and display progressive hyperplasia in the same endocrine cells that required Cdk4 expression to proliferate: pancreatic □ cells, Leydig cells and adenohypophysis cells[39, 41, 42]. This hyperplastic growth often results in the appearance of insulinomas, Leydig cell tumours and pituitary tumours after longer latencies (10 to 18 months). In addition, Cdk4 R24C mice develop a wide range of other tumours that include epithelial (lung and liver tumours), mesenchymal (hemangiosarcomas) and lymphoid malignancies (Figure 2)[40, 41]. As expected, the major malignancies observed in Cdk4 R24C mice also occur in mice lacking one or more INK4 inhibitors. For instance, soft-tissue sarcomas —responsible for more than half of the deaths in Cdk4 R24C mice— are also the most frequent tumour type in p15[INK4b]-deficient animals[43] and p16[INK4a]-null mice[44]. Similarly, pituitary tumours develop in most p18[INK4c] knock-out mice[43, 45]. Hematopoietic hyperproliferative disorders as well as renal cysts and mammary gland ectasia observed in p16[INK4a], p15[INK4b] and p18[INK4c] have also been observed in Cdk4 R24C mice[41, 43, 44].

Cdk4 R24C mice are also highly susceptible to tumour development upon carcinogenic insult. For instance, treatment of Cdk4 R24C mice with the classical DMBA/TPA skin tumorigenesis protocol results in more abundant and more aggressive skin carcinomas[42]. This suggests that the Cdk4 mutation harbors the propensity to act in concert with distinct oncogenic or chemical carcinogenic events to further worsen the cancerous state. In fact, this treatment leads to the rapid onset of invasive melanomas[42], a malignancy that we have not observed in untreated Cdk4 R24C mice. In a parallel treatment, p15[INK4b]- or p18[INK4c]-deficient mice did not develop invasive melanomas although p18[INK4c]-null mice showed premalignant lesions and faster proliferation of melanocytes[42]. p16[INK4a]-deficient mice were subjected to similar carcinogenic protocols with DMBA alone, resulting in a lower incidence of melanomas[44, 46]. Unfortunately, the differences in the carcinogenic protocol make difficult the direct comparison of the melanoma susceptibility between Cdk4 R24C and p16[INK4a]-deficient mice. However, the fact that the absence of p18[INK4c] favors melanocyte proliferation suggests a compensatory role for INK4 proteins in preventing melanoma development.

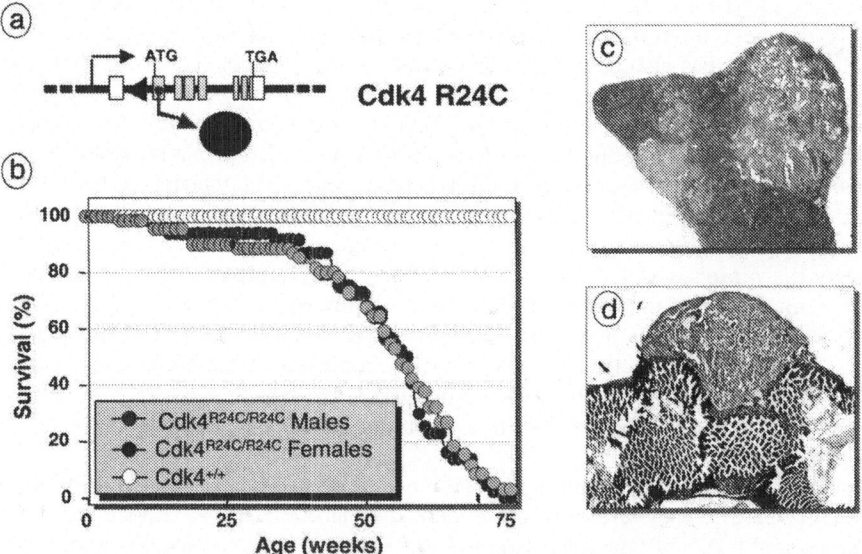

Figure 2. The Cdk4 R24C knock in mice. a, The normal Cdk4 allele was substituted by a R24C mutant in the endogenous locus that is therefore driven by the normal Cdk4 regulatory sequences. The triangle in intron 1 represents a loxP site (34 bp) as a result of the targeting strategy. b, Survival curve of Cdk4 R24C mice compared to wild-type animals. c, Representative sarcoma of the spleen in Cdk4 R24C knock in mice. d, Metastasis of a sarcoma in the gut.

CONCLUDING REMARKS

Lessons from the molecular analysis of human tumours as well as from the generation of gene targeted mice have taught us that minor alterations in the balance that controls the activity of some cell cycle regulators almost invariably result in neoplastic proliferation. In general, most, if not all, neoplasias show a deregulated cell cycle. Imbalances in the specific molecular sensors that control the progression through G1 and the G1/S transition, such as loss of cell cycle inhibitors or overexpression of cyclins, may cooperate to trigger malignant transformation. Some of the alterations, such as overexpression of cyclin E1 or inactivation of p27[Kip1] —which have prognostic value— have an unknown genetic origin and the identification of the mechanistic basis for these defects is a challenge for the next years. All these observations strongly implicate that G1 and G1/S Cdk activity should be a primary target to control neoplastic proliferation[4]. Targeting the cell cycle regulatory machinery, and specifically the Cdks, is being currently explored in both academia and pharmaceutical companies to develop new anticancer drugs. However, in spite of the extensive molecular characterisation of cell cycle control mechanisms, we still do not know whether the "ideal" therapeutic drug should target Cdk4/6, Cdk2, or even Cdk1 activity or a combination of them. Recently, a few "first generation" compounds have entered clinical trials with promising results although their specificity is not well defined[47].

From human tumours and mouse models, it is now clear that misregulation of Cdk4/6 activity by either overexpression of D-type cyclins or loss of INK4 proteins almost invariably leads to hyperproliferative defects and eventually to tumour development. First, many genetic mutations in human tumours affect Cdk4/6 regulation. Second, knock-in mice expressing a deregulated Cdk4 develop a wide spectrum of spontaneous tumours confirming the central role of Cdk4 in the entry into the cell cycle. Moreover, since this mutation only affects the ability of INK4 proteins to inhibit Cdk4, these results suggest the importance of this inhibition in maintaining the postmitotic state in adult cells. These observations, taken together, illustrate that regardless of whether Cdk4 is essential or not for G1 progression (see above), its deregulation dramatically affects those requirements that allow cells to enter the cell cycle.

Acknowledgements

This work was supported by grants from the Comunidad de Madrid, and the Fundación Ramón Areces (to M.M.) and Spanish Ministerio de Ciencia y Tecnología (to M.M. and M.B.).

References

1. Hanahan, D. and Weinberg, R.A. (2000) The hallmarks of cancer. Cell 100, 57-70.
2. Sherr, C.J. and Roberts, J.M. (1999) CDK inhibitors: positive and negative regulators of G1-phase progression. Genes Dev. 13, 1501-1512.
3. Sherr, C.J. (2000) Cancer cell cycles revisited. Cancer Res. 60, 3689-3695.
4. Malumbres, M. and Barbacid, M. (2001) To cycle or not to cycle: a critical decision in cancer. Nat. Rev. Cancer 1, 222-231.
5. Hartwell, L.H. and Weinert, T.A. (1989) Checkpoints: controls that ensure the order of cell cycle events. Science 246, 629-634.
6. Paulovich, A.G., Toczyski, D.P. and Hartwell, L.H. (1997) When checkpoints fail. Cell 88, 315-321.
7. Dyson, N. (1998) The regulation of E2F by pRB-family proteins. Genes Dev. 12, 2245-2262

8. Harbour, J.W. and Dean, D.C. (2000) The pRb/E2F pathway: expanding roles and emerging paradigms. Genes Dev. 14, 2393-2409.
9. Nevins, J.R. (2001) The Rb/E2F pathway and cancer. Hum. Mol. Genet. 10, 699-703.
10. Morgan, D.O. and De Bondt, H.L. (1994) Protein kinase regulation: insights from crystal structure analysis. Curr. Opin. Cell Biol. 6, 239-246.
11. Pavletich, N.P. (1999) Mechanisms of cyclin-dependent kinase regulation: structures of cdks, their cyclin activators, and Cip and INK4 inhibitors. J. Mol. Biol. 287, 821-828.
12. Carnero, A. and Hannon, G.J. (1998) The INK4 family of CDK inhibitors. Curr. Top. Microbiol. Immunol. 227, 43-55.
13. Blain, S.W., Montalvo, E. and Massagué, J. (1997) Differential interaction of the cyclin-dependent kinase (Cdk) inhibitor p27Kip1 with cyclin A-Cdk2 and cyclin D2-Cdk4. J. Biol. Chem. 272, 25863-25872.
14. Cheng, M., Olivier, P., Diehl, J.A., Fero, M., Roussel, M.F., Roberts, J.M. and Sherr, C.J. (1999) The p21Cip1 and p27Kip1 Cdk inhibitors are essential activators of cyclin D-dependent kinases in murine fibroblasts. EMBO J. 18, 1571-1583.
15. LaBaer, J., Garrett, M.D., Stevenson, L.F., Slingerland, J.M., Sandhu, C., Chou, H.S., Fattaey, A. and Harlow, E. (1997). New functional activities for the p21 family of CDK inhibitors. Genes Dev. 11, 847-862.
16. Geng, Y., Whoriskey, W., Park, M.Y., Bronson, R.T., Medema, R.H., Li, T., Weinberg, R.A. and Sicinski, P. (1999) Rescue of cyclin D1 deficiency by knockin cyclin E. Cell 97, 767-777.
17. Geng, Y., Yu, Q., Sicinska, E., Das, M., Bronson, R.T. and Sicinski, P. (2001) Deletion of the p27[Kip1] gene restores normal development in cyclin D1-deficient mice. Proc. Natl. Acad. Sci. USA 98, 194-199.
18. Tong, W. and Pollard, J.W. (2001) Genetic evidence for the interactions of cyclin D1 and p27[Kip1] in mice. Mol. Cell. Biol. 21, 1319-1328.
19. Weinberg, R.A. (1995) The retinoblastoma protein and cell cycle control. Cell 81, 323-330.
20. Malumbres, M. and Carnero, A. (2002) Cell cycle deregulation: a common motif in cancer. Prog. Cell Cycle Res. 5, in press.
21. Ortega, S., Malumbres, M. and Barbacid, M. (2002) Cyclin D-dependent kinases, INK4 inhibitors and cancer.Biochim. Biophys. Acta 1602, 73-87.
22. Philipp-Staheli, J., Payne, S.R. and Kemp, C.J. (2001) p27(Kip1): regulation and function of a haploinsufficient tumor suppressor and its misregulation in cancer.Exp. Cell Res. 264, 148-168.
23. Malek, N.P., Sundberg, H., McGrew, S., Nakayama, K., Kyriakides, T.R., Roberts, J.M. and Kyriakidis, T.R. (2001) A mouse knock-in model exposes sequential proteolytic pathways that regulate p27Kip1 in G1 and S phase. Nature 413, 323-7.
24. Latres, E., Chiarle, R., Schulman, B.A., Pavletich, N.P., Pellicer, A., Inghirami, G. and Pagano, M. (2001) Role of the F-box protein Skp2 in lymphomagenesis. Proc. Natl. Acad. Sci. USA 98, 2515-20.
25. Gstaiger, M., Jordan, R., Lim, M.,, Catzavelos, C,, Mestan, J., Slingerland, J. and Krek, W. (2001). Skp2 is oncogenic and overexpressed in human cancers. Proc. Natl. Acad. Sci. USA 98, 5043-5048.
26. Moberg, K.H., Bell, D.W., Wahrer, D.C., Haber, D.A. and Hariharan, I.K. (2001) Archipelago regulates Cyclin E levels in Drosophila and is mutated in human cancer cell lines. Nature 413, 311-6.
27. Strohmaier, H., Spruck, C.H., Kaiser, P., Won, K.A., Sangfelt, O. and Reed, S.I. (2001) Human F-box protein hCdc4 targets cyclin E for proteolysis and is mutated in a breast cancer cell line. Nature 413, 316-22.
28. Paggi, M.G. and Giordano, A. (2001) Who is the boss in the retinoblastoma family? The point of view of Rb2/p130, the little brother. Cancer Res. 61, 4651-4654.
29. Mulligan, G. and Jacks, T. (1998) The retinoblastoma gene family: cousins with overlapping interests. Trends Genet. 14, 223-229.
30. Jallepalli, P.V. and Lengauer, C. (2001) Chromosome segregation and cancer: cutting through the mystery. Nat Rev. Cancer 1,109-117.
31. Malumbres, M., Ortega, S. and Barbacid, M. (2000) Genetic analysis of mammalian cyclin-dependent kinases and their inhibitors. Biol. Chem. 381, 827-838 .
32. Classon, M. and Dyson, N. (2001) p107 and p130: versatile proteins with interesting pockets. Exp. Cell Res. 264, 135-147.
33. Gomez Lahoz, E., Liegeois, N.J., Zhang, P. et al. (1999) Cyclin D- and E-dependent kinases and the p57[KIP2] inhibitor: cooperative interactions in vivo. Mol. Cell. Biol. 19, 353-363.
34. Miliani de Marval, P.L., Gimenez-Conti, I.B., LaCava, M. et al. (2001). Transgenic expression of cyclin-dependent kinase 4 results in epidermal hyperplasia, hypertrophy, and severe dermal fibrosis. Am. J. Pathol. 159, 369-379.

35. Robles, A.I., Larcher, F. and Whalin, R.B. (1996) Expression of cyclin D1 in epithelial tissues of transgenic mice results in epidermal hyperproliferation and severe thymic hyperplasia. Proc. Natl. Acad. Sci. USA 93, 7634-7638.
36. Rodriguez-Puebla, M.L., LaCava, M., Miliani de Marval, P.L. et al. (2000). Cyclin D2 overexpression in transgenic mice induces thymic and epidermal hyperplasia whereas cyclin D3 expression results only in epidermal hyperplasia. Am. J. Pathol. 157, 1039-1050.
37. Wolfel, T., Hauer, M., Schneider, J., Serrano, M., Wolfel, C., Klehmann-Hieb, E., De Plaen, E., Hankeln, T., Meyer zum Buschenfelde, K.H. and Beach, D. (1995) A p16Ink4a – insensitive Cdk4 mutant targeted by cytolytic T lymphocytes in a human melanoma. Science 269, 1281-1284.
38. Zuo, L., Weger, J., Yang, Q., Goldstein, A.M., Tucker, M.A., Walker, G.J., Hayward, N. and Dracopoli, N.C. (1996). Germline mutations in the p16INK4a binding domain of Cdk4 in familial melanoma. Nat. Genet. 12, 97-99.
39. Rane, S.G., Dubus, P., Mettus, R.V., Galbreath, E.J., Boden, G., Reddy, E.P. and Barbacid, M. (1999) Loss of Cdk4 expression causes insulin-deficient diabetes and Cdk4 activation results in ß-cell hyperplasia. Nat. Genet. 22, 44-52.
40. Rane SG, Cosenza SC, Mettus RV, Reddy EP. (2002) Germ line transmission of the Cdk4(R24C) mutation facilitates tumorigenesis and escape from cellular senescence. Mol. Cell. Biol. 22, 644-56.
41. Sotillo, S., Dubus, P., Martín, J., de la Cueva, E., Ortega, S., Malumbres, M. and Barbacid, M. (2001) Wide spectrum of tumors in knock-in mice carrying a Cdk4 protein insensitive to INK4 inhibitors. EMBO J. 20, 6637-6647.
42. Sotillo, R., García, J. F., Ortega, S., Martín, J., Dubus, P., Barbacid, M and Malumbres M. (2001) Invasive melanoma in Cdk4-targeted mice. Proc. Natl. Acad. Sci. USA 98, 13312-13317.
43. Latres, E., Malumbres, M., Sotillo, R., Martín, J., Ortega, S., Martín-Caballero, J., Flores, J.M., Cordón-Cardo, C. and Barbacid, M. (2000) Limited overlapping roles of p15[INK4b] and p18[INK4c] cell cycle inhibitors in proliferation and tumorigenesis. EMBO J. 19, 3496-3506.
44. Sharpless, N.E., Bardeesy, N., Lee, K.H., Carrasco, D., Castrillon, D.H., Aguirre, A.J., Wu, E.A., Horner, J.W. and DePinho, R.A. (2001) Loss of p16[INK4a] with retention of p19[ARF] predisposes to tumorigenesis. Nature 413, 86-91.
45. Franklin, D. S. Godfrey, V.L., Lee, H., Kovalev, G.I., Schoonhoven, R., Chen-Kiang, S., Su, L. and Xiong, Y. (1998). Cdk inhibitors p18INK4c and p27Kip1 mediate two separate pathways to collaborative suppress pituitary tumorigenesis. Genes Dev. 12, 2899-2911.
46. Krimpenfort, P., Quon, K. C., Mooi, W. J., Loonstra, A. and Berns, A. (2001) Loss of p16Ink4a confers susceptibility to metastatic melanoma in mice. Nature 413, 83-86.
47. Senderowicz, A.M. and Sausville, E.A. (2000) Preclinical and clinical development of cyclin-dependent kinase modulators. J. Natl. Cancer Inst. 92, 376-387.

PROLIFERATION: THE CELL CYCLE

Manuel Serrano

EMBO Member, Department of Immunology and Oncology, Spanish National Center of Biotechnology, Campus de Cantoblanco, Madrid E-28049. SPAIN.

Normal cells possess mechanisms that protect them from the action of oncogenes. Thus, normal primary cells are not affected by neoplastic transformations, whereas the majority of immortal cells used in laboratory cultures have acquired mutations during the immortalization process and are susceptible to being transformed. Our main interest is the study of the molecular mechanisms which signal anti-tumor responses as well as the impact these anti-tumor responses have upon the cell cycle.

THE p16^{INK4a}/Rb TUMOR SUPPRESOR PATHWAY

P16^{INK4a} is the founding member of a family of cyclin dependent kinases inhibitors CDK4 y CDK6, hence their name "INhibitors of CDK4" (Serrano et al., 1993). The four members of this family are p16^{INK4a}, p15^{INK4b}, p18^{INK4c}, and p19^{INK4d}. In general, the endogenous levels of these inhibitors are extremely low and make cell proliferation possible, even if in the presence of certain specific to the INK4 family, these levels may increase bringing the proliferation process to an end.

CDK4 and CDK6 kinases are part of the cell cycle machinery. Their activity is essential for cells to overcome the block often imposed on them by the Rb tumor suppressor during the early G1 phase. In fact, CDK4 and CDK6 are regarded as the site at which the irreversible entry into a new cell division cycle is decided depending on the balance between proliferating and non-proliferating signals.

Although Rb regulation is extremely complex and requires the involvement of a large number of proteins, it is a fact that p16^{INK4a}/CDK4/cyclin D1/Rb make up an extremely important regulating pathway in neoplastic transformation (Fig. 1). This pathway comprises two tumor suppressing negative regulators, p16^{INK4a} and Rb as well as two positive

New Trends in Cancer for the 21st Century, edited by
Llombart-Bosch and Felipo, Kluwer Academic/Plenum Publishers, 2003

13

regulators, CDK4 and cyclin D1, which become oncogenic when hyperactivated. The alteration of this pathway is regarded as a landmark of tumor cells. Alterations may affect one or several members of the pathway and the loss of p16[INK4a] is the most frequent alteration, occurring in about 40% of human aggressive tumors regardless of their type. Rb loss is common in retinoblastomas, osteosarcomas and lung cancers. CDK4 hyperactivation is common in sarcomas and gliomas. And finally, D1 cyclin hyperactivation is common in breast cancer.

Using targeted mutagenesis techniques, we have recently identified the binding site of p16[INK4a] in CDK4 and CDK6 (see Brotherton et al., 1998). This information has been useful to interpret the tridimensional structure of p19[INK4d] bound to CDK6, which has recently been resolved thanks to the a cooperation effort between several research centers led by Ernest Laue (Brotherton et al., 1998).

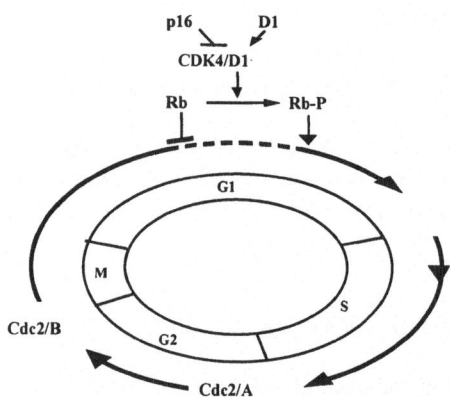

Figure 1. The cell-cycle and its regulation by the p16/CDK4/cyclin D1/Rb pathway.

THE p19[ARF]/p53 TUMOR SUPPRESOR PATHWAY

P19[ARF] is associated to tumor suppressor p53 and its negative regulator, oncogene MDM2. In the presence of high levels of p19[ARF], p53 is protected from MDM2 mediated degradation and gains full competencies as a transcriptional activator.

Again, of all regulators involved in the activation of p53 and of all the genes which become activated by p53, there are a few which often undergo alterations in human aggressive tumors. These genes and their products make up the p53/MDM2/p19[ARF] pathway (Fig. 2). This pathway is composed by two tumor suppressing negative regulators of the cell cycle, p53 and p19[ARF], and by a positive regulator, MDM2, which is oncogenic when hyperactivated. Alteration of this pathway, like that of the p16/Rb pathway, is a landmark of tumor cells. About 50% of all human tumors have suffered a loss of p53, whereas other tumors show a loss of p19[ARF] or hyperactivation of the MDM2 oncogene.

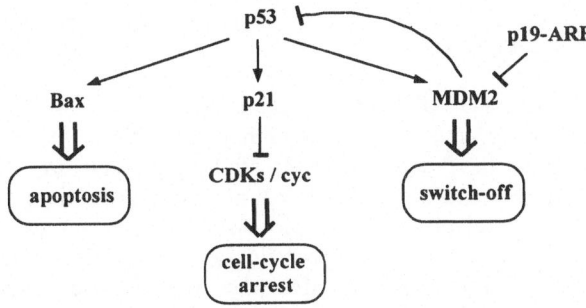

Figure 2. Genes regulated by p53 and their function, and the p19/MDM2/p53 pathway.

THE SAME GENETIC LOCUS CODES FOR p16^{INK4a} AND p19^{ARF}

The INK4a-ARF genomic locus is placed in position 9p21, which corresponds to one of the most frequently altered sites in human tumors from a cytogenetic point of view. This locus codes for the two tumor suppressor proteins p16^{INK4a} and p19^{ARF} in a way which is both unusual and complex, involving two different promoters, two different 5' exons, common internal and 3' exons and different reading frames (Fig. 3). The final result is two proteins which are not related in terms of their aminoacid sequences but which probably share some features related to their transcriptional regulation. The importance of p16^{INK4a} and p19^{ARF} for tumor prevention is web documented: about 40% of all human tumors, regardless of their type, have selected inactivating mutations at the INK4a-ARF locus; all alterations affect the function of p16^{INK4a}, whereas half (20% of total) affect the function of p19^{ARF}. In addition, the germline acquisition of mutated INK4a-ARF alleles increases susceptibility to the development of tumors both in humans and in mice (Serrano et al., 1996; revised in Serrano, 1997).

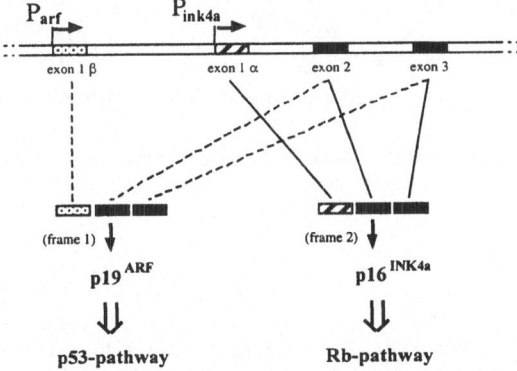

Figure 3. Genomic structure of the INK4a-ARF locus and involvement of its gene products, p16^{INK4a} and p19^{ARF}, in the regulation of the Rb- and p53-pathways, respectively.

THE INK4a-ARF LOCUS ACTS AS A SENSOR OF ONCOGENIC STRESSES AND PREVENTS NEOPLASTIC TRANSFORMATION

Expression of INK4a and ARF genes is ubiquitous and very weak, detectable in the majority of tissues only by means of methods requiring PCR. In addition, genetically manipulated mice which have deficient levels of these proteins are viable but develop tumors at an early age (Serrano et al., 1996). All of this suggests that p16^{INK4a} and p19^{ARF} are not essential for normal physiological processes but they *are* essential however to prevent neoplastic transformation. In collaboration with David Beach and Scott Lowe we have found that p16^{INK4a} and p53 levels rise when the Ras oncogene is introduced in primary cells (Serrano et al., 1997). We have extended these findings and discovered that p19^{ARF} levels also increase in response to the Ras oncogene and that this induction is necessary for the subsequent activation of p53 (Palmero et al., 1998). In short, it can be argued that the aberrant activity of the Ras oncogene in primary cells is initially detected by the INK4a-ARF locus, which increases the levels of p16^{INK4a} and p19^{ARF} which, in turn, activate tumor suppressors Rb and p53, thus bringing permanent proliferation to an end. Primary cells derived from genetically deficient mice in the INK4a-ARF locus are susceptible to the action of the Ras oncogene and, as a consequence, are efficiently transformed.

Other researchers have obtained similar findings by introducing in the cells other oncogenes whose behavior is different from that of the Ras oncogene, such as the Myc oncogene (Fig. 4).

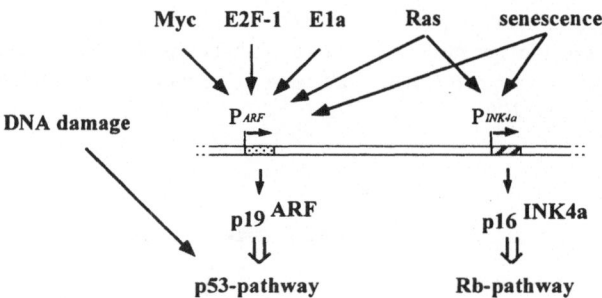

Figure 4. The INK4a/ARF locus as a sensor of oncogenic stresses.

References

Brotherton, D. H., Dhanaraj, V., Wick, S., Brizuela, L., Domaille, P. J., Volyanik, E., Xu, X., Parisini, E., Smith, B. O., Archer, S. J., Serrano, M., Brenner, S. L., Blundell, T. L., and Laue, E. D. (1998). Crystal structure of the complex of the cyclin D-dependent kinase Cdk6 bound to the cell-cycle inhibitor p19^{INK4d}. *Nature* **395**, 244-250

Palmero, I., Pantoja, C., and Serrano, M. (1998). P19^{ARF} links the tumour suppressor p53 to Ras. *Nature* **395**, 125-126

Serrano, M., Lin, A. W., McCurrach, M. E., Beach, D., and Lowe, S. W. (1997). Oncogenic *ras* provokes premature cell senescence associated with accumulation of p53 and p16^{INK4a}. *Cell* **88**, 593-602

Serrano, M., Lee, H.-W., Chin, L., Cordon-Cardo, C., Beach, D. and DePinho, R. A. (1996). Role of the *INK4a* locus in tumor suppression and cell mortality. *Cell*, **85**, 27-37

Serrano, M., Hannon, G. and Beach, D. (1993). A New Regulatory Motif in Cell-cycle Control Causing Specific Inhibition of Cyclin D/CDK4. *Nature*, **336**, 704-707

Serrano, M. (1997). The Tumor Suppressor Protein p16^{INK4a}. *Exp. Cell Res.* **237**, 7-13.

MOLECULAR ANALYSIS OF GENE EXPRESSION IN TUMOR PATHOLOGY

Heinz Höfler[1], Katja Specht, and Karl-Friedrich Becker

Institut für Pathologie, Technische Univeristät München and GSF-Forschungszentrum für Umwelt und Gesundheit Neuherberg, Germany

ABSTRACT

Human cancers are diverse in their pathology and responsiveness to clinical treatment. This diversity is at least in part due to variations in cellular gene expression programs. Although the analyis of proteins - the key players in cells and potential drug targets - is advancing rapidly, there are situations in which the analysis of RNA rather than proteins can provide valuable information for the diagnosis of cancer. These situations include absense of an antibody for the protein of interest, expression of functionally defective proteins, expressed small nucleotide polymorphisms (SNPs), analysis of alternatively or abnormally spliced molecules, and functional analysis of splice site mutations. In this chapter we will focus on the analysis of RNA from clinical samples and will summarize how gene expression studies on the RNA level using a variety of new tools can be useful for discovering new classes of tumors, for predicting clinical outcome or therapy response, and for designing novel personalized clinical interventions that can not be achieved with histology alone.

CONTROL OF GENE EXPRESSION: PURPOSES AND GENERAL PRINCIPLES

Critical factors determining the types and amounts of various proteins within cells are the frequency at which the protein′s coding mRNA is synthesized, the concentration and stability of the mRNA and the stability and activity of the protein itself. The term "gene expression" commonly refers to the entire process by which the genetic information encoded by a particular gene is decoded into the corresponding protein. The initial RNA transcript within the nucleus is processed by 5′-capping, 3′-addition of a poly(A) tail, and splicing, generating a functional mRNA. The mRNA is then transported into the cytoplasm where translation occurs (Table 1). Thus, the level of an

---

[1] Heinz Höfler, Institut für Pathologie, Technische Univeristät München, Trogerstrasse 18, D-81675 München-Germany. Tel.: ++49 89 4140 4160. FAX: ++49 89 4140 4865. hoefler@lrz.tum.de

New Trends in Cancer for the 21st Century, edited by
Llombart-Bosch and Felipo, Kluwer Academic/Plenum Publishers, 2003

mRNA in the cytoplasm is determined by the rate at which the mRNA precursor is synthesized in the nucleus and the rates of nuclear RNA processing and export and cytoplasmic mRNA degradation[1].

Basically, regulation at any one of the various steps in this process could lead to *differential* gene expression, resulting in an extraordinary complex pattern of cell characteristics. In contrast to single-celled organisms, cells of multicellular organisms live in a rather constant environment, i.e. they are protected from immediate outside influences. The execution of precise developmental decisions is the most critical requirement of gene control in multicellular organisms. It is most important that the right genes are activated in the right cells at the right time during development. Generally, in most cases a developmental step is not reversed once it has been taken. Many differentiated cells walk down a specific pathway until final death, leaving no progeny behind.

Table 1. Steps involved in Gene expression

• **RNA transcription**
• **5′- capping**
• **3′- addition of poly(A)**
• **splicing**
• **transport in the cytoplasm**
• **translation (and functional activation)**
• **degradation/inactivation**

CLINICAL SIGNIFICANCE FOR MOLECULAR ANALYSIS OF GENE EXPRESSION

Today, classification of human tumors and pathological diagnosis in general is largely based on conventional histopathological and morphological features. However, it is anticipated that whole genome expression monitoring of pathologically altered tissues and the identification of recurrent genetic alterations will expand our understanding of the etiologies and pathogenesis of human disease processes and will eventually lead to a definition of molecular disease entities and a molecular taxonomy of tumors. Importantly, a gene expression – based classification system will not only complement conventional histopathology, but identify targets for specific therapeutic intervention and predict outcome and response to therapy. Numerous research groups are utilizing gene expression profiling technologies to stratify tumors into different subclasses. Alizadeh et al.[2], and Scherf et al.[3] for example, succeeded in defining clinical subsets of diffuse large B-cell lymphoma (DLBL) having dramatically different disease outcome and very recently, two other studies[4, 5] linked gene expression profiles of lymph node negative breast cancer to clinical outcome.

STRATEGIES FOR DNA, RNA AND PROTEIN DETECTION

In the center for molecular diagnosis of cancer is the analysis of DNA, RNA, and proteins isolated from tissues or body fluids. Here we summarize possibilities for RNA analysis and only briefly touch DNA- and protein-based applications. The genetic alterations that arise during tumor development can be used to detect and characterize tumor cells in clinical samples[6]. *DNA* is well suited for clinical analysis as it can survive the often uncontrolled conditions by which such samples for molecular analysis are aquired. In addition, it can be amplifed by PCR-based techniques and subsequently analyzed often within one day, which is important to provide clinicians with fast and accurate informations. Since there are amplification methods available, the amount of starting material may be low, e.g. a few thousands cells may be sufficient in many situations. Not only mutations in oncogenes or tumor suppressor genes can be analyzed using genomic DNA-based techniques but also determination of changes in DNA repeat sequences (micosatellites) can be used as markers for clonal evolution of tumor cells (e.g. for the analysis of loss of heterozygosity, LOH).

The functional defects due to mutations in oncogene and tumor suppressor genes can result in significant changes in expression of many other genes. These changes in gene expression in tumor cells can be determined at the *RNA* level. Measuring the transcription rates of multiple genes in several cell types has demonstrated that regulation of *transcription initiation* is the most widespread mechanism of gene control in eukaryotes although examples of regulation at each of the steps mentioned above have been described. The most *direct method* of measuring gene transcription is by exposing cells for a short period of time to a labeled RNA precursor and then performing hybridization to a cloned DNA probe for determination of the amount of the labeled nuclear RNA. A second method, run-on analysis, has widely been used for accurately measuring transcription rates. Here, isolated nuclei are allowed to incorporate radiolabeled ribonucleoside tripshosphates directly into growing RNA chains, resulting in the formation of highly labeled RNA samples. Obviously, these direct techniques are impractical for tumor analysis in a clinical setting but have been extensively used for analysis of gene transcription in cultered cells. Consequently, most other techniques for clinical analysis do not measure the transcription rate but rather the *amount of mRNA* for a specifc gene at a certain time point. Methods used for RNA expression analysis are listed in Table 2. Some of the techniques allow the assignment to histology. Other methods are based on RNA detection after disruption of cells or tissues and isloation of RNA for subsequent analysis. A widely used method has been Northern blotting, separation of RNA in an electric field, transfer to a membrane an hybridization using a probe that is specific for a particular gene. Here expression of several genes can be analyzed and compared to a housekeeping gene whose expression is expected not to change significantly. This technique has been very valuable for the analysis of a limited number of genes. Other strategies to analyze gene transcripts are based on cDNA rather than on RNA. Using reverse transcriptase, RNA isolated from clinical samples is converted into cDNA which then can be analyzed using PCR amplification techniques (reverse transcription PCR, RT-PCR. For quantification of the amount of cDNA in a certain sample, a quantitative method has been established, quantitative real time RT-PCR.

Several methods have been devised to study *gene expression on a large scale*: cDNA subtraction, differential display, representational difference analysis (RDA), expressed sequence tag (EST) sequencing, serial analysis of gene expression (SAGE), and differential hybridization on either high-density chips, potted nylon filters or glass microarrays[6].

However, a crucial factor for the reliability of the results of most of these techniques is the use of morphologically well defined cell populations. Tissues are a complex mixture of various types of interacting cell populations and tumors contain an abundance of reactive stromal and inflammatory cells, which may outnumber the neoplastic population. Since the cell population of interest might constitute only a minute fraction of the total tissue volume, the problem of cellular heterogeneity has been a major barrier to the molecular analysis of normal versus diseased tissue. In expression profiling of bulk tissue, admixed cell populations can potentially obscure tumor-specific signatures and can make message assignment to specific cell types impossible. Furthermore, early pathologic lesions, such as dysplasia or carcinoma in situ, are frequently inaccessible for conventional molecular analysis.

Table 2. Methods used for RNA expression analysis

• **Northern blot** • **Dot blot** • **Nuclease protection assay** • **Subtractive hybridization** • **(Q) RT-PCR** • **Differential display** • **SAGE** • **cDNA/oligonucleotide arrays** • **Large scale sequencing**	• **No morphology assignment**
• **in situ hybridization** • **in situ PCR**	• **Morphology assignment possible**

To circumvent these problems and to obtain more homogeneous cell populations for molecular analysis, manual and micromanipulator-based *microdissection techniques* have been developed during the last decade[7, 8]. The development of easy-to-handle, laser-assisted technologies such as laser capture microdissection (LCM) or laser microbeam microdissection (LMM) allows rapid and highly precise procurement of purified cell populations suitable for a variety of downstream analyses.

PREREQUISITES FOR CLINICALLY RELEVANT RNA ANALYSIS

Due to the rapid evolution of genomic and proteomic techniques, the demands for handling and preserving clinical tissue samples are changing. Formalin fixation and snap freezing of tissue are the two main ways of preserving tissue, both having limitations for downstream molecular analysis. Whereas the quality of RNA in snap-frozen tissue is usually excellent, the tissue architecture is not satisfactory. On the other hand, the formalin fixation process results in an excellent preservation of morphology, but the fixatives and chemical reagents used in the paraffin process have a severe impact on RNA integrity. However, very recently, we demonstrated that quantitative RT-PCR can be applied to study gene expression in microdissected tissue samples from archival formalin-fixed tissues[9]. The influence of several RNA extraction techniques, formalin-fixation and laser-assisted microdissection on mRNA quantitation was assessed and it was demonstrated that expression level determinations from archival tissues were comparable to matched frozen specimens when using small target sequences in a range of 60 -100 bp for real-time RT-PCR amplification. Furthermore, it was shown that mRNA quantitation could be reliably performed from as few as 50 microdissected formalin-fixed cells.

Another problem in the clinical setting relies to the quantity of tissue. Until recently, the application of cDNA array techniques has been limited to mRNA isolated from millions or, at very best, several thousand cells thereby restricting the study of small samples and complex tissues. Since the total RNA content of mammalian cells is in the range of 20 – 40 pg and mRNA accounts for only 1-5% of the cellular RNA, any attempt at single-cell profiling must be capable of dealing with a total of $10^5 - 10^6$ mRNA molecules.

However, linear RNA amplification is increasingly used in combination with microarray technology to overcome these limitations.

WHEN IS RNA ANALYSIS USEFUL – EXAMPLES

There are several situations in which the analysis of RNA rather than DNA or protein can provide valuable clinical information:

(A) *Absense of antibody.* If there are no antibodies available reacting specifically with a protein of interest, it is possible to measure RNA transcripts for analysis of gene-specific expression. An example here is the analysis of the transcription factors involved in downregulation of the cell adhesion molecule and tumor suppressor gene E-cadherin. Recently, it could be demonstrated that epithelial-mesenchymal-transition (EMT) regulators such as the transcription factors snail and sip1 directly repress E-cadherin at the transcriptional level. There are no antibodies available for the analysis of these factors in tissue samples. We used quantitative real time RT-PCR (see above) for evaluation of snail and sip1 expression in gastric cancer and found a relationship between snail and sip1 for diffuse-type and intestinal-type gastric cancer, respectively[10].

(B) *Effect of splice site mutations.* A "simple" heterozygous point mutation in the coding region of a gene detected at the genomic level that is expected to result in an amino acid change may instead activate a cryptic splice site resulting in mRNA alterations and subsequent protein truncation leading to a dominant negative form. Thus, at the genomic DNA level this mutation would be interpreted as a nucleotide exchange; however, at the RNA level the messenger RNA coding for the protein would be found to be altered as part of it is removed by mutation-induced altered splicing. An E-cadherin mutation in a colon cancer[11] can serve as example for the activation of a novel splice-site (Fig. 1). Consequently, without analysis of RNA it is often not possible to predict whether a point mutation affects regular splicing and what kinds of RNA are generated due to the alteration. Abnormal transcripts due to sequence changes causing splice-site errors have recently been analyzed by allele separation in somatic cell hybrids ("conversion" technology)[12].

(C) *Alterations of marker genes.* In a usually heterogenous clinical sample of a resected tumor specimen, cancer cell-specific detection of genetic alterations may be difficult. This is especially a challenge if tumor cells account for less than 10% of the cells in a certain sample as is the case for many scattered cell carcinomas, e.g. diffuse-type gastric cancer. To detect gene mutations in the epithelial marker gene E-cadherin, we used RNA rather than DNA for mutation analysis as E-cadherin mRNA is synthezied only by epithelial cells and absent in stromal cells (fibroblasts, endothelial cells, lymphocytes etc.). We succeeded in identifying E-cadherin gene mutations in 50% of the gastric cancer samples, demonstrating E-cadherin gene mutations as the hallmark for diffuse-type gastric cancer[13, 14]. Moreover, using mutation-specific monoclonal antibodies it is even possible to detect a mutant E-cadherin protein in cancerous tissues that may have been missed using general antibodies due to a change in the epitope recognized by the general antibody[15] (Fig. 2). The special kind of E-cadherin alterations in gastric cancer, mainly in-frame exon deletions, were the basis for the development for a rapid E-cadherin mutation detection method for patient with peritoneal cancer cell dissemination[16], providing clinically valuable molecular pathological data within one day.

E-cadherin genomic DNA

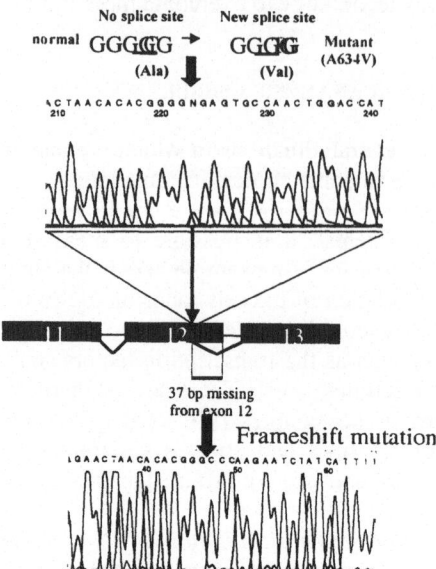

Figure 1. Difference between DNA and RNA level in the analysis of critical gene mutations: an E-cadherin gene mutation in a colon cancer activates a novel splice-site, resulting in a frame-shift mutation (37 base pair deletion, cDNA level) rather than an amino acid exchange (A634V, DNA level).

E-cadherin cDNA

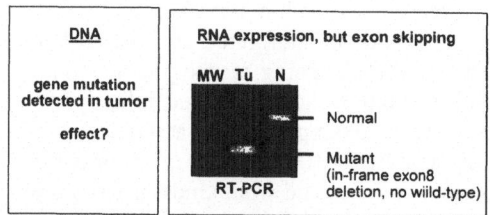

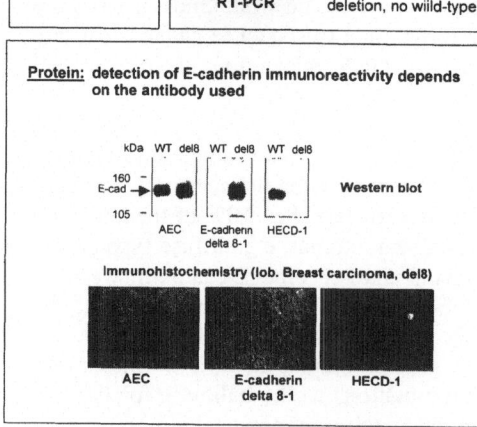

Figure 2. Allele-specific gene expression on the RNA and protein level. Gene mutations affecting the splice site at the intron 7/exon8 border of the E-cadherin gene result in in-frame skipping of exon 8 (RNA level). Using monoclonal antibodies specific for the normal or mutant form, respectively, it is possible to differentiate between the two variants even at the protein level in carcinomas harbouring such splice-site gene mutations. Note that expression of the wild-type allele is lost in the tumor (no reactivity with HECD-1).

Antibodies: AEC, anti-E-cadherin (epitope located outside of exon 8, Transduction Laboratories, Lexington, KT, USA); delta 8-1, monoclonal antibody reacting specifically with the exon 8 deletion mutant; HECD-1, epitope at least partially located within exon 8 (Ref. 15).

(D) *Allele-specific gene expression.* Very recently, quantitative measures of gene expression demonstrated that a constitutional decrease in expression of one adenomatous polyposis coli tumor suppressor gene (APC) allele can lead to the development of familial adenomatous polyposis[17]. Remarkably, no sequence variations, except the known polymorphisms, were detected in either allele that may have caused the reduction. The authors used digital SNP-analysis to quantify the relative levels of each APC allele. In this technique, dilution of reverse transcribed mRNA (cDNA) template, resulting in approximately one template molecule per well of a multititer well plate, is quantified with fluorescent probes that discriminate between the two alleles. Yan et al found that genomic DNA from FAP probands had the expected 50% allelic ratio; however, using cDNA from lymphoblastoid cells, the ratio was 66%. Linkage analysis then demonstrated that the allele that was expressed at a lower amount was the one that was linked to disease. Moreover, loss of heterozygosity in benign tumors was detected in 23 out of 28 tumors analysed. The allele that was lost in the tumors was the one that was expressed at relatively higher levels and not linked to disease! The normal allele ratios were observed in individuals without FAP. The genetic basis for the reduced expression of the affected allele was not evident. Presumably, colon-specific transcription factors or mutations deep within an intron may have been responsible for the reduced expression. These results are in line with the hypothesis of a finely balanced threshold for APC synthesis to suppress intestinal tumorigenesis.

CONCLUSION

Although several innovative therapies have found their way into the clinic, simple and effective treatments for most common cancers are still the exception. However, cell biological mechanisms responsible for clinical behavior of many malignancies are being identified at the transcriptional level. The genetic alterations that have been characterized so far and will be characterized in the future provide the molecular pathologist and clinical oncologist with a variety of (potential) new markers and tools that may markedly redefine the current criteria for tumor diagnosis. In addition, new ways for early detection of malignat cells may be designed. More specific and accurate molecular tumor diagnosis is preceeding molecular treatments, resulting in a change of the way cancer patients are treated using current therapies.

References

1. Lodish et al. Molecular Cell Biology, 4th Edition, Freeman and Company New York 2000
2. Alizadeh AA, Eisen MB, Davis RE, Ma C, Lossos IS, Rosenwald A, Boldrick JC, Sabet H, Tran T, Yu X, Powell JI, Yang L, Marti GE, Moore T, Hudson J Jr, Lu L, Lewis DB, Tibshirani R, Sherlock G, Chan WC, Greiner TC, Weisenburger DD, Armitage JO, Warnke R, Staudt LM, et al.: Distinct types of diffuse large B-cell lymphoma identified by gene expression profiling. Nature 2000 Feb 3;403(6769):503-11
3. Scherf U, Ross DT, Waltham M, Smith LH, Lee JK, Tanabe L, Kohn KW, Reinhold WC, Myers TG, Andrews DT, Scudiero DA, Eisen MB, Sausville EA, Pommier Y, Botstein D, Brown PO, Weinstein JN. A gene expression database for the molecular pharmacology of cancer. Nat Genet. 2000 Mar;24(3):236-44
4. Sorlie T, Perou CM, Tibshirani R, Aas T, Geisler S, Johnsen H, Hastie T, Eisen MB, van de Rijn M, Jeffrey SS, Thorsen T, Quist H, Matese JC, Brown PO, Botstein D, Eystein Lonning P, Borresen-Dale AL. Gene expression patterns of breast carcinomas distinguish tumor subclasses with clinical implications. Proc Natl Acad Sci U S A 2001 Sep 11;98(19):10869-74
5. van 't Veer LJ, Dai H, van de Vijver MJ, He YD, Hart AA, Mao M, Peterse HL, van der Kooy K, Marton MJ, Witteveen AT, Schreiber GJ, Kerkhoven RM, Roberts C, Linsley PS, Bernards R, Friend SH. Gene expression profiling predicts clinical outcome of breast cancer. Nature. 2002 Jan 31;415(6871):530-6.
6. Sidransky D. Nucleic acid-based methods for the detection of cancer. Science. 1997 Nov 7;278(5340):1054-9.
7. Best CJ, Emmert-Buck MR. Molecular profiling of tissue samples using laser capture microdissection. Expert Rev Mol Diagn. 2001 May;1(1):53-60

8. Schutze K, Posl H, Lahr G. Laser micromanipulation systems as universal tools in cellular and molecular biology and in medicine. Cell Mol Biol (Noisy-le-grand). 1998 Jul;44(5):735-46
9. Specht K, Richter T, Muller U, Walch A, Werner M, Höfler H: Quantitative Gene Expression Analysis in Microdissected Archival Formalin-Fixed and Paraffin-Embedded Tumor Tissue. Am. J. Pathol. (2001) 158 (2): 419-429
10. Rosivatz E, Becker I, Specht K, Fricke E, Luber B, Busch R, Hofler H, Becker KF. Differential Expression of the Epithelial-Mesenchymal Transition Regulators Snail, SIP1, and Twist in Gastric Cancer. Am J Pathol. 2002 Nov;161(5):1881-91.
11. Vecsey-Semjen B, Becker KF, Sinski A, Blennow E, Vietor I, Zatloukal K, Beug H, Wagner E, Huber LA. Novel colon cancer cell lines leading to better understanding of the diversity of respective primary cancers. Oncogene. 2002 Jul 11;21(30):4646-62
12. Nakagawa H, Yan H, Lockman J, Hampel H, Kinzler KW, Vogelstein B, De La Chapelle A. Allele separation facilitates interpretation of potential splicing alterations and genomic rearrangements. Cancer Res. 2002 Aug 15;62(16):4579-82
13. Becker KF, Atkinson MJ, Reich U, Becker I, Nekarda H, Siewert JR, Hofler H. E-cadherin gene mutations provide clues to diffuse type gastric carcinomas. Cancer Res. 1994 Jul 15;54(14):3845-52
14. Becker KF, Reich U, Schott C, Becker I, Berx G, van Roy F, Hofler H. Identification of eleven novel tumor-associated E-cadherin mutations. Mutations in brief no. 215. Online. Hum Mutat. 1999;13(2):171
15. Becker KF, Kremmer E, Eulitz M, Schulz S, Mages J, Handschuh G, Wheelock MJ, Cleton-Jansen AM, Hofler H, Becker I. Functional allelic loss detected at the protein level in archival human tumours using allele-specific E-cadherin monoclonal antibodies. J Pathol. 2002 Aug;197(5):567-74
16. Schuhmacher C, Becker KF, Reich U, Schenk U, Mueller J, Siewert JR, Hofler H. Rapid detection of mutated E-cadherin in peritoneal lavage specimens from patients with diffuse-type gastric carcinoma. Diagn Mol Pathol. 1999 Jun;8(2):66-70.
17. Yan H, Dobbie Z, Gruber SB, Markowitz S, Romans K, Giardiello FM, Kinzler KW, Vogelstein B. Small changes in expression affect predisposition to tumorigenesis. Nat Genet. 2002 Jan;30(1):25-6

EWING TUMOR BIOLOGY: PERSPECTIVES FOR INNOVATIVE TREATMENT APPROACHES

Heinrich Kovar

Children´s Cancer Research Institute, St. Anna Kinderspital, Vienna

ABSTRACT

The Ewing´s sarcoma family of tumors (EFT) is a group of malignancies affecting bone and soft tissue in adolescents. It is characterized by a unique gene rearrangement between the *EWS* gene and an *ets* transcription factor gene. EFT can be cured with conventional multi modal treatment, however, about 40% of patients still succumb to the disease. Relapses can be observed more than 5 years after the end of primary treatment suggesting persistence of minimal residual disease (MRD). Due to the still enigmatic nature of EFT histogenesis the phenotype of EFT stem cells and of dormant tumor cells remains unknown. The most frequent fusion product associated with EFT, EWS-FLI1, is the founding member of a whole class of similarly structured chimeric proteins associated with a variety of human sarcomas and also specific leukemias. The corresponding gene rearrangement constitutes a rate limiting step in oncogenesis as implied by the high association of EFT with *EWS-ETS* fusions, strong selective pressure for maintenance of a correct reading frame in the tumors, and by experimental data confirming the transforming and tumorigenic potential of EWS-FLI1. Understanding the biology of *EWS-ETS* gene fusions and its interplay with essential cellular pathways regulating cell growth, apoptosis, differentiation, genomic integrity, and treatment resistance may unravel specifically vulnerable sites for therapeutic targeting. This review summarizes the current knowledge about the EWS-FLI1 pathway in EFT and provides some ideas as to how this knowledge may be translated into innovative treatment approaches.

A NEED FOR NOVEL THERAPEUTICS IN THE TREATMENT OF EWING´S SARCOMA FAMILY TUMORS

Ewing´s sarcoma family tumors (EFT) (Ewing´s sarcoma, peripheral primitive neuroectodermal tumor/neuroepithelioma, Askin tumor) are a group of poorly differentiated primitive tumors affecting bone and soft tissue in children and young adults. The mean age of diagnosis is 13.5 years with a slight male preponderance. The annual incidence rate in Caucasians is 3 per 1 million children <15 years of age. Thus, EFT constitutes about 10 to 15% of malignant bone tumors. The disease is extremely rare in black and Chinese people. The tissue of origin is still an enigma. Due to limited neuroglial differentiation a neuroectodermal descent is discussed. This view is further

New Trends in Cancer for the 21st Century, edited by
Llombart-Bosch and Felipo, Kluwer Academic/Plenum Publishers, 2003

27

supported by preliminary gene expression profiling results. Clinically, EFT appears as very aggressive neoplasms with a high tendency for dissemination. In the pre-chemotherapy era with local treatment alone, almost all patients succumbed to the disease due to the development of distant metastases. Today, combination therapy regimens that include multi-agent chemotherapy and local control by wide resection and radiotherapy result in cure of about 60% of patients with localized disease. However, patients presenting with clinically detectable metastases at diagnosis, patients not responding to therapy and patients with disease relapse still have an adverse prognosis with less than 20% cure rate even using myeloablative approaches with stem cell reinfusion. Although the majority of events are usually observed during the first year after the end of primary treatment, late relapses may occur more than 5 years later compatible with the persistence of dormant disease. Thus, despite significant advances during the last two decades in the cure of cancer patients using "conventional" therapeutic regimens, treatment results for EFT patients are still not satisfactory. The success stories of the antibody Herceptin targeting the epidermal growth factor receptor 2 in breast cancer, the tyrosine kinase inhibitor Imatinib interfering with BCR-ABL signaling in chronic myeloid leukemia, and the *E1B* gene defective oncolytic adenovirus ONYX-O15 selectively replicating in cancer cells with p53/p14[ARF] deficiencies, have raised great hopes as to the use of "smart drugs" in other cancers as well. Potential targets should be i) largely tumor specific and not present/active in normal tissue, ii) expressed in all (including dormant and disseminated) tumor cells of the specific cancer and in all patients suffering from this cancer. The first step in the definition of such a target comes from the cytogenetic identification of a chromosomal aberration consistently associated with the disease. For EFT, this is the translocation t(11;22)(q24;q12)[1] that leads to the fusion between the Ewing´s sarcoma gene *EWS* and the *ets* transcription factor gene *FLI1* in about 85% of patients[2]. In the majority of the remaining histopathologically classified EFT cases, variant gene rearrangements between *EWS* and other *ets* genes (*ERG, ETV1, FEV, E1AF*) have been observed (reviewed in Kovar et al., 1999[3]).

THE EWS-ETS FUSION PROTEIN, A CANDIDATE THERAPEUTIC TARGET?

The EWS-FLI1 gene rearrangement in EFT can be considered prototypic for *TET*-transcription factor gene fusions in human cancer. Ectopic expression of EWS-FLI1 is toxic to the majority of cell types. Loss of the p16 or the p53/p14[ARF] pathways was found to induce tolerance to EWS-FLI1 expression[4], which, in NIH3T3 cells, results in in-vitro transformation and tumorigenicity in nude mice[5]. An intact IGF1 receptor pathway was found to be essential for the transformation and tumorigenicity of fibroblasts[6,7]. The transforming ability of EWS-FLI1 is minimally dependent on the presence of the first 82 amino terminal amino acids of EWS, the very C-terminus of FLI1, and the DNA binding domain[5,8,9]. However, mutations of the DNA-binding domain do not completely abolish the transforming potential of EWS-FLI1[10,11], and the minimal EWS transforming domain is distinct from the domain with the highest transactivating potential. These findings are compatible with additional, transcription-independent functions of EWS-FLI1 and possibly other TET fusion proteins in oncogenesis.

Since *EWS-ets* gene rearrangements are associated with at least 95% of EFT, these gene rearrangements are considered to be causative for the disease. In addition, comparison between the genomic breakpoints and the structure of the fusion mRNA revealed selective pressure for maintenance of a correct reading frame (skipping of out-of-frame exons)[12,13]. In fact, antisense DNA studies confirmed that continuous EWS-FLI1 expression is required for EFT cell proliferation in-vitro and tumorigenicity in vivo[14-17]. In contrast, ectopic expression of EWS-FLI1 in heterologous cellular systems results in cell death. Here, rescue from apoptosis requires loss of the *p53/INK4A* gene pathways. However, in EFT, *p53* mutations and *INK4A* deletions are rare accounting for only 10% and 20-30% of cases, respectively[18,19]. Thus, most EFT appear to be permissive for EWS-FLI1 expression in the absence of p53/INK4A pathway alterations. The importance of the cellular context is further underlined by gene expression profiling studies. Several genes have been found to be activated in EWS-FLI1 transgenic NIH3T3 cells (reviewed in Arvand et al.[20]). However, for none of them could consistent expression be confirmed in EFT. Vice versa, genes whose expression is tightly linked with the EFT phenotype did not show-up in the expression profiles of EWS-FLI1 transformed NIH3T3 cells. Most recently, however, using hTERT immortalized human fibroblasts, Lessnick at al. detected up-regulation of CD99 – a hallmark of EFT [21,22]. Using NIH3T3 cells for ectopic EWS-FLI1 expression, up-regulation of cyclinD1 has been observed[23], however, this gene is not consistently activated in EFT[19]. While in rodent fibroblasts IGF1 receptor expression has been demonstrated to enable EWS-FLI1 expression[6,7], a functional bFGF receptor pathway is required for EWS-FLI1 expression in EFT [24].

In order to evaluate the potential of EWS-FLI1 and its variants to serve as therapeutic targets, we have to understand the cellular processes and mechanisms in which not only these fusion proteins but also their normal counterparts are involved. An understanding of the biological role of EWS-FLI1 comes only after observing the phenotypic consequences of altering its expression/function within the authentic living cell. In the absence of any animal model for EFT, EFT cell lines remain the only relevant model to account for an authentic cellular context when studying EWS-FLI1.

FUNCTION OF TET PROTEINS AND THEIR ONCOGENIC FUSIONS

EWS belongs to the *TET* family of genes encoding for the putative RNA binding proteins EWS, TLS, and TAF$_{II}$68 (TAF15, TAF2N, RPB56). *TET* genes are not only rearranged in EFT but also involved in other chromosomal translocations in solid tumors and acute leukemia (Table 1). TET proteins share common structural motifs, including copies of the degenerate hexapeptide motif SYGQQS in varying numbers, and a unique RNA-binding domain comprised of a RNP motif and RGG boxes. TET gene rearrangements uniformly lead to the replacement of the C-terminal RNA binding domain of the TET protein by the DNA binding domain of a transcription factor. The amino terminal TET portion (NTD) provides a strong transcriptional activation domain to the novel chimeric DNA binding protein. While the NTD is functionally largely interchangeable between the different TET family fusion proteins, the C-terminal transcription factor moiety determines the tumor phenotype and appears to be disease-specific[25].

The normal function of TLS, EWS, and TAF$_{II}$68 is only partly known. All three proteins have been found in association with the TF$_{II}$D general transcription factor complex [26,27]. In addition, interactions with core polymerase II components (RPB3, 5, 7)[27,28] and with splicing factors U1C, SR, SF1 and YB1[29-33] have been described (Fig. 1). Furthermore, TLS has been found to be identical to the pre-mRNA associated factor hnRNP P2[34]. Thus, it is assumed that TET proteins serve as a bridge between transcription and RNA processing. Interestingly, expression profiling on EWS-FLI1 transgenic NIH3T3 cells revealed a similar number of repressed as activated genes[9]. In fact, the only confirmed target gene of EWS-ets fusion proteins in EFT is the gene for the TGFβ type 2 receptor (*TGFβRII*)[35] (Fig. 2). The mechanism of target gene repression by TET-fusion proteins remains elusive, but may involve altered RNA processing. Interaction of EWS-FLI1 with U1C, for example, represses EWS-FLI1 mediated transactivation in-vitro[30]. While communication with RNA polymerase II occurs via the N-terminal domain present in the normal and the rearranged TET proteins, interaction with the splicing apparatus involves both, the N-terminus (U1C, SF1) and the C-terminus (YB1, SR splicing factors). In in-vitro splicing assays, oncogenic TLS-ERG and EWS-FLI1 fusion proteins interfere with YB1 and SR protein mediated splicing[29,32,36] and EWS-FLI1 as well as EWS-NOR fusion proteins were demonstrated to alter 5′splice site selection presumably via their interaction with U1C[37,38]. In addition, we recently identified interaction of EWS and EWS-FLI1 via the minimal transforming domain with BARD1[39], a protein involved in the inhibition of RNA maturation in response to DNA damage[40,41]. Since BARD1 complexes with the breast cancer susceptibility gene BRCA1, which serves as a platform for the binding of several DNA repair and cell cycle regulatory proteins (Venkitaraman, 2001[42]), and which functions in recombination repair of DNA double strand breaks, a role for normal and/or aberrant TET proteins in DNA repair and/or checkpoint control cannot be excluded. Interestingly, TLS has a DNA-pairing activity and TLS deficient mice are characterized by pronounced genomic instability, radiation sensitivity, and impaired meiosis[43,44]. Of note, poly (ADP-ribose) polymerase (PARP) expression, which is regulated by ets transcription factors[45] and which plays an important role in the radiation response, is significantly increased in EFT cells[46]. Furthermore, the transactivation domain containing the amino terminal half of TLS was found to bind to nuclear receptors for steroid and thyroid hormones, and retinoids[47]. TLS serves as a co-activator in nuclear factor-kappa B p65-mediated transcription[48]. Protein interaction studies imply that TET proteins and potentially their oncogenic fusions may be targeted by several signaling pathways via phosphorylation by v-Src, Pyk, and Bruton´s tyrosine kinase, and protein kinase C[49-53] (Fig. 3). However, the actual status of post-translational modification of the TET proteins and their oncogenic fusions as well as its functional relevance is largely unknown. A recent report describes the presence of N-acetylglucosamin moieties on at least a fraction of cellular EWS. Interestingly, the glycosylation level of EWS was found to change during the neural differentiation of P19 cells[54]. The recent finding of a heavily methylated form of EWS exposed on the cell surface indicates a further level of complexity for TET protein function[55].

Table 1. Rearrangements of the EWS family members

EWS family member	Transcription factor (type)	Neoplasm
EWS	FLI1 (ETS)	Ewing tumor (85%)
EWS	ERG (ETS)	Ewing tumor (10%)
EWS	ETV1 (ETS)	Ewing tumor (<1%)
EWS	E1AF (ETS)	Ewing tumor (<1%)
EWS	FEV (ETS)	Ewing tumor (<1%)
EWS	ZSG (zinc finger)	Askin-like, CD99 neg.
TLS	ERG (ETS)	AML
EWS	CIZ/NMP4 (zinc finger)	cALL, AUL
TAFII68	CIZ/NMP4 (zinc finger)	AML, ALL
EWS	CHOP (bZIP)	Myxoid liposarcoma
TLS	CHOP (bZIP)	Myxoid liposarcoma
EWS	ATF1 (bZIP)	Melanoma of soft parts
EWS	WT1 (zinc finger)	Desmoplastic small round cell tumor
EWS	TEC/CHN (Steroid R)	Extraskeletal myxoid chondrosarcoma
TAFII68	TEC/CHN (Steroid R)	Extraskeletal myxoid chondrosarcoma

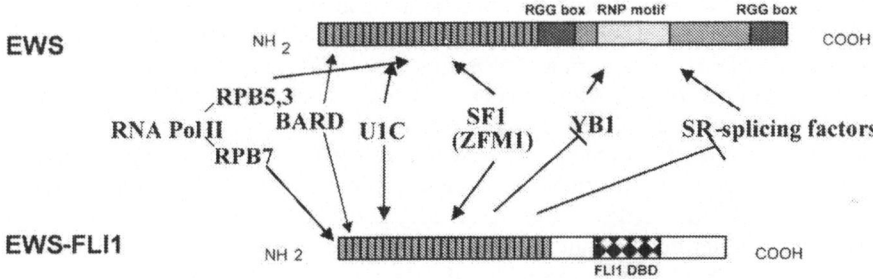

Figure 1 Proteins interacting with EWS and EWS-FLI1.

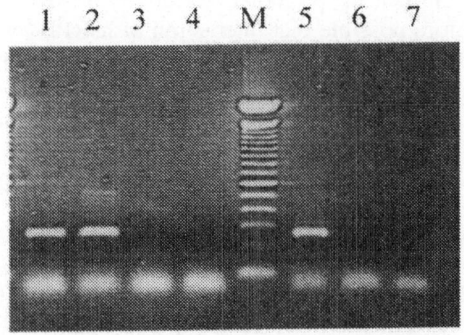

Figure 2 Demonstration by chromatin immuno precipitation of direct binding of EWS-FLI1 to the TGFβRII promoter in an EFT cell line lacking EWS expression. The TGFβRII promoter sequence bound in EWS-FLI1 containing complexes is detected by PCR. 1 and 2: EWS specific antibodies; 3 irrelevant antibody; 4 no antibody; M size marker; 5 positive and 6 and 7 negative PCR controls.

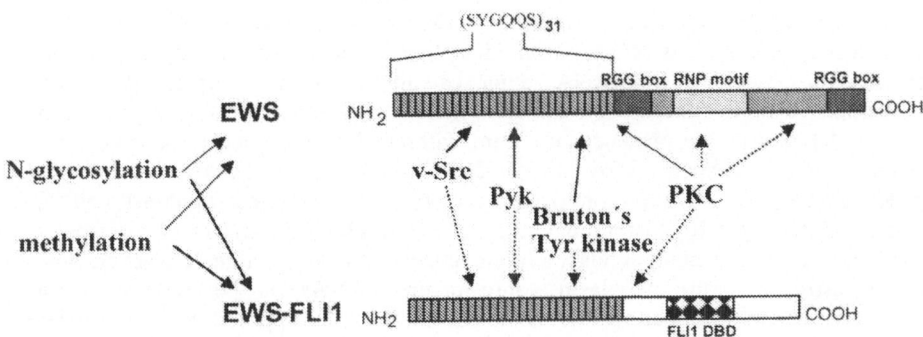

Figure 3 Post transcriptional modifications targeting EWS and possibly (stippeled arrows) also EWS-FLI1.

TET proteins are constitutively expressed at high levels in most, if not all tissues. In protein interaction studies we recently identified homo- and heterodimerization of EWS and EWS-FLI1 proteins in vitro and in the living cell (unpublished). Thus it is possible that EWS-FLI1 interferes with normal EWS function. However, this interaction is unlikely to play a general role in fusion protein mediated oncogenesis, since we recently described an EFT cell line lacking germline EWS expression[56].

In addition to interfering with the normal functions of their constituents TET fusion proteins may acquire new functions. The interaction of the EWS N-terminal transforming domain with hsRPB7 was observed exclusively in the context of the fusion protein[28] or a C-terminally truncated EWS[27], but not in the context of full length EWS. Since the EWS-FLI1 interaction with hsRPB7 was not only observed between endogenous proteins but also between bacterially expressed recombinant proteins, post-translational modification is unlikely to account for the specificity of the interaction. Rather, loss of the C-terminal EWS domain due to gene fusion results in a structural change at the EWS amino terminus exposing previously not accessible epitopes for protein interaction within the context of the oncogenic fusion protein. In yeast, RPB7, in complex with RPB4, influences promoter selectivity of RNA Pol II under stress conditions[57]. It is therefore possible that interaction of hsRPB7 with EWS-FLI1 affects target gene selection of the oncogenic fusion protein. A functional role for the protein structure in EWS fusion proteins is further confirmed in studies by Kevin Lee, who demonstrated that the presence of the EWS C-terminus suppresses the transactivation activity of the EWS N-terminal domain[58].

SITES WITHIN THE EWS-FLI1 PATHWAY FOR POSSIBLE THERAPEUTIC ATTACK

The requirement for continuous EWS-FLI1 expression to sustain EFT cell proliferation makes it an attractive target for therapeutic intervention. As shown in Figure 4, the pathway may be attacked at several sites: Antisense approaches, although resulting in some useful information, have proved rather inefficient and laborious in this respect[14-17]. However, they provided evidence that downregulation of EWS-FLI1 expression can inhibit EFT growth in a nude mouse model[59]. Preliminary studies indicate that RNA interference (RNAi) may provide a potent alternative to modulate EWS-FLI1 expression in EFT (Fig 5). RNAi is based on post-transcriptional degradation of a specific mRNA by a ribonuclease complex (the RNA induced silencing complex RISC) that uses short interfering double stranded RNA (siRNA) as a guide to target and degrade the complementary mRNA. Only perfectly matched RNA sequences will be recognized[60]. Thus RNAi is an ideal tool to target specifically mutant and chimeric RNA sequences. SiRNA duplexes appear to be surprisingly stable. Modifications, such as fluorine-derivatization increase resistance to RNases[61] and allow for direct delivery in the presence of serum without the requirement for lipofection. Efficient in-vivo gene silencing by either injected synthetic siRNA or siRNA expressed from RNA polymerase III driven retroviral vectors has already been demonstrated[62-64]. Targeting of the specific fusion region of EWS-ets chimeric RNAs by therapeutic siRNA or siRNA-like compounds therefore appears to be feasible. However, since RNAi is restricted to the cytoplasm[65] only mature mRNAs can be attacked. It may happen that under sustained RNAi-mediated EWS-FLI1 suppression EFT develop resistance to a specific siRNA through alternative splicing. This problem may be specifically but not exclusively important in cases with non-type 1 EWS-FLI1 fusion products. The presence of several minor splicing variants in EFT in addition to the major fusion product has previously been documented for an EWS exon 9/FLI1 exon 4 fusion[66]. Also, a significant percentage of EFT express a functional EWS exon 7/FLI1 exon 6 fusion protein despite an out-of-frame genomic EWS intron 8/FLI1 intron 5 rearrangement due to exon skipping[12,13]. Since the minimal transforming domains of EWS-FLI1 are encoded by EWS exons 1 to 7 and FLI1 exon 9, which are also minimally included in the fusion products observed in EFT, there is a chance that selective pressure may result in post-transcriptional switching of the chimeric mRNA structure to an EWS exon 7 to FLI1 exon 8 or exon 9 fusion by alternative splicing. Consequently, the capability of siRNA to down-regulate EWS-FLI1 expression may only be transient. However, since antisense studies suggested that down regulation of EWS-FLI1 expression may increase the chemosensitivity of EFT[67], one could think of using siRNA in a combination treatment regimen with conventional cytotoxic drugs.

RNAi approaches will also be of use to identify the downstream genes of TET fusion proteins, which are considered to mediate their oncogenic activity, and will therefore indirectly contribute to the identification of novel therapeutic targets as well. EWS-FLI1 expression or tolerance appear to be dependent on growth factor receptor signaling. Both, the IGF1 and bFGF receptors have been implicated in EWS-FLI1 regulation[6,7,24], although the mechanism of this regulation remains unclear. Signaling by many growth factors including IGF1 involves N-linked glycosylation. Interestingly, inhibition of both 3-hydroxy-3-methylglutaryl coenzyme A (HMG-CoA) reductase by lovastatin and N-linked glycosylation by tunicamycin drastically decreased the expression of the EWS-FLI1 fusion protein and consequently proliferation of EFT cells in-vitro[68]. These results may pave the way to the development of more specific therapeutically useful small molecules targeting growth factor receptor pathways in EFT.

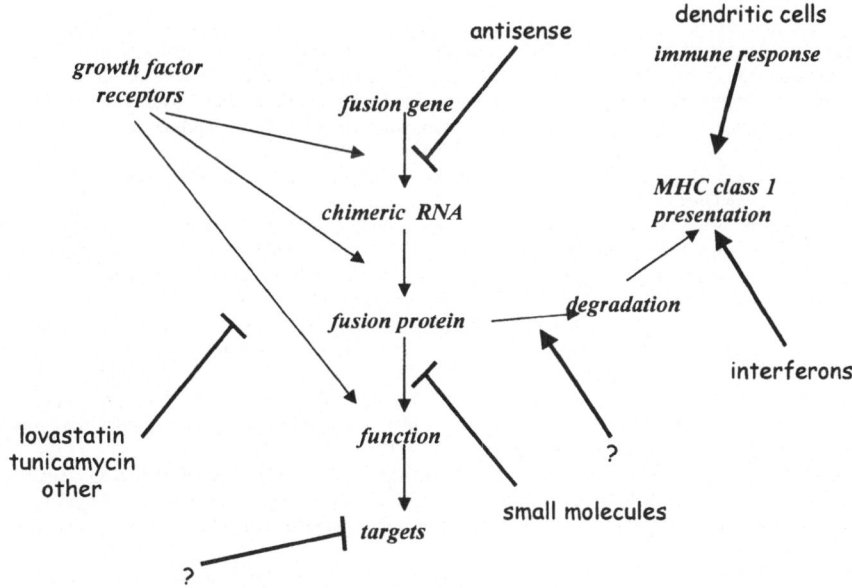

Figure 4. Sites of possible intervention in the EWS-FLI1 fusion gene pathway.

Figure 5. Modulation of EWS-FLI expression by RNA interference. EFT cells were transfected with a GFP expression vector plus either an RNA Pol III driven siRNA expression vector (pSUPERshEF4) or empty control vector (pSUPER). Cells were sorted according to their GFP positivity and the expression of endogenous EWS-FLI1 as compared to the vector encoded control gene NPT was evaluated in a multi-primer PCR reaction. Clearly, EWS-FLI1 expression is modulated in EFT cells expressing siRNA. Also shown is the up-regulation of TGFβRII expression upon modulation of EWS-FLI1. β-actin expression served as a control.

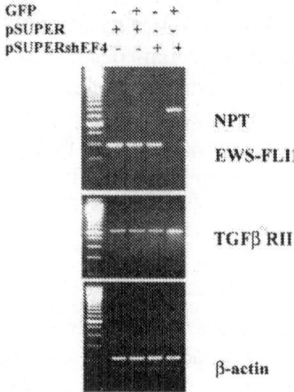

The fusion proteins resulting from chromosomal translocations in tumor cells may be envisaged as neoantigens and consequently as tumor markers. Among the proteasomal break-down products peptides spanning the fusion region should be new to the immune system if presented in an adequate MHC context. In contrast, EFT escape immuno surveillance of the patients. Preliminary studies using fusion peptide pulsed dendritic cells as a tumor vaccine gave disappointing results[69]. Intense research into the mechanisms of tolerance/anergy towards the fusion antigen is required to further develop immuno therapeutic strategies against EFT.

References

1. Turc Carel, C., Aurias, A., Mugneret, F., Lizard, S., Sidaner, I., Volk, C., Thiery, J. P., Olschwang, S., Philip, I., Berger, M. P., and et al Chromosomes in Ewing's sarcoma. I. An evaluation of 85 cases of remarkable consistency of t(11;22)(q24;q12). Cancer Genet.Cytogenet., *32*: 229-238, 1988.
2. Delattre, O., Zucman, J., Plougastel, B., Desmaze, C., Melot, T., Peter, M., Kovar, H., Joubert, I., De Jong, P., Rouleau, G., and et al Gene fusion with an ETS DNA-binding domain caused by chromosome translocation in human tumours. Nature, *359*: 162-165, 1992.
3. Kovar, H., Aryee, D., and Zoubek, A. The Ewing family of tumors and the search for the Achilles' heel. Curr.Opin.Oncol, *11*: 275-284, 1999.
4. Deneen, B. and Denny, C. T. Loss of p16 pathways stabilizes EWS/FLI1 expression and complements EWS/FLI1 mediated transformation. Oncogene, *20*: 6731-6741, 2001.
5. Lessnick, S. L., Braun, B. S., Denny, C. T., and May, W. A. Multiple domains mediate transformation by the Ewing's sarcoma EWS/FLI-1 fusion gene. Oncogene, *10*: 423-431, 1995.
6. Toretsky, J. A., Kalebic, T., Blakesley, V., LeRoith, D., and Helman, L. J. The insulin-like growth factor-I receptor is required for EWS/FLI-1 transformation of fibroblasts [In Process Citation]. J.Biol.Chem., *272*: 30822-30827, 1997.
7. Scotlandi, K., Benini, S., Nanni, P., Lollini, P. L., Nicoletti, G., Landuzzi, L., Serra, M., Manara, M. C., Picci, P., and Baldini, N. Blockage of insulin-like growth factor-I receptor inhibits the growth of Ewing's sarcoma in athymic mice. Cancer Res., *58*: 4127-4131, 1998.
8. May, W. A., Gishizky, M. L., Lessnick, S. L., Lunsford, L. B., Lewis, B. C., Delattre, O., Zucman, J., Thomas, G., and Denny, C. T. Ewing sarcoma 11;22 translocation produces a chimeric transcription factor that requires the DNA-binding domain encoded by FLI1 for transformation. Proc.Natl.Acad.Sci.U.S.A., *90*: 5752-5756, 1993.
9. Arvand, A., Welford, S. M., Teitell, M. A., and Denny, C. T. The COOH-terminal domain of FLI-1 is necessary for full tumorigenesis and transcriptional modulation by EWS/FLI-1. Cancer Res., *61* : 5311-5317, 2001.

10. Jaishankar, S., Zhang, J., Roussel, M. F., and Baker, S. J. Transforming activity of EWS/FLI is not strictly dependent upon DNA- binding activity [In Process Citation]. Oncogene, *18*: 5592-5597, 1999.

11. Welford, S. M., Hebert, S. P., Deneen, B., Arvand, A., and Denny, C. T. DNA binding domain-independent pathways are involved in EWS/FLI1-mediated oncogenesis. J.Biol.Chem., *276*: 41977-41984, 2001.

12. Zucman-Rossi, J., Legoix, P., Victor, J. M., Lopez, B., and Thomas, G. Chromosome translocation based on illegitimate recombination in human tumors. Proc.Natl.Acad.Sci.U.S.A., *95*: 11786-11791, 1998.

13. Zucman, J., Melot, T., Desmaze, C., Ghysdael, J., Plougastel, B., Peter, M., Zucker, J. M., Triche, T. J., Sheer, D., Turc Carel, C., and et al Combinatorial generation of variable fusion proteins in the Ewing family of tumours. EMBO J., *12*: 4481-4487, 1993.

14. Kovar, H., Aryee, D. N., Jug, G., Henockl, C., Schemper, M., Delattre, O., Thomas, G., and Gadner, H. EWS/FLI-1 antagonists induce growth inhibition of Ewing tumor cells in vitro. Cell Growth Differ., *7*: 429-437, 1996.

15. Ouchida, M., Ohno, T., Fujimura, Y., Rao, V. N., and Reddy, E. S. Loss of tumorigenicity of Ewing's sarcoma cells expressing antisense RNA to EWS-fusion transcripts. Oncogene, *11*: 1049-1054, 1995.

16. Tanaka, K., Iwakuma, T., Harimaya, K., Sato, H., and Iwamoto, Y. EWS-Fli1 antisense oligodeoxynucleotide inhibits proliferation of human Ewing's sarcoma and primitive neuroectodermal tumor cells. J.Clin.Invest., *99*: 239-247, 1997.

17. Toretsky, J. A., Connell, Y., Neckers, L., and Bhat, N. K. Inhibition of EWS-FLI-1 fusion protein with antisense oligodeoxynucleotides. J.Neurooncol., *31*: 9-16, 1997.

18. Kovar, H., Auinger, A., Jug, G., Aryee, D., Zoubek, A., Salzer Kuntschik, M., and Gadner, H. Narrow spectrum of infrequent p53 mutations and absence of MDM2 amplification in Ewing tumours. Oncogene, *8*: 2683-2690, 1993.

19. Kovar, H., Jug, G., Aryee, D. N. T., Zoubek, A., Ambros, P., Gruber, B., Windhager, R., and Gadner, H. Among genes involved in the RB dependent cell cycle regulatory cascade, the p16 tumor suppressor gene is frequently lost in the Ewing family of tumors. Oncogene, *15*: 1997.

20. Arvand, A. and Denny, C. T. Biology of EWS/ETS fusions in Ewing's family tumors. Oncogene, *20*: 5747-5754, 2001.

21. Kovar, H., Dworzak, M., Strehl, S., Schnell, E., Ambros, I. M., Ambros, P. F., and Gadner, H. Overexpression of the pseudoautosomal gene MIC2 in Ewing's sarcoma and peripheral primitive neuroectodermal tumor. Oncogene, *5*: 1067-1070, 1990.

22. Lessnick, S. L., Dacwag, C. S., and Golub, T. R. The Ewing's sarcoma oncoprotein EWS/FLI induces a p53-dependent growth arrest in primary human fibroblasts. Cancer Cell 1, 393-401. 2002. Ref Type: Generic

23. Matsumoto, Y., Tanaka, K., Nakatani, F., Matsunobu, T., Matsuda, S., and Iwamoto, Y. Downregulation and forced expression of EWS-Fli1 fusion gene results in changes in the expression of G(1)regulatory genes. Br.J.Cancer, *84*: 768-775, 2001.

24. Girnita, L., Girnita, A., Wang, M., Meis-Kindblom, J. M., Kindblom, L. G., and Larsson, O. A link between basic fibroblast growth factor (bFGF) and EWS/FLI-1 in Ewing's sarcoma cells. Oncogene, *19*: 4298-4301, 2000.

25. Thompson, A. D., Teitell, M. A., Arvand, A., and Denny, C. T. Divergent Ewing's sarcoma EWS/ETS fusions confer a common tumorigenic phenotype on NIH3T3 cells [In Process Citation]. Oncogene, *18*: 5506-5513, 1999.

26. Bertolotti, A., Lutz, Y., Heard, D. J., Chambon, P., and Tora, L. hTAF(II)68, a novel RNA/ssDNA-binding protein with homology to the pro-oncoproteins TLS/FUS and EWS is associated with both TFIID and RNA polymerase II. EMBO J., *15*: 5022-5031, 1996.

27. Bertolotti, A., Melot, T., Acker, J., Vigneron, M., Delattre, O., and Tora, L. EWS, but not EWS-FLI-1, is associated with both TFIID and RNA polymerase II: interactions between two members of the TET family, EWS and hTAFII68, and subunits of TFIID and RNA polymerase II complexes [In Process Citation]. Mol.Cell Biol., *18*: 1489-1497, 1998.

28. Petermann, R., Mossier, B. M., Aryee, D. N., Khazak, V., Golemis, E. A., and Kovar, H. Oncogenic EWS-Fli1 interacts with hsRPB7, a subunit of human RNA polymerase II [In Process Citation]. Oncogene, *17*: 603-610, 1998.

29. Chansky, H. A., Hu, M., Hickstein, D. D., and Yang, L. Oncogenic TLS/ERG and EWS/Fli-1 fusion proteins inhibit RNA splicing mediated by YB-1 protein. Cancer Res., *61*: 3586-3590, 2001.

30. Knoop, L. L. and Baker, S. J. The splicing factor U1C represses EWS/FLI-mediated transactivation. J.Biol.Chem., *275*: 24865-24871, 2000.

31. Yang, L., Embree, L. J., Tsai, S., and Hickstein, D. D. Oncoprotein TLS interacts with serine-arginine proteins involved in RNA splicing. J.Biol.Chem., 273: 27761-27764, 1998.

32. Yang, L., Chansky, H. A., and Hickstein, D. D. EWS[middle dot]Fli-1 fusion protein interacts with hyperphosphorylated RNA polymerase II and interferes with serine-arginine protein-mediated RNA splicing. J.Biol.Chem., 275: 37612-37618, 2000.

33. Zhang, D., Paley, A. J., and Childs, G. The transcriptional repressor ZFM1 interacts with and modulates the ability of EWS to activate transcription. J.Biol.Chem., 273: 18086-18091, 1998.

34. Calvio, C., Neubauer, G., Mann, M., and Lamond, A. I. Identification of hnRNP P2 as TLS/FUS using electrospray mass spectrometry. RNA., 1: 724-733, 1995.

35. Hahm, K. B., Cho, K., Lee, C., Im, Y. H., Chang, J., Choi, S. G., Sorensen, P. H., Thiele, C. J., and Kim, S. J. Repression of the gene encoding the TGF-beta type II receptor is a major target of the EWS-FLI1 oncoprotein. Nat.Genet., 23: 222-227, 1999.

36. Yang, L., Embree, L. J., and Hickstein, D. D. TLS-ERG leukemia fusion protein inhibits RNA splicing mediated by serine-arginine proteins. Mol.Cell Biol., 20: 3345-3354, 2000.

37. Knoop, L. L. and Baker, S. J. EWS/FLI alters 5'-splice site selection. J.Biol.Chem., 276: 22317-22322, 2001.

38. Ohkura, N., Yaguchi, H., Tsukada, T., and Yamaguchi, K. The EWS/NOR1 fusion gene product gains a novel activity affecting pre-mRNA splicing. J.Biol.Chem., 277: 535-543, 2002.

39. Spahn, L., Petermann, R., Siligan, C., Schmid, J. A., Aryee, D. N., and Kovar, H. Interaction of the EWS NH2 terminus with BARD1 links the Ewing's sarcoma gene to a common tumor suppressor pathway. Cancer Res., 62: 4583-4587, 2002.

40. Kleiman, F. E. and Manley, J. L. Functional interaction of BRCA1-associated BARD1 with polyadenylation factor CstF-50. Science, 285: 1576-1579, 1999.

41. Kleiman, F. E. and Manley, J. L. The BARD1-CstF-50 Interaction Links mRNA 3' End Formation to DNA Damage and Tumor Suppression. Cell, 104: 743-753, 2001.

42. Venkitaraman, A. R. Functions of BRCA1 and BRCA2 in the biological response to DNA damage. J.Cell Sci., 114: 3591-3598, 2001.

43. Hicks, G. G., Singh, N., Nashabi, A., Mai, S., Bozek, G., Klewes, L., Arapovic, D., White, E. K., Koury, M. J., Oltz, E. M., Van Kaer, L., and Ruley, H. E. Fus deficiency in mice results in defective B-lymphocyte development and activation, high levels of chromosomal instability and perinatal death. Nat.Genet., 24: 175-179, 2000.

44. Kuroda, M., Sok, J., Webb, L., Baechtold, H., Urano, F., Yin, Y., Chung, P., de Rooij, D. G., Akhmedov, A., Ashley, T., and Ron, D. Male sterility and enhanced radiation sensitivity in TLS(-/-) mice. EMBO J., 19: 453-462, 2000.

45. Soldatenkov, V. A., Trofimova, I. N., Rouzaut, A., McDermott, F., Dritschilo, A., and Notario, V. Differential regulation of the response to DNA damage in Ewing's sarcoma cells by ETS1 and EWS/FLI-1. Oncogene, 21: 2890-2895, 2002.

46. Prasad, S. C., Thraves, P. J., Bhatia, K. G., Smulson, M. E., and Dritschilo, A. Enhanced poly(adenosine diphosphate ribose) polymerase activity and gene expression in Ewing's sarcoma cells. Cancer Res., 50: 38-43, 1990.

47. Powers, C. A., Mathur, M., Raaka, B. M., Ron, D., and Samuels, H. H. TLS (translocated-in-liposarcoma) is a high-affinity interactor for steroid, thyroid hormone, and retinoid receptors. Mol.Endocrinol., 12: 4-18, 1998.

48. Uranıshi, H., Tetsuka, T., Yamashita, M., Asamitsu, K., Shimizu, M., Itoh, M., and Okamoto, T. Involvement of the pro-oncoprotein TLS (translocated in liposarcoma) in nuclear factor-kappa B p65-mediated transcription as a coactivator. J.Biol.Chem., 276: 13395-13401, 2001.

49. Deloulme, J. C., Prichard, L., Delattre, O., and Storm, D. R. The prooncoprotein EWS binds calmodulin and is phosphorylated by protein kinase C through an IQ domain [In Process Citation]. J.Biol.Chem., 272: 27369-27377, 1997.

50. Felsch, J. S., Lane, W. S., and Peralta, E. G. Tyrosine kinase Pyk2 mediates G-protein-coupled receptor regulation of the Ewing sarcoma RNA-binding protein EWS. Curr.Biol., 9: 485-488, 1999.

51. Guinamard, R., Fougereau, M., and Seckinger, P. The SH3 domain of Bruton's tyrosine kinase interacts with Vav, Sam68 and EWS. Scand.J.Immunol., 45: 587-595, 1997.

52. Olsen, R. J. and Hinrichs, S. H. Phosphorylation of the EWS IQ domain regulates transcriptional activity of the EWS/ATF1 and EWS/FLI1 fusion proteins. Oncogene, 20: 1756-1764, 2001.

53. Kim, J., Lee, J. M., Branton, P. E., and Pelletier, J. Modulation of EWS/WT1 activity by the v-Src protein tyrosine kinase. FEBS Lett., 474: 121-128, 2000.

54. Matsuoka, Y., Matsuoka, Y., Shibata, S., Yasuhara, N., and Yoneda, Y. Identification of Ewing's Sarcoma Gene Product as a Glycoprotein Using a Monoclonal Antibody that Recognizes an

Immunodeterminant Containing O-Linked N-Acetylglucosamine Moiety. Hybrid.Hybridomics., *21*: 233-236, 2002.

55. Belyanskaya, L. L., Gehrig, P. M., and Gehring, H. Exposure on cell surface and extensive arginine methylation of EWS protein. J.Biol.Chem., .: 2001.

56. Kovar, H., Jug, G., Hattinger, C., Spahn, L., Aryee, D. N., Ambros, P. F., Zoubek, A., and Gadner, H. The ews protein is dispensable for ewing tumor growth. Cancer Res., *61*: 5992-5997, 2001.

57. Khazak, V., Sadhale, P. P., Woychik, N. A., Brent, R., and Golemis, E. A. Human RNA polymerase II subunit hsRPB7 functions in yeast and influences stress survival and cell morphology. Mol.Biol.Cell, *6*: 759-775, 1995.

58. Li, K. K. and Lee, K. A. Transcriptional activation by the Ewing's sarcoma (EWS) oncogene can be cis-repressed by the EWS RNA-binding domain. J.Biol.Chem., *275*: 23053-23058, 2000.

59. Lambert, G., Bertrand, J. R., Fattal, E., Subra, F., Pinto-Alphandary, H., Malvy, C., Auclair, C., and Couvreur, P. EWS fli-1 antisense nanocapsules inhibits ewing sarcoma-related tumor in mice. Biochem.Biophys.Res.Commun., *279*: 401-406, 2000.

60. McManus, M. T. and Sharp, P. A. Gene silencing in mammals by small interfering RNAs. Nat.Rev.Genet., *3*: 737-747, 2002.

61. Capodici, J., Kariko, K., and Weissman, D. Inhibition of HIV-1 Infection by Small Interfering RNA-Mediated RNA Interference. J.Immunol., *169*: 5196-5201, 2002.

62. Xia, H., Mao, Q., Paulson, H. L., and Davidson, B. L. siRNA-mediated gene silencing in vitro and in vivo. Nat.Biotechnol., *20*: 1006-1010, 2002.

63. Lewis, D. L., Hagstrom, J. E., Loomis, A. G., Wolff, J. A., and Herweijer, H. Efficient delivery of siRNA for inhibition of gene expression in postnatal mice. Nat.Genet., *32*: 107-108, 2002.

64. Brummelkamp, T., Bernards, R., and Agami, R. Stable suppression of tumorigenicity by virus-mediated RNA interference. Cancer Cell, *2*: 243, 2002.

65. Zeng, Y. and Cullen, B. R. RNA interference in human cells is restricted to the cytoplasm. RNA., *8*: 855-860, 2002.

66. Zoubek, A., Pfleiderer, C., Salzer-Kuntschik, M., Amann, G., Windhager, R., Fink, F. M., Koscielniak, E., Delattre, O., Strehl, S., and Ambros, P. F. Variability of EWS chimaeric transcripts in Ewing tumours: a comparison of clinical and molecular data. Br.J.Cancer, *70*: 908-913, 1994.

67. Yi, H., Fujimura, Y., Ouchida, M., Prasad, D. D., Rao, V. N., and Reddy, E. S. Inhibition of apoptosis by normal and aberrant Fli-1 and erg proteins involved in human solid tumors and leukemias. Oncogene, *14*: 1259-1268, 1997.

68. Wang, M., Xie, Y., Girnita, L., Nilsson, G., Dricu, A., Wejde, J., and Larsson, O. Regulatory Role of Mevalonate and N-Linked Glycosylation in Proliferation and Expression of the EWS/FLI-1 Fusion Protein in Ewing's Sarcoma Cells. Exp.Cell Res., *246*: 38-46, 1999.

69. Mackall, C., Berzofsky, J., and Helman, L. J. Targeting tumor specific translocations in sarcomas in pediatric patients for immunotherapy. Clin.Orthop., *275*: 25-31, 2000.

CANCER EPIGENETICS: DNA METHYLATION AND CHROMATIN ALTERATIONS IN HUMAN CANCER

Manel Esteller

Cancer Epigenetics Laboratory, Spanish National Cancer Center (CNIO), Melchor Fernandez Almagro 3, 28029 Madrid, Spain

ABSTRACT

Aberrations in the DNA methylation patterns are nowadays recognized as a hallmark of human cancer. One of the most characteristic changes is the hypermethylation of CpG islands of tumor suppressor genes associated with their transcriptional silencing. The target genes are distributed in all cellular pathways (apoptosis, DNA repair, cell cycle, cell adherence, etc.). They are "classical" tumor suppressor genes with associated familial cancers (BRCA1, hMLH1, p16^{INK4a}, VHL, etc.) and putative new tumor suppressor genes which loss may contribute to the transformed phenotype (MGMT, p14^{ARF}, GSTP1, RARB2, etc.). A tumor-type specific profile of CpG island hypermethylation exist in human cancer that allows the use of these aberrantly hypermethylated loci as biomarkers of the malignant disease. The irruption of new technologies for the careful study of the DNA methylation patterns, and their genetic partners in accomplishing gene silencing, it may also provide us with new drugs for the epigenetic treatment of human tumors.

GENE INACTIVATION BY PROMOTER HYPERMETHYLATION IN HUMAN CANCER: CONCEPTS

The inheritance of information based on gene expression levels is known as epigenetics, as opposed to genetics, which refers to information transmitted on the basis of gene sequence. The main epigenetic modification in mammals, and in particular in humans, is the methylation in the cytosine nucleotide residue. We can consider than about 3-4% of all cytosines are methylated in normal human DNA. Gross alterations such as the aneuploidy state, deletions (loss of heterozigosity) or gains (gene amplification) of genomic material,

New Trends in Cancer for the 21st Century, edited by
Llombart-Bosch and Felipo, Kluwer Academic/Plenum Publishers, 2003

and small changes (point mutations, small insertions or deletions) in multiple genes are present through the genome of a neoplastic cell. But the malignant cell has also adquired a different epigenotype. In a healthy cell, the DNA methylation patterns are conserved through cell divisions allowing the expression of the particular set of cellular genes necessary for that cell type and blocking the expression of exogenous inserted sequences.

The presence of the CpG dinucleotide in the human genome is suppressed by a statistical criterion[1]. The evolutionary proposed reason for this lack of CpGs in our genome is to avoid spontaneous deamination in the germline. However, approximately half of the human gene promoter regions contain CpG-rich regions, known as "CpG islands"[1]. Although the majority of CpG islands are associated with "house-keeping" genes, some of them are located in "tissue-specific genes". It should also be noted that although the most significant proportion of CpG islands is located in the 5´-unstranslated regions and the first exon of the genes, certain CpG islands could occasionally be found within the body of the gene, or even in the 3'-region. CpG islands in these atypical locations are more prone to methylation[2]. Hypermethylation of CpG islands located in the promoter regions of tumor suppressor genes is now definitely established as an important mechanism for gene inactivation.

CpG island hypermethylation has been described in every tumor type. Many cellular pathways are inactivated by this type of epigenetic lesion: DNA repair (hMLH1, MGMT), cell cycle (p16^{INK4a}, p15^{INK4b}, p14^{ARF}), cell adherence (CDH1, CDH13), apoptosis (DAPK), detoxification (GSTP1), hormonal response (RARB2, ER). etc...[3]. However, we still do not know the mechanisms of aberrant methylation and why certain genes are selected over others. Hypermethylation is not an isolated layer of epigenetic control, but is linked to the other pieces of the puzzle such as methyl-binding proteins, DNA methyltransferases, histone deacetylases and histone methyltransferases, but our understanding of the degree of specificity of these epigenetic layers in the silencing of specific tumor suppressor genes remains incomplete. Careful functional and genetic studies are necessary to determine which hypermethylation events are truthfully relevant for human tumorigenesis. The development of CpG island hypermethylation profiles for every form of human tumors has yielded valuable pilot clinical data in monitoring and treating cancer patients based in our knowledge of DNA methylation.

SUMMARIZING THE HISTORY OF CpG ISLAND HYPERMETHYLATION

The first discovery of methylation in a CpG island of a tumor suppressor gene in a human cancer was that of the Retinoblastoma (Rb) gene in 1989[4], only a few years after the first oncogene mutation (H-ras) was discovered in a human primary tumor. In 1994 was born the idea that CpG island promoter hypermethylation could be a mechanism to inactivate genes in cancer fully restored as a result of the discovery that the Von Hippel-Lindau (VHL) gene also undergoes methylation-associated inactivation[5]. However, the true origin of the current period of research in cancer epigenetic silencing was perhaps the discovery that CpG island hypermethylation was a common mechanism of inactivation of the tumor suppressor gene p16^{INK4a} in human cancer[6, 7, 8]. The introduction of powerful and accessible techniques, such as sodium bisulfite modification[9] and Methylation-Specific PCR[10], provided keys to start the game. From that time, the list of candidate genes with putative aberrant methylation of their CpG islands has grown exponentially[3].

A TUMOR-TYPE SPECIFIC GENE HYPERMETHYLATION PROFILE OF HUMAN CANCER

We know that cancer is a disease of multiple pathways and genetic lesions and all of them are necessary to develop a fully established tumor The existence of genetic alterations affecting genes involved in cellular proliferation and death, such as *p53* and *K-ras*, is one of the most common features of tumor cells. Recently, the inactivation of tumor suppressor genes by promoter hypermethylation has been added to this scenario. The presence of CpG island promoter hypermethylation affects genes involved in cell cycle (p16^{INK4a}, p15^{INK4b}, Rb, p14^{ARF}), DNA repair (BRCA1, hMLH1, MGMT), cell-adherence (CDH1, CDH13), apoptosis (DAPK, TMS1), carcinogen-metabolism (GSTP1), hormonal response (RARB2, ER), etc. (Figure 3) shows the most relevant hypermethylated genes in human cancer reported so far and their chromosomal localization. In most of cases, methylation involves loss of expression, absence of a coding mutation and restoration of transcription by the use of demethylating agents.

A profile of CpG island hypermethylation exists according to the tumor type[3]. For example BRCA1 hypermethylation is characteristic of breast and ovarian tumors[11], but it does not occur in other tumor types[3]. Or hMLH1 methylation-mediated silencing occurs in colorectal, gastric and endometrial neoplasms, but in almost none of the other solid tumors[3]. This cautiously respected pattern of epigenetic inactivation is not only a property of the sporadic tumors, but also that neoplasms appearing in inherited cancer syndromes display CpG island hypermethylation specific to the tumor type[11]. We can call this the "Methylotype", for the pattern of analogy with the genetic term "Genotype". There are also tumor types that have more methylation of the known CpG islands than others: for example the most hypermethylated tumor types are originated from the gastrointestinal tract (esophagus, stomach, colon), while significantly less hypermethylation has been reported in other types such as ovarian tumors[3]. There is a clear gradient of the distribution of tumors with different degrees of CpG island methylation: from tumors with few hypermethylated CpG islands until neoplasms with a very high number of hypermethylated islands. This is the rate expected for events occurring randomly and being selected because they confer advantage to the cancer cell, excluding the existence of any significant methylator phenotype.

DNA METHYLATION HITS IN A CANCER CELL

The epigenetic balance of the cell suffers a dramatic alteration in cancer: transcriptional silencing of tumor suppressor genes by CpG island hypermethylation and histone deacetylation, global genomic hypomethylation and genetic defects in chromatin-related genes.

Not every gene is methylated in every tumor type. There is a delicate profile of hypermethylation that occurs in human tumors, but CpG island methylation affects all cellular pathways. The growing list of genes inactivated by promoter region hypermethylation provides an opportunity to examine the patterns of inactivation of such genes among different tumors. Usually one or more genes are hypermethylated in every tumor type. However, the profile of promoter hypermethylation for the genes differs for each cancer type providing a tumor-type and gene specific profile. In each case and tumor type, this epigenetic lesion occurs in the absence of a genetic lesion.

If we look at our gene hypermethylation profile from the tumor type point of view, the picture is particularly interesting. Gastrointestinal tumors (colon and gastric) share a set of genes undergoing hypermethylation characterized by $p16^{INK4a}$, $p14^{ARF}$, MGMT, APC and hMLH1, while other aerodigestive tumor types, such as lung and head and neck, have a different pattern of hypermethylated genes including DAPK, MGMT, $p16^{INK4a}$ but not hMLH1 or $p14^{ARF}$. Similarly, breast and ovarian cancers be inclined to methylate certain genes including BRCA1, GSTP1 and $p16^{INK4a}$. This gene hypermethylation profile of human cancer is consistent with the data of particular "methylotypes" proposed for single tumor types.

In a cancer cell there is a clear distortion in the expression profiles and the presence of a dramatic change in the methylation patterns is one of the guilty parts. First, there is a disregulation in the methylating enzymes. Second, there is a global hypomethylation when compare to a normal cell; this is achieved due to a generalized demethylation in the CpGs dotted in the body of the genes and may be involved in causing global genomic fragility and reexpresion of inserted viral sequences. And third and finally, there are local and discrete regions normally devoid of methylation that suffer an intense hypermethylation.

HYPERMETHYLATION AND MUTATION: THE STRANGE COUPLE

When the first genetic mutation was discovered in a human cancer, the idea that a large number of genes would be found mutated in all tumors was everywhere. However, twenty years later only two genes, the oncogene K-ras and the tumor suppressor p53 have found to be consistently mutated in a high proportion of tumors. This concept of how to transform expectations to reality could also be applied to CpG island hypermethylation.

One of the most critical steps in giving CpG island methylation its accurate value is the fact that it should occur in the absence of gene mutations. Both events (genetic and epigenetic) abolish normal gene function. The selective advantage of promoter hypermethylation in this context is provided by multiple examples. The cell cycle inhibitor $p16^{INK4a}$ in one allele of the HCT-116 colorectal cancer cell line has a genetic mutation while the other is wild-type: p16INK4a hypermethylation occurs only on the wild-type allele, while the mutated allele is kept unmethylated[12]. Examples like that put CpG island hypermethylation evenly balanced with gene mutation for accomplishing selective gene inactivation.

A subset of human tumors display a bizarre genetic phenotype defined by the microsatellite instability (MSI) phenomena. MSI+ tumors are defined because they show aberrant insertions or deletions of mono- or dinucleotides repeats when the tumors are compared with their normal counterparts. The tumor types mainly involved in the disease are colorectal, endometrial and gastric carcinoma. In these HNPCC families the defect is attributed to germline mutations in the DNA mismatch-repair (MMR) genes, mainly hMLH1 and hMSH2, while other components of the MMR pathway such as hMSH3, hMSH6, hPMS1 and hPMS2 seem to play a minor role in the disease. MSI positive tumors were also observed in spontaneous cases, however, MMR mutations were found in less than 10% of sporadic MSI+ tumors. The explanation of this data is that the presence of MSI is due to transcriptional inactivation of hMLH1 by promoter hypermethylation[13,14].

Other exciting example of how promoter hypermethylation affects the genome of the cancer cell is provided by the DNA repair gene O^6-methylguanine DNA methyltransferase

(*MGMT*). The DNA repair gene *MGMT* is transcriptionally silenced by promoter hypermethylation in primary human tumors[15]. These tumors then accumulate a considerable number of G to A transition mutations affecting key genes such as *p53* and *K-ras*, in a similar way that loss of the *hMLH1* mismatch repair gene by methylation targets other genes.

Two more genes related to potential DNA lesions undergo inactivation by promoter hypermethylation, the glutathione S-transferase P1 (*GSTP1*) and the breast cancer familial gene *BRCA1*. Changes of *GSTP1* expression may prevent DNA damage, but its cause was imprecise until aberrant methylation of the *GSTP1* CpG island in prostate, breast and kidney carcinoma was reported[16,17]. The case of the tumor suppressor gene *BRCA1* gene, responsible for almost half of the cases of inherited breast cancer and ovarian cancer, is also relevant. *BRCA1* promoter hypermethylation leading to *BRCA1* loss of function is present in breast and ovarian primary tumors and cell lines[18,11]. What are the link between changes in *BRCA1* protein levels and DNA damage? Two hypothesis were defended: BRCA1 cooperate with the RNA helicase A and the histone deacetylase complex in the transcriptional regulation of DNA integrity maintain genes and BRCA1 play an important role in DNA repair forming supercomplexes with proteins like *ATM*, *RAD51* and *hMSH2*.

Now, let´s check the other side of the coin. We could mention different examples where a link between genetic modification that causes epigenetic fluctuations is established: ATRX, ICF syndrome, PML-RAR fusion protein and Methyl-group Metabolism genes. Mutations in *ATRX* give rise to characteristic developmental abnormalities including severe mental retardation, facial dysmorphism, urogenital abnormalities and alfa-thalasaemia. Mutations in *ATRX* give rise to changes in the pattern of methylation of several highly repeated sequences. ATRX is localized to pericentromeric heterochromatin and might exert chromatin-mediated effects in the nucleus and act as a transcriptional regulator through an effect on chromatin. A human genetic disorder (ICF syndrome) is caused by mutations in the DNA methyltransferase 3B (DNMT3B) gene. A second human disorder (Rett syndrome) has been found to result from mutations in the MECP2 gene, which encodes a protein that binds to methylated DNA. Global genome demethylation caused by targeted mutations in the DNA methyltransferase-1 (Dnmt1) gene has shown that cytosine methylation plays essential roles in X-inactivation, genomic imprinting and genome stabilization. The leukemia-promoting PML-RAR fusion protein induces gene hypermethylation and silencing by recruiting DNA methyltransferases to target promoters and that hypermethylation contributes to its leukemogenic potential[19,20]. Retinoic acid treatment induces promoter demethylation, gene reexpression, and reversion of the transformed phenotype. Furthermore, germline variants in the methyl-group metabolism genes involved in the regeneration of the universal methyl-donor SAM (S-adenosyl-methionine) are also associated with different DNA methylation patterns in the cancer cell[21]. These results establish a mechanistic link between genetic and epigenetic changes during transformation and suggest that hypermethylation contributes to the early steps of carcinogenesis.

WHY DO CERTAIN CpG ISLANDS BECOME SUSCEPTIBLE TO HYPERMETHYLATION?

The CpG island are usually unmethylated in all normal tissues and span the 5' end of genes. If transcription factors are available and the island remains in an unmethylated state with open chromatin configuration-associated with hyperacetylated histones, transcription will occur. Certain CpG islands are normally methylated: imprinted genes and genes of one X-chromosome in women. DNA methylation has also a role in repressing parasitic DNA sequences.

In the transformed or malignant cell certain CpG islands of tumor suppressor genes (real or putative) will become hypermethylated[22, 23]. This is probably a progressive process, in contrast to the sudden appearance of a gene mutation. Perhaps several "steps" of disregulated methylation will be necessary to produce the dense hypermethylation necessary for transcriptionally silencing that particular promoter anchored in the CpG island. Two obvious theories can be postulated for this aberrant de *novo* methylation. First, the cancer methylation spreads from normal methylation-centers surrounding the methylation-free CpG island, for example from Alu regions[24]. Second, a basal status of methylation exists and certain single CpG dinucleotides in the island became methylated and subsequently this "be a magnet for" more methylation. This process has a positive cooperative effect until hypermethylation is achieved. A model that combines prior gene silencing with "seeds" of methylation has been proposed for the GSTP1 in prostate cancer[25]. Both hypotheses are plausible and compatible. However, there is not definitive support for either.

Another question on why certain CpG islands became hypermethylated. It has been known for a long time that an overall increase in the enzymatic DNA methyltransferase activity occurs in tumors versus normal tissues (reviewed [23]). This finding has been supported as a result of the molecular characterization of the genes encoding several DNA methyltranferases (DNMT1, DNMT3a, DNMT3b, DNMT3L and DNMT2), which has shown that the mRNA transcripts of DNMT1 (the classical methylation maintenance enzyme) and DNMT3b (the de novo methylation enzyme) are increased in several solid and hematological[26].

However, the most critical question still unclear: why do certain CpG islands become hypermethylated while others remain unmethylated in a cancer cell? Certain CpG islands become hypermethylated rather than others because they confer a selective advantage for the survival of that particular cancer cell. For example BRCA1 undergoes promoter hypermethylation only in breast and ovarian tumors[3,18] because only in these tumors types does the lack of this transcript have important cellular consequences. This Darwinian concept is supported by the classical genetic studies of familial tumors: carriers of BRCA1 germline mutations develop predominantly breast and ovarian tumors and carriers of hMLH1 germline mutations mostly develop colorectal, gastric and endometrial tumors. There is a perfect match between the genetic and epigenetic worlds.

DNA HYPOMETHYLATION OCCURS IN A WORLD OF CpG ISLAND HYPERMETHYLATION

CpG islands become hypermethylated but the genome of the cancer cell undergoes a dramatic global hypomethylation: 20-60% less genomic 5mC accomplished from the hypomethylation of the "body" of genes and repetitive DNA sequences. Global DNA hypomethylation may contribute to carcinogenesis causing chromosomal instability, reactivation of transposable elements and loss of imprinting.

The presence of alterations in the profile of DNA methylation in cancer was initially thought to be exclusively a global hypomethylation of the genome[27, 28] that would possibly lead to massive overexpression of oncogenes whose CpG islands were normally hypermethylated. Nowadays, this is considered to be an unlikely or, at best, incomplete scenario. The idea that the genome of the cancer cell undergoes a reduction of its 5-methylcytosine content in comparison to the normal tissue from which it originated is essentially correct, as also corroborated in a large survey of sporadic and inherited breast and colon tumors[11].

The popularity of the concept of demethylation of oncogenes leading to their activation is in clear decadency. The first experiments supporting this hypothesis effectively demonstrated DNA hypomethylation, but as only certain methyl-sensitive restriction sites were used a significant amount of this "demethylation" was present in the "body" of the genes (internal exons and introns) rather than in the canonical CpG island. In fact, the vast majority of CpG islands are completely unmethylated in normal tissues[1], with the logical exceptions of imprinted genes and X-chromosome genes in females.

HOW CpG ISLAND HYPERMETHYLATION DRIVES TO TRANSCRIPTIONAL GENE SILENCING? MOLECULAR STEPS

Throughout the last twenty years research on cell signaling has carefully characterized the components involved in the transmission of signals. The same molecular dissection should now be applied to elucidate how CpG island hypermethylation leads to transcriptional gene silencing. Perhaps, each step of this chain is specific to each gene or group of genes. One clue to unscrambling the enigma was the discovery that DNA methylation results in the formation of nuclease-resistant chromatin and the subsequent repression of gene activity[29].

Nowadays the most widely accepted explanation of events starts with the binding of certain methyl-binding proteins (MBDs) to the methylated CpG dinucleotides of the densely hypermethylated CpG island. The search for proteins with different binding properties for methylated and unmethylated DNA initially yielded two activities which were named MeCP1 and MeCP2, the first being a complex of proteins and the second a single polipeptide[30]. Further database searches revealed novel MBD-containing proteins, MBD1, MBD2, MBD3 and MBD4. A new question then arises: are there MBDs specific for subgroups of hypermethylated CpG island of tumor suppressor genes in cancer? Different methylation densities may attract different MBDs for example. Two recent reports have addressed this problem in one of the most interesting epigenetics spots in the human genome: the p15^{INK4b}/ p16^{INK4a}/p14^{ARF} locus in the 9p21 chromosomal region. These studies demonstrate that MeCP2[2] and MBD2[31] bind to the hypermethylated CpG islands of p14^{ARF} and p16^{INK4a}. If we improve the instrumental tools, it will signal that it is time to start mapping all the CpG island promoters of tumor suppressor genes for their MBD binding patterns.

Another critical result was the association of MeCP2 and histone deacetylase (HDAC) activity in repressing transcription[32, 33]. The remaining MBDs have also proved to be members of similar HDAC complexes. Thus, the current model propose that MBDs recruit HDAC activities to methylated promoters which, in turn deacetylate histones, leading to a chromatin-repressed state of gene transcription. Considering the CpG islands that undergo hypermethylation in the cancer cell, the association of hypoacetylated histones H3 and H4 with a hypermethylated CpG island has now been demonstrated for the p16^{INK4a}, p14^{ARF},

BRCA1, COX-2 and TMS1 genes. Thus, CpG island hypermethylation and histone hypoacetylation seems to be firmly associated[34].

TRANSLATIONAL STUDIES OF CpG ISLAND HYPERMETHYLATION: FROM THE BENCH TO THE BEDSIDE

Great expectations have been raised by the large amount of genetic information regarding cancer biology that has been gathered in the past two decades. CpG island hypermethylation of tumor suppressor genes may be a very valuable tool. One obvious advantage over genetic markers is that the detection of hypermethylation is a "positive" signal that can be accomplished in the context of a group of normal cells, while certain genetic changes such as homozygous deletions are not going to be detected in a background of normal DNA. Furthermore, while mutations occur at multiple sites and can be of very different types, promoter hypermethylation occurs within the same region of a given gene in each form of cancer, thus we do not need to test the methylation status first to assay the marker in serum or a distal site. Three major clinical areas can benefit from hypermethylation-based markers: detection, tumor behavior and treatment.

a) Detection of cancer cells using CpG island hypermethylation as a marker. If we want to use these epigenetic markers, we will need to use quick, easy, non-radioactive and sensitive ways to detected hypermethylation in CpG islands of tumor suppressor genes, such as methylation-specific PCR technique. The detection of DNA hypermethylation in biological fluids of cancer patients (and even patients at risk of cancer) should lead to create consortiums of different institutions to develop comprehensive studies to validate the use of these markers in the clinical environment. We open a new avenue of research in 1999 with the demonstration that it was possible to detect the presense of hypermethylated CpG islands of tumor suppressor genes in the serum DNA of cancer patients[35].

b) CpG island hypermethylation as a marker for tumor behavior. There are two components: prognostic and predictive factors. Prognostic factors will give us information about the virulence of the tumors. For example, Death Associated Protein Kinase (DAPK) and p16[INK4a] hypermethylation has been linked to aggressive tumors in lung and colorectal cancer patients[36, 37]. The second component is the group of factors that predict response to therapy. For example, the response to alkylating agents (BCNU and cyclophosphamide) is enhanced in those human primary tumors (gliomas and lymphomas, respectively) where the DNA repair gene MGMT is hypermethylated[38, 39].

c) CpG island hypermethylation as target for therapy. We have been able to reactivate hypermethylated genes in vitro. One obstacle to the transfer of this technique to human primary cancers is the lack of specificity of the drugs used. Demethylating agents such as 5-azacytidine or 5-aza-2-deoxicytidine (Decitabine) inhibits the DNMTs and cause global hypomethylation, and we cannot reactivate exclusively the particular gene we would wish to. If we consider that only tumor suppressor genes are hypermethylated this would not be a great problem. However, we do not know if we have disrupted some essential methylation at certain sites, and global hypomethylation may be associated with even greater chromosomal instability. Another disadvantage is the toxicity to normal cells. However, these compounds and their derivatives have been used in the clinic with some therapeutic benefit, especially in hematopoietic malignancies[40, 41]. The discovery that lower doses of 5-azacytidine associated with inhibitors of HDACs may also reactivate tumor suppressor genes was hopeful. Nertheless, we are still left with the obstacle of non-specificity.

CONCLUSIONS

Epigenetic changes have become established in recent years as being one of the most important molecular signatures of human tumors. The discovery of hypermethylation of the CpG islands of certain tumor suppressor genes in cancer links DNA methylation to the classic genetic lesions with the disruption of many cell pathways, from DNA repair to apoptosis, cell cycle and cell adherence. Promoter hypermethylation is now considered to be a bona-fide mechanism for gene inactivation.

The picture that has emerged in recent years have shown us that cancer is a poligenetic disease but also a poliepigenetic disease, where genes involved through multiple pathways from cell cycle to apoptosis, from cellular adhesion to hormonal response are inactivated by promoter hypermethylation. The patterns of epigenetic lesions are extremely specific in human cancer and reflect the idiosyncrasy of each cell type. The analysis of candidate genes can be seen as only a part of the methylation changes in cancer. First, there are certainly still numerous genes that undergo epigenetic inactivation waiting to be discovered. The completion of the human genome sequence and the use of several described techniques to find new genes with differential methylation will be extremely useful for this purpose. The spectrum of epigenetic alterations for a relatively small subset of genes provides a potentially powerful system of biomarkers for developing molecular detection strategies for virtually every form of human cancer.

References

1. Bird, A.P. CpG-rich islands and the function of DNA methylation. Nature 1986, 321:209-213.
2. Nguyen C, Liang G, Nguyen TT, Tsao-Wei D, Groshen S, Lubbert M, Zhou JH, Benedict WF, Jones PA. Susceptibility of nonpromoter CpG islands to de novo methylation in normal and neoplastic cells. J Natl Cancer Inst. 2001, 93,1465-72.
3. Esteller, M., Corn, P.G., Baylin, S.B., and Herman, J.G. A gene hypermethylation profile of human cancer. Cancer Res, 2001, 61, 3225-3229.
4. Greger V, Passarge E, Hopping W, Messmer E, Horsthemke B. Epigenetic changes may contribute to the formation and spontaneous regression of retinoblastoma. Hum Genet. 1989, 83,155-8.
5. Herman JG, Latif F, Weng Y, Lerman MI, Zbar B, Liu S, Samid D, Duan DS, Gnarra JR, Linehan WM. Silencing of the VHL tumor-suppressor gene by DNA methylation in renal carcinoma. Proc Natl Acad Sci U S A. 1994, 91,9700-4.
6. Merlo, A,, Herman, J.G., Mao, L., Lee, D.J., Gabrielson, E., Burger, P.C., Baylin, S.B., and Sidransky, D.
5. CpG island methylation is associated with transcriptional silencing of the tumour suppressor p16/CDKN2/MTS1 in human cancers. Nat. Med. 1995, 1: 686-692,
7. Herman JG, Merlo A, Mao L, Lapidus RG, Issa JP, Davidson NE, Sidransky D, Baylin SB. Inactivation of the CDKN2/p16/MTS1 gene is frequently associated with aberrant DNA methylation in all common human cancers. Cancer Res. 1995, 55,4525-30.
8. Gonzalez-Zulueta, M., Bender, C.M., Yang, A.S., Nguyen, T., Beart, R.W., Van Tornout, J.M., and Jones PA. Methylation of the 5' CpG island of the p16/CDKN2 tumor suppressor gene in normal and transformed human tissues correlates with gene silencing.
9. Clark, S.J., J. Harrison, C.L. Paul and M. Frommer. High sensitivity mapping of methylated cytosines. Nucleic Acids Res 1994, 22:2990-2997.

10. Herman JG, Graff JR, Myohanen S, Nelkin BD, Baylin SB. Methylation-specific PCR: a novel PCR assay for methylation status of CpG islands. Proc Natl Acad Sci U S A. 1996, 93,9821-6.

11. Esteller M, Fraga MF, Guo M, Garcia-Foncillas J, Hedelfank I, Godwin AK, Trojan J, Vaurs-Barrière C, Bignon Y-J, Ramus S, Benitez J, Akiyama Y, Caldes T, Canal MJ, Rodriguez R, Capella G, Peinado MA, Borg A, Aaltonen LA, Ponder BA, Baylin SB, Herman JG. DNA methylation patterns in hereditary human cancers mimic sporadic tumorigenesis. Human Molecular Genetics , 2001, 10, 3001-7.

12. Myohanen SK, Baylin SB, Herman JG. Hypermethylation can selectively silence individual p16ink4A alleles in neoplasia. Cancer Res. 1998, 58,591-3.

13. Herman, J.G., Umar, A., Polyak, K., Graff, J.R., Ahuja, N., Issa, J.P., Markowitz, S., Willson, J.K., Hamilton, S.R., Kinzler, K.W., Kane, M.F., Kolodner, R.D., Vogelstein, B., Kunkel, T.A, and Baylin, S.B. Incidence and functional consequences of hMLH1 promoter hypermethylation in colorectal carcinoma. Proc. Natl. Acad. Sci. U S A. 1998, 95: 6870-6875,

14. Esteller M, Levine R, Baylin SB, Ellenson LH, Herman JG. MLH1 promoter hypermethylation is associated with the microsatellite instability phenotype in sporadic endometrial carcinomas. Oncogene, 1998, 17, 2413-2417.

15. Esteller M, Hamilton SR, Burger PC, Baylin SB, Herman JG. Inactivation of the DNA repair gene O6-methylguanine-DNA methyltransferase by promoter hypermethylation is a common event in primary human neoplasia. Cancer Research, 1999, 59, 793-797.

16. Lee WH, Morton RA, Epstein JI, Brooks JD, Campbell PA, Bova GS, Hsieh WS, Isaacs WB, Nelson WG. Cytidine methylation of regulatory sequences near the pi-class glutathione S-transferase gene accompanies human prostatic carcinogenesis. Proc Natl Acad Sci U S A. 1994, 91,11733-7.

17. Esteller M, Corn PG, Urena JM, Gabrielson E, Baylin SB, Herman JG. Inactivation of glutathione S-transferase P1 gene by promoter hypermethylation in human neoplasia. Cancer Research , 1998, 58, 4515-4518.

18. Esteller M, Silva JM, Dominguez G, Bonilla F, Matias-Guiu X, Bussaglia E, Lerma E, Prat J, Harkes IC, Repasky EA, Gabrielson E, Schutte M, Baylin SB, Herman JG. Promoter hypermethylation and BRCA1 inactivation in sporadic breast and ovarian tumors. Journal of the National Cancer Institute 2000, 92, 564-9.

19. Di Croce L, Raker VA, Corsaro M, Fazi F, Fanelli M, Faretta M, Fuks F, Lo Coco F, Kouzarides T, Nervi C, Minucci S, Pelicci PG. Methyltransferase recruitment and DNA hypermethylation of target promoters by an oncogenic transcription factor. Science 2002, 295, 1079-1082.

20. Esteller M, Fraga MF, Paz MF, Campo E, Colomer D, Novo FJ, Calsanz MJ, Galm O, Guo M, Benitez J, Herman JG. Cancer epigenetics and methylation. Science 2002, 297, 1807-1808.

21. Paz MF, Avila S, Fraga MF, Pollan M, Capella G, Peinado MA, Sanchez-Cespedes M, Herman JG, Esteller M. Germ-line variants in methyl-group metabolism genes and susceptibility to DNA methylation in normal tissues and human primary tumors. Cancer Res. 2002, 62, 4519-4524.

22. Jones PA, Laird PW. Cancer epigenetics comes of age. Nat Genet 1999, 21,163-7.

23. Baylin SB, Esteller M, Rountree MR, Bachman KE, Schuebel K, Herman JG. Aberrant patterns of DNA methylation, chromatin formation and gene expression in cancer. Hum Mol Genet. 2001, 10, 687-92.

24. Graff JR, Herman JG, Myohanen S, Baylin SB, Vertino PM. Mapping patterns of CpG island methylation in normal and neoplastic cells implicates both upstream and downstream regions in de novo methylation. J Biol Chem. 1997, 272: 22322-9

25. Song JZ, Stirzaker C, Harrison J, Melki JR, Clark SJ. Hypermethylation trigger of the glutathione-S-transferase gene (GSTP1) in prostate cancer cells. Oncogene 2002, 21, 1048-61.

26. Robertson KD, Uzvolgyi E, Liang G, Talmadge C, Sumegi J, Gonzales FA, Jones PA. The human DNA methyltransferases (DNMTs) 1, 3a and 3b: coordinate mRNA expression in normal tissues and overexpression in tumors. Nucleic Acids Res. 1999, 27,2291-8.

27. Feinberg AP, Vogelstein B. Hypomethylation distinguishes genes of some human cancers from their normal counterparts. Nature. 1983, 301,89-92.

28. Ehrlich M. DNA hypomethylation and cancer. In: DNA alterations in cancer: genetic and epigenetic changes. Edited by Melanie Ehrlich, Eaton Publishing, Natick, Pages 273-291, 2000.

29. Keshet, I., Lieman-Hurwitz, J. and Cedar, H. DNA methylation affects the formation of active chromatin. Cell 1986, 44, 535-543.

30. Lewis, J.D., Meehan, R.R., Henzel, W.J., Maurer-Fogy, I., Jeppesen, P., Klein, F. and Bird A. Purification, sequence, and cellular localization of a novel chromosomal protein that binds to methylated DNA. Cell 1992, 69, 905-914.

31. Magdinier, F. and Wolffe, A.P. Selective association of the methyl-CpG binding protein MBD2 with the silent p14/p16 locus in human neoplasia. Proc. Natl. Acad. Sci. U.S.A. 2001, 98, 4990-4995.
32. Nan, X., Ng, H.H., Johnson, C.A., Laherty, C.D., Turner, B.M., Eisenman, R.N. and Bird. A. Transcriptional repression by the methyl-CpG-binding protein MeCP2 involves a histone deacetylase complex. Nature 1998, 393, 386-389.
33. Jones, P.L., Veenstra, G.J., Wade, P.A., Vermaak, D., Kass, S.U., Landsberger, N., Strouboulis, J. and Wolffe, A.P. Methylated DNA and MeCP2 recruit histone deacetylase to repress transcription. Nat Genet., 1989, 19, 187-191.
34. Ballestar E and Esteller M. The impact of chromatin in human cancer: linking DNA methylation to gene silencing. Carcinogenesis 2002, 23: 1103-9.
35. Esteller M, Sanchez-Cespedes M, Rosell R, Sidransky D, Baylin SB, Herman JG. Detection of aberrant promoter hypermethylation of tumor suppressor genes in serum DNA from non-small cell lung cancer patients. Cancer Research, 1999, 59, 67-70.
36. Tang X, Khuri FR, Lee JJ, Kemp BL, Liu D, Hong WK, Mao L. Hypermethylation of the death-associated protein (DAP) kinase promoter and aggressiveness in stage I non-small-cell lung cancer. J Natl Cancer Inst. 2000, 92,1511-6.
37. Esteller M, Gonzalez S, Risques RA, Marcuello E, Mangues R, Germa JR, Herman JG, Capella G, Peinado MA. K-ras and p16 aberrations confer poor prognosis in human colorectal cancer. J Clin Oncol, 2001,19, 299-304.
38. Esteller M, Garcia-Foncillas J, Andion E, Goodman SN, Hidalgo OF, Vanaclocha V, Baylin SB, Herman JG. Inactivation of the DNA-repair gene MGMT and the clinical response of gliomas to alkylating agents. N Engl J Med, 2000, 343, 1350-1354.
39. Esteller M, Gaidano G, Goodman SN, Zagonel V, Capello D, Botto B, Rossi D, Gloghini A, Vitolo U, Carbone A, Baylin SB, Herman JG. Hypermethylation of the DNA repair gene O(6)-methylguanine DNA methyltransferase and survival of patients with diffuse large B-cell lymphoma. J Natl Cancer Inst 2002, 94, 6-7.
40. Wijermans PW, Krulder JW, Huijgens PC, Neve P. Continuous infusion of low-dose 5-Aza-2'-deoxycytidine in elderly patients with high-risk myelodysplastic syndrome. Leukemia. 1997, 11,1-5.
41. Schwartsmann G, Fernandes MS, Schaan MD, Moschen M, Gerhardt LM, Di Leone L, Loitzembauer B, Kalakun L. Decitabine (5-Aza-2'-deoxycytidine; DAC) plus daunorubicin as a first line treatment in patients with acute myeloid leukemia: preliminary observations. Leukemia. 1997, 11 Suppl 1:S28-31.

MOLECULAR ANALYSIS OF CANCER USING DNA AND PROTEIN MICROARRAYS

Juan Madoz-Gurpide and Sam M. Hanash[*]

INTRODUCTION

Substantial progress has been made in our understanding of cancer as a multistep, complex disease that involves progressive changes in the genome and proteome. Various types of cancers share similarities as well as exhibit differences in cellular, biochemical and molecular traits. Microarray technologies have the potential of providing valuable insight regarding disease processes. The array format is now an established method for global analysis of nucleic acids, and in the past few years this approach has been adapted for protein studies (Table 1). Microarrays allow profiling of tumors' genomes, transcriptomes and proteomes at a scale unattainable previously.

Table 1. Reported and potential medical applications of DNA and protein microarrays in cancer research

DNA microarrays	Protein microarrays
Gene expression	Profiling of sera and body fluids
Mutation screening	Biomarker discovery
Genomic imbalance screening	Biochemical activities
Polymosphism genotyping	Protein-protein interactions
Diagnostics	Protein-DNA/RNA interactions
	Protein-drugs interactions
	Phenotype analysis
	Epitope mapping
	Diagnostics

CANCER PROFILING USING DNA MICROARRAYS

Genomics studies, especially profiling gene expression, using DNA array have had a tremendous impact on biomedical research, resulting in well over 1,000 published reports in 2002 alone. A substantial number of published studies dealt with cancer. Disease related

---

[*] Department of Pediatrics. Comprehnsive Cancer Center. University of Michigan. Ann Arbor 48109-094 USA

New Trends in Cancer for the 21st Century, edited by
Llombart-Bosch and Felipo, Kluwer Academic/Plenum Publishers, 2003

51

applications of DNA microarrays include uncovering unsuspected associations between genes and specific clinical features of disease that are helping devise novel molecular based disease classifications. Most published tumor studies using DNA microarrays have either examined a pathologically homogeneous set of tumors to identify clinically relevant subtypes, for example survivors vs non-survivors, or pathologically distinct subtypes belonging to the same lineage, for example limited stage vs advanced stage tumors to identify molecular correlates, or tumors of different lineages to identify molecular signatures for each lineage.

One of the landmark studies that have attracted much interest with respect to the potential contribution of DNA microarrays to uncover novel classes of tumors, is an analysis of diffuse large B-cell lymphoma, the most common subtype of non-Hodgkin's lymphoma[24]. Large B-cell lymphoma is a clinically heterogeneous disease. Only 40% of patients have a good response to current therapy with a prolonged survival. A systematic characterization of gene expression in this disease using DNA microarrays uncovered a diversity in gene expression that reflected variation in tumor proliferation rate, host response and differentiation state of the tumor. Two molecularly distinct forms of diffuse large B-cell lymphoma were uncovered which had gene expression patterns indicative of different stages of B-cell differentiation. One type expressed genes characteristic of germinal center B cells and had a significantly better overall survival than the second type, which expressed genes normally induced during in vitro activation of peripheral blood B cells. The analysis therefore identified previously undetected and clinically significant subtypes of lymphoma.

Studies to classify breast carcinomas based on gene expression profiles revealed that the tumors could be classified into a basal epithelial-like group, an ERBB2-overexpressing group and a normal breast-like group[25, 26]. A luminal epithelial/estrogen receptor-positive group could be divided into at least two subgroups, each with a distinctive expression profile. Survival analyses on a subcohort of patients with locally advanced breast cancer uniformly treated, in a prospective study, showed significantly different outcomes for patients belonging to the various groups, including a poor prognosis for the basal-like subtype and a significant difference in outcome for the two estrogen receptor-positive groups. In an independent study of 38 invasive breast cancers, striking molecular differences between ductal carcinoma specimens were uncovered that led to a suggested new classification for estrogen-receptor negative breast cancer[27]. Similarly, a study of 58 node-negative breast carcinomas discordant for ER status also uncovered a list of genes which discriminated tumors according to ER status[28]. Artificial neural networks could accurately predict ER status even after excluding top discriminator genes, including ER itself. Only a small proportion of the 100 most important ER discriminator genes are regulated by estradiol in MCF-7 cells.

An informative approach to analyze DNA microarray data in clinical studies is to divide such data into a training set to uncover associations between specific genes and certain clinical features of the disease, and a testing set to validate these associations. However since both training and testing sets are derived from the same pool of patients whose samples were available to the investigators, the extent to which such associations may apply to other patients not included in the study, who may have different characteristics, cannot be inferred. Beer et al. have undertaken a study of lung cancer in which the association they observed between a set of genes and patient survival was validated with a testing set of tumors they had available and further validated with an independent set of tumors for which microarray data was collected by another group not associated with that study[29]. Such extensive validation clearly indicated the robustness of the association uncovered between a set of genes and survival in lung adenocarcinoma.

The numerous published studies using DNA microarrays justify the use of this technology for uncovering patterns of gene expression that are clinically informative. However it is substantially more difficult to develop an understanding of disease at a mechanistic level using DNA microarrays. For most of the published studies it is unclear how well RNA levels reported correlate with protein levels. A lack of correlation may imply that the predictive property of the gene(s) is independent of gene function. In studies of lung cancer, Chen et al. collected both DNA microarray and 2-D PAGE data, which allowed them to compare mRNA and protein levels in the same tumors[30]. The integrated intensities of 165 protein spots representing protein products of 98 genes were analyzed in 76 lung adenocarcinomas and 9 unaffected lung tissues using 2-D gels. For the same 85 samples, mRNA levels were determined using oligonucleotide microarrays. Only 21 of 98 genes (21.4%) had a statistically significant correlation between protein and mRNA levels ($r > 0.2445$; $P < 0.05$). The mRNA/protein correlation coefficients also varied between isoforms of the same protein, indicating potentially isoform-specific mechanisms for the regulation of protein abundance.

PROTEIN MICROARRAYS IN CANCER RESEARCH

Despite the advances in our understanding of the molecular basis of cancer, substantial gaps remain both in our understanding of cancer pathogenesis and in the development of effective strategies for early diagnosis and for treatment. A proteomic approach to investigating diseases such as cancer may overcome some of the limitations of other approaches[1]. DNA microarrays have limited utility for the analysis of biological fluids and for uncovering directly in the fluid, assayable biomarkers. Numerous alterations may occur in proteins that are not reflected in changes at the RNA level.

Unlike DNA microarrays that provide one measure of gene expression, namely RNA levels, there is a need to implement protein microarray strategies that address the many different features of proteins including determination of their levels in biological samples, and determination of their selective interactions with other proteins, antibodies, drugs or various small ligands. Arrays that incorporate antibodies[32-39] or recombinant proteins obtained using cDNA expression libraries[40-42] or phage-display libraries[43] have been utilized for different types of protein based assays. With other types of microarrays, whole tissue-derived samples have been directly arrayed onto slides, to assess the reactivity of total protein lysates with specific ligand[44-46]. Two practical applications of protein microarrays were presented by Kodadek[60], designated protein function array and protein-detecting array. With protein function arrays, a large amount of protein is spotted on a solid support at a defined location and tested to characterize either a biochemical activity or a molecular interaction. The protein-detecting array consists of an arrayed set of protein ligands used to profile gene expression and draw signatures indicative of the cellular state. The whole process of assembling the protein array requires considerations related to the nature of the support, the type of immobilization, as well as the molecular architecture of the particle being attached. Four main different supports have been optimized to perform assays of this magnitude: chemically modified glass slides (poly-L-lysines, polyaldehides, boronic acid derivatives, chelates to poly-Histidines, etc.), nitrocellulose membranes or polyacrylamide gel on glass slides, and microwell plates. Each type of support exhibits advantages and disadvantages, as recently noted by Zhu and Snyder[61].

One of the limitations of most of the current protein microarray technologies is the lack of control over orientation in the immobilization process. It has been shown repeatedly that optimization of physical interactions between immobilized macromolecules, e.g., antigens, antibodies, peptides, and their corresponding target ligands affects sensitivity[64, 65]. There is currently a substantial variety of procedures for oriented immobilization: ionic interaction, specific covalent binding, apoenzyme reconstituted on the surface that binds to a prostetic group, receptor/ligand interactions, specific affinity motifs engineered into the surface of proteins, etc. In most cases it has been shown that optimal binding of protein to solid supports requires hydrophilic spacers[66]. Further optimization of the arraying approach should include coupling of protein separation technologies with techniques for orientational control, that would permit different surface orientations of a given protein to interact with other proteins or ligands, to enhance efficiency and reproducibility.

The compelling need for protein chips has led numerous biotechnology companies to devise novel strategies for producing biochips for various applications. New classes of capture agents include aptamers (SomaLogic, http://www.somalogic.com/), ribozymes (Archemix, http://www.archemix.com/), partial-molecule imprints (Aspira Biosystems, http://www.aspirabio.com) and modified binding proteins (Phylos, http://www.phylos.com). For assays of protein interaction, biochips that contain either peptides or proteins are being produced. Peptides may be synthesized in very large numbers directly on the chip[47] (Figure 1). Alternatively, recombinant proteins may be arrayed and effort is underway to assemble large sets of purified recombinant proteins for microarrays and other applications. As an example of innovative approaches in protein biochips, a bioanalytical system based on a planar waveguide technology has been developed which allows multiplexed, quantitative biomolecular interaction analyses to be performed with high sensitivity in a microarray format. The analytical system comprises microarray chips with integrated microfluidics and a highly sensitive fluorescence reader[48]. Applications of such a system include both protein expression profiling and studies of protein-protein interactions. Important requirements for protein biochips include ability of the capture agents to bind their ligands linearly across the entire set of capture agents deposited or synthesized on the chip, and with adequate sensitivity and dynamic range.

There is intense interest in applying proteomics to disease marker identification. Approaches to that effect include comparative analysis of protein expression in normal and cancer tissues to identify aberrantly expressed proteins that may represent novel markers, analysis of secreted proteins in cell lines and primary cultures and direct serum protein profiling to uncover potential markers. There has been recently substantial interest in the potential of mass spectrometry to yield comprehensive profiles of peptides and proteins in biological fluids without the need to first carry out protein separations. In principle, such an approach is highly suited for marker identification because of reduced sample requirements and high throughput. This approach is currently popularized, particularly for serum analysis, by the technology referred to as surface-enhanced laser-desorption ionization (SELDI)[1]. Microlitre quantities of serum from many samples are applied to the surface of a protein-binding plate, with properties to bind a class of proteins. The bound proteins are treated and analyzed by matrix-assisted laser-desorption ionization (MALDI). The mass spectra patterns obtained for different samples reflect the protein and peptide contents of these samples. Patterns that distinguish between cancer patients and normal subjects with remarkable accuracy, have been reported for several types of cancer[1]. The coupling of protein arrays with mass spectrometry technologies is likely to become a powerful analytic tool with which to profile protein expression. Such an approach, known as ProteinChip (Ciphergen Inc, USA), was successfully applied to study prostate and ovarian cancers[60] and, more recently, head and neck cancers[60]. Results from these studies revealed the involvement of proteins in carcinogenesis processes and specifically identified protein fingerprints from which cancer biomarkers were extracted. The major drawbacks of direct analysis of tissues or biological fluids by MALDI is the preferential detection of proteins with a lower molecular mass and the difficulty in identifying the proteins corresponding to the masses observed. Further technological improvements could enhance the utility of direct mass spectrometric analysis of tissues and biological fluids.

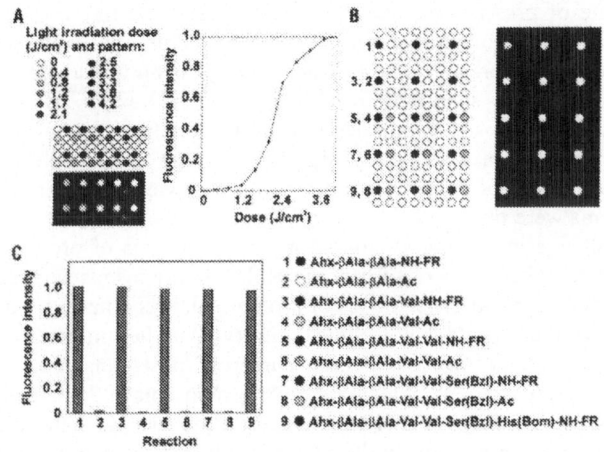

Figure 1. Representative experiments for optimization of PGA deprotection. (Reproduced from Pellois *et al.*, 2002).

Cancer tissue profiling studies that have utilized protein microarrays are beginning to emerge. As a model to better understand how patterns of protein expression shape the tissue microenvironment, Knezevic et al. analyzed protein expression in tissue derived from squamous cell carcinomas of the oral cavity through an antibody microarray approach for high-throughput proteomic analysis[49]. Utilizing laser capture microdissection to procure total protein from specific microscopic cellular populations, they demonstrated that quantitative, and potentially qualitative, differences in expression patterns of multiple proteins within epithelial cells reproducibly correlated with oral cavity tumor progression. Differential expression of multiple proteins was found in stromal cells surrounding and adjacent to regions of diseased epithelium that directly correlated with tumor progression of the epithelium. Most of the proteins identified in both cell types were involved in signal transduction pathways. They hypothesized therefore that extensive molecular communications involving complex cellular signaling between epithelium and stroma play a key role in driving oral cavity cancer progression.

A clinically relevant application of protein microarrays is the identification of proteins that induce an antibody response in autoimmune disorders[50]. Microarrays were produced by attaching several hundred proteins and peptides to the surface of derivatized glass slides. Arrays were incubated with patient serum, and fluorescent labels were used to detect autoantibody binding to specific proteins in autoimmune diseases, including systemic lupus erythematosus and rheumatoid arthritis. Such microarrays represent a powerful tool to study immune responses, in a variety of diseases including cancer.

A reverse phase protein array approach that immobilizes the whole repertoire of a tissue's proteins has been developed[46]. A high degree of sensitivity, precision and linearity was achieved, making it possible to quantify the phosphorylated status of signal proteins in human tissue cell subpopulations. Using this approach Paweletz et al.[46] have longitudinally analyzed the state of pro-survival checkpoint proteins at the microscopic transition stage from patient matched histologically normal prostate epithelium to prostate intraepithelial neoplasia and to invasive prostate cancer. Cancer progression was associated with increased phosphorylation of Akt, suppression of apoptosis pathways, as well as decreased phosphorylation of ERK. At the transition from histologically normal epithelium to intraepithelial neoplasia, a statistically significant surge in phosphorylated Akt and a concomitant suppression of downstream apoptosis pathways preceding the transition into invasive carcinoma were observed.

A major challenge in making biochips for global analysis of protein expression is the current lack of comprehensive sets of genome scale capture agents such as antibodies. As a result, biochips that target specific classes of proteins such as kinases or cytokines are much easier to produce, that would have clinical utility. Another important consideration in protein microarrays is that proteins undergo numerous post-translational modifications eg phosphorylations, glycosylations, which are highly important to their functions, as they can determine activity, stability, localization and turnover. To address the need for comprehensive analysis of proteins in their modified forms, several approaches to the liquid based separation of cell and tissue lysates were investigated in order to obtain protein fractions with reduced complexity or pure individual proteins[51]. The separation products can be arrayed in a manner that allows the probing of protein constituents of cells and tissues to uncover specific targets. For example, using a combination of anion exchange and reverse phase LC, Madoz-Gurpide et al. have obtained some 2000 individual protein fractions that have been utilized to produce microarrays that interrogate cancer cell proteomes. Fractions that react with specific probes are within the reach of chromatographic and gel based separation techniques for resolving their individual protein constituents and of mass spectrometric techniques for identification of their constituent proteins. The LC procedures allow sufficient protein amounts to be resolved for the construction of large numbers of microarrays from a given cell or tissue source.

Protein microarrays of different types are likely to become commercially available for assays of broad sets of proteins and may well rival or at least complement DNA microarrays as tools for global expression analysis.

SUMMARY

In conclusion, array-based technologies have emerged that contribute to profiling tissues at the genomic, transcriptomic and proteomic levels. Analytical tools are needed to mine the vast amount of data generated. Ultimately the molecular analysis of cancer at a genome and proteome scale will allow better classification of disease and tailored individualized therapy for individual patients.

References

1. Petricoin, E.F., Zoon, K.C., Kohn, E.C., Barrett, J.C. & Liotta, L.A. Clinical proteomics: translating benchside promise into bedside reality. *Nature Reviews Drug Discovery* **1**, 683-695 (2002).
24. Alizadeh, A.A. *et al.* Distinct types of diffuse large B-cell lymphoma identified by gene expression profiling. *Nature* **403**, 503-511 (2000).
25. Perou, C.M. *et al.* Molecular portraits of human breast tumours. *Nature* **406**, 747-752 (2000).
26. Sorlie, T. *et al.* Gene expression patterns of breast carcinomas distinguish tumor subclasses with clinical implications. *Proceedings of the National Academy of Sciences, USA* **98**, 10869-10874 (2001).
27. Brenton, J.D., Aparicio, S.A. & Caldas, C. Molecular profiling of breast cancer: portraits but not physiognomy. *Breast Cancer Research* **3**, 77-80 (2001).
28. Gruvberger, S. *et al.* Estrogen receptor status in breast cancer is associated with remarkably distinct gene expression patterns. *Cancer Research* **61**, 5979-5984 (2001).
29. Beer, D.G. *et al.* Gene-expression profiles predict survival of patients with lung adenocarcinomas. *Nature Medicine* **8**, 816-824 (2002).
30. Chen, G. *et al.* Proteomic analysis of lung adenocarcinoma: identification of a highly expressed set of proteins in tumors. *Clinical Cancer Research* **8**, 2290-2305 (2002).
31. Microarray standards at last. *Nature* **419**, 323 (2002).
32. Ge, H. UPA, a universal protein array system for quantitative detection of protein-protein, protein-DNA, protein-RNA and protein-ligand interactions. *Nucleic Acids Research* **28**, e3 (2000).
33. Rowe, C.A., Scruggs, S.B., Feldstein, M.J., Golden, J.P. & Ligler, F.S. An array immunosensor for simultaneous detection of clinical analytes. *Analytical Biochemistry* **71**, 433-439 (1999).
34. Mendoza, L.G. *et al.* High-throughput microarray-based enzyme-linked immunosorbent assay (ELISA). *Biotechniques* **27**, 778-780, 782-786, 788 (1999).
35. Silzel, J.W., Cercek, B., Dodson, C., Tsay, T. & Obremski, R.J. Mass-sensing, multianalyte microarray immunoassay with imaging detection. *Clinical Chemistry* **44**, 2036-2043 (1998).
36. Arenkov, P. *et al.* Protein microchips: use for immunoassay and enzymatic reactions. *Analytical Biochemistry* **278**, 123-131 (2000).
37. Haab, B.B., Dunham, M.J. & Brown, P.O. Protein microarrays for highly parallel detection and quantitation of specific proteins and antibodies in complex solutions. *GenomeBiology* **2**, Research0004.1-0004.13 (2001).
38. MacBeath, G. & Schreiber, S.L. Printing proteins as microarrays for high-throughput function determination. *Science* **289**, 1760-1763 (2000).
39. Schweitzer, B. *et al.* Inaugural article: immunoassays with rolling circle DNA amplification: a versatile platform for ultrasensitive antigen detection. *Proceedings of the National Academy of Sciences, USA* **97**, 10113-10119 (2000).
40. Bussow, K. *et al.* A method for global protein expression and antibody screening on high-density filters of an arrayed cDNA library. *Nucleic Acids Research* **26**, 5007-5008 (1998).
41. Lueking, A. *et al.* Protein microarrays for gene expression and antibody screening. *Analytical Biochemistry* **270**, 103-111 (1999).
42. Zhu, H. *et al.* Analysis of yeast protein kinases using protein chips. *Nature Genetics* **26**, 283-289 (2000).
43. DeWildt, R.M.T., Mundy, C.R., Gorick, B.D. & Tomlinson, I.M. Antibody arrays for high-throughtput screening of antibody-antigen interactions. *Nature Biotechnology* **18**, 989-994 (2001).
44. Kononen, J. *et al.* Tissue microarrays for high-throughput molecular profiling of tumor specimens. *Nature Medicine* **4**, 844-847 (1998).

45. Kallioniemi, O.P., Wagner, U., Kononen, J. & Sauter, G. Tissue microarray technology for high-throughput molecular profiling of cancer. *Human Molecular Genetics* **10**, 657-662 (2001).
46. Paweletz, C.P. *et al.* Reverse phase protein microarrays which capture disease progression show activation of pro-survival pathways at the cancer invasion front. *Oncogene* **20**, 1981-1989 (2001).
47. Pellois, J.P. *et al.* Individually addressable parallel peptide synthesis on microchips. *Nature Biotechnology* **20**, 922-926 (2002).
48. Pawlak, M. *et al.* Zeptosens' protein microarrays: a novel high performance microarray platform for low abundance protein analysis. *Proteomics* **2**, 383-393 (2002).
49. Knezevic, V. *et al.* Proteomic profiling of the cancer microenvironment by antibody arrays. *Proteomics* **1**, 1271-1278 (2001).
50. Robinson, W.H. *et al.* Autoantigen microarrays for multiplex characterization of autoantibody responses. *Nature Medicine* **8**, 295-301 (2002).
51. Madoz-Gurpide, J., Wang, H., Misek, D.E., Brichory, F. & Hanash, S.M. Protein based microarrays: A tool for probing the proteome of cancer cells and tissues. *Proteomics* **1**, 1279-1287 (2001).
52. Yamamoto, A. *et al.* Infrequent presence of anti-c-Myc antibodies and absence of c-Myce oncoprotein in sera from lung cancer patients. *Oncology* **56**, 129-133 (1999).
53. Stockert, E. *et al.* A survey of the humoral immune response of cancer patients to a panel of human tumor antigens. *Journal of Experimental Medicine* **187**, 1349-1354 (1998).
54. Gourevitch, M.M. *et al.* Polymorphic epithelial mucin (MUC-1)-containing circulating immune complexes in carcinoma patients. *British Journal of Cancer* **72**, 934-938 (1995).
55. Gure, A.O. *et al.* Human lung cancer antigens recognized by autologous antibodies: Definition of a novel cDNA derived from the tumor suppressor gene locus on chromosome 3p21.3. *Cancer Research* **58**, 1034-1341 (1998).
56. Yamamoto, A., Shimizu, E., Ogura, T. & Sone, S. Detection of auto-antibodies against L-myc oncogene products in sera from lung cancer patients. *International Journal of Cancer* **22**, 283-289 (1996).
57. Soussi, T. The humoral response to the tumor-suppressor gene product p53 in human cancer: Implications for diagnosis and therapy. *Immunology Today* **17**, 354-356 (1996).
58. Old, L.J. & Chen, Y.T. New paths in human cancer serology. *Journal of Experimental Medicine* **187**, 1163-1167 (1998).
59. Le Naour, F. *et al.* A distinct repertoire of autoantibodies in hepatocellular carcinoma identified by proteomic analysis. *Molecular and Cellular Proteomics* **1**, 197-203 (2002).
60. Kodadek, T. Protein microarrays: Prospects and problems. *Chemical Biology* **8**, 105-115 (2001).
61. Zhu, H. *et al.* Protein arrays and microarrays. *Current Opinion in Chemical Biology* **5**, 40-45 (2001).
    Senior, K. Fingerprinting disease with protein chip arrays. *Molecular Medicine Today* **5**, 326-327 (1999).
63. Eggeling, F. *et al.* Tissue-specific microdissection coupled with ProteinChip array technologies. Applications in cancer research. *Biotechniques* **29**, 1066-1070 (2000).
64. Madoz-Gúrpide, J. *et al.* Modulation of electroenzymatic NADPH oxidation through oriented immobilization of ferredoxin : NADP(+) reductase onto modified gold electrodes. *Journal of the American Chemical Society* **122**, 9808-9817 (2000).
65. Delamarche, E. *et al.* Immobilization of antibodies on a photoactive self-assembled monolayer on gold. *Langmuir*, **12**, 1997-2006 (1996).
66. Muller, W. *et al.* Attempts to mimic docking processes of the immune system: recognition-induced formation of protein multilayers. *Science* **262**, 1706-1708 (1993).

PROTEOMIC APPROACHES TO THE DIAGNOSIS, TREATMENT, AND MONITORING OF CANCER

Julia D. Wulfkuhle[1, *], Cloud P. Paweletz[1, Υ], Patricia S. Steeg[2], Emanuel F. Petricoin III[3], and Lance Liotta[1]

[1]FDA/NCI Clinical Proteomics Program, Laboratory of Pathology, Center for Cancer Research, National Cancer Institute, Bethesda, MD 20892. [2]Women's Cancers Section, Laboratory of Pathology, Center for Cancer Research, National Cancer Institute, Bethesda, MD 20892. [3]FDA/NCI Clinical Proteomics Program, Center for Biologics Evaluation and Research, Food and Drug Administration, Bethesda, MD 20892

ABSTRACT

The field of proteomics holds promise for the discovery of new biomarkers for the early detection and diagnosis of disease, molecular targets for therapy and markers for therapeutic efficacy and toxicity. A variety of proteomics approaches may be used to address these goals. Two-dimensional gel electrophoresis (2D-PAGE) is the cornerstone of many discovery-based proteomics studies. Technologies such as laser capture microdissection (LCM) and highly sensitive MS methods are currently being used together to identify greater numbers of lower abundance proteins that are differentially expressed between defined cell populations. Newer technologies such as reverse phase protein arrays will enable the identification and profiling of target pathways in small biopsy specimens. Surface-enhanced laser desorption/ionization time-of-flight (SELDI-TOF) analysis enables the high throughput characterization of lysates from very few tumor cells or body fluids and may be best suited for diagnosis and monitoring of disease. Such technologies are expected to supplement our arsenal of mRNA-based assays, and we believe that in the future, entire cellular networks and not just a single deregulated protein will be the target of therapeutics and that we will soon be able to monitor the status of these pathways in diseased cells before, during and after therapy.

* To whom correspondence should be addressed: Julia Wulfkuhle, Ph.D., CBER/FDA, Bldg. 29A/2B20, HFM 535, 8800 Rockville Pike, Bethesda, MD 20892; Phone: 301-402-0211; e-mail: wulfkuhle@cber.fda.gov

Υ Current address: Department of Anatomy, Physiology, and Genetics, Institute for Molecular Medicine, Uniformed Services School of Medicine, Bethesda, MD 20814

New Trends in Cancer for the 21st Century, edited by
Llombart-Bosch and Felipo, Kluwer Academic/Plenum Publishers, 2003

59

INTRODUCTION

As we enter into the post-genomic era, proteomics-based approaches promise to revolutionize the study and treatment of individual disease processes. While genomics and mRNA expression-based technologies will continue to contribute substantially to biology and medicine, there are limits to the type and amount of information such studies can provide. Genes "work" at the protein level, and comparisons of transcript and corresponding protein expression have shown that mRNA and protein levels are not necessarily highly correlative[1, 2]. In addition to providing quantitative data, proteomics can provide additional qualitative information that transcriptional analyses cannot. This includes post-translational modifications such as acetylation, ubiquitination, phosphorylation[3, 4], or glycosylation[5, 6]. Proteomics of subcellular organs have been reported, including the mitochondrion and the cell membrane[7, 9]. Most recently, attempts at functional proteomics have been reported[10, 14]. Protein-protein and protein-DNA interactions can be described via analysis of the proteome. Moreover, since almost all therapeutic intervention strategies involve targeting and modulating protein function and activity, it is imperative that analyses of mechanisms underlying tumorigenesis include proteomics.

The molecular events that underlie neoplastic progression are complex and diverse, and they remain incompletely characterized. The identification, quantification, classification, and functional assignment of proteins will be essential to the full understanding of these molecular events. Such information will prove to be crucial in cancer prognostics, diagnostics, prevention and therapeutics, with the ultimate goals being therapeutic target discovery, rational drug design, and the identification of early detection surrogate biomarkers[1, 2, 15-17].

Proteomic studies offer the potential to revolutionize cancer diagnosis and treatment. Two- dimensional gel analyses combined with LCM and MS sequencing can identify new targets for therapy and prevention of disease. Technologies such as surface enhanced laser desorption/ ionization time of flight (SELDI-TOF) and multiplexed protein arrays can examine complex protein expression patterns, and will be valuable for diagnostic and predictive studies as well as for the development of patient-tailored treatment strategies.

LCM-BASED DISCOVERY PROTEOMICS IN BREAST CANCER

LCM technology has made it possible to carry out proteomics studies with pure cell populations harvested directly from frozen tumor sections[18]. Defined cell populations are precisely acquired by use of an infrared laser that melts an ethylene vinyl acetate polymer film over selected cells. This thermoplastic film forms a solid composite with the tissue at the targeted sites such that when the film is lifted from the tissue section, only cells of interest remain on the film's surface. These cells can be lysed directly from the film surface for protein analysis. LCM does not disrupt the histological architecture of the tissue, and it preserves the state of the in vivo cellular molecules.

The application of such a precise and non-disruptive technology becomes particularly important in the proteomic comparison of normal and malignant breast tissue. Because breast cancer typically arises from the epithelium of the terminal ductal lobular unit (TDLU), the epithelial component of normal breast tissue is often substantially smaller than that found in malignant breast lesions. The clusters of TDLUs are frequently small and widely dispersed within tissue sections, thus making LCM vital to the accurate procurement and enrichment of normal epithelial cells for comparative analyses with malignant cells.

We have performed breast cancer proteomic studies using LCM-derived cell populations[19]. Figure 1 presents 2D gels of a breast ductal carcinoma in situ (DCIS) tumor. The left panel shows the proteomic profile of whole cryostat sections, and the right panel represents approximately 50,000 LCM-procured breast tumor epithelial cells (10,000 laser pulses) from the same specimen. Several examples of protein spots enriched in the gel of microdissected tissue are indicated. Studies in other cancers have confirmed that LCM offers a different proteomics image than whole tumors[20, 21, 22].

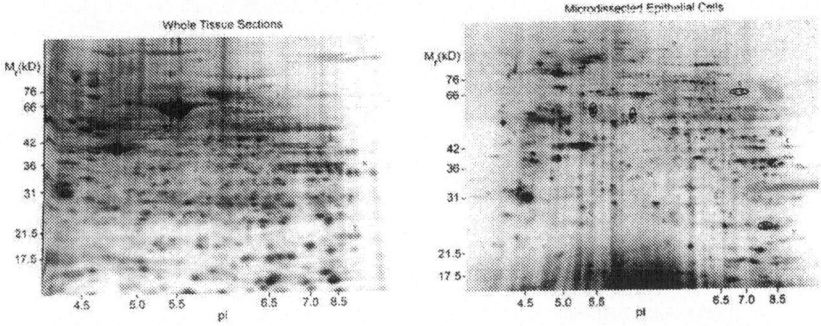

Figure 1. Enrichment of specific proteins in 2D-gels of microdissected tumor epithelial cells. Samples containing whole cryostat sections (left) or 50,000 microdissected DCIS epithelial cells (right) from the same tumor were separated by 2D-PAGE using a pH 3-10 nonlinear first dimension and gradient SDS-PAGE second dimension. Examples of protein spots enriched in the gels of microdissected material are indicated with circles.

Several technical considerations of using LCM for breast cancer proteomics should be noted. Factors such as the time between surgical removal and tissue processing are vitally important to the success of proteomic analysis. Ethanol-fixed, frozen breast tissue may provide the best quality protein with concomitant cellular morphology preservation for pathologic analysis[23]. Numerous tissue sections are often required to obtain an adequate number of LCM-captured cells for 2D-PAGE, especially if large-format SDS-gels are used in lieu of minigels. This is particularly true of normal ductal/lobular tissue, in which the epithelial component depends on the density and cellularity of the ductal tree, which in turn is dependent on biological factors such as age, parity and menstrual cycle. Once the 2D-gels are run, they must be stained for protein visualization. We routinely use silver-stain to analyze gels of microdissected material, which provides the highest sensitivity and enables the resolution of many protein spots, but will not permit routine MS sequencing. We therefore use our microdissected 2D-gels only for analysis of differential protein expression. The spots of interest are identified and excised from 2D-gels of whole cryostat sections stained with Sypro Red (Molecular Probes, Eugene, OR) or colloidal Coomassie blue. These stains are suitable for MS sequencing, and the gels often have sufficient protein for sequencing of many that are considered to be "low abundance".

Our studies comparing patient-matched, LCM-procured normal ductal/lobular and DCIS epithelial cells identified a number of differentially expressed proteins between normal and diseased tissue involved in a variety of cell biological processes such as cytoskeletal regulation, subcellular trafficking, oxidative damage control, and protein stability (Table 1;)[19]. The molecular alterations that accompany DCIS, the earliest detectable form of breast cancer, represent prime molecular targets for the exploring the origins and prevention of breast cancer. With further analysis, a number of proteins identified in this study may also point to potential pathways for targeted therapy.

Table 1. Selected Targets Identified in 2D-PAGE Comparisons of Human Breast Normal Ductal/Lobular Epithelium and DCIS Tissue

Protein:	Trend:
Cytoskeletal Regulation:	
Transgelin	N>DCIS[1]
Cofilin	DCIS>N
Macrophage capping protein (CapG)	DCIS>N
Arp3b	DCIS>N
L-plastin	DCIS>N
Stathmin	DCIS>N
Oxidative Damage:	
Peroxiredoxins 1 and 2	DCIS>N
Subcellular Trafficking:	
Cellular retinoic acid binding protein 2	DCIS>N
Rab 11a	DCIS>N
Fatty acid binding protein 3	N>DCIS
Fatty acid binding protein 5	DCIS>N
Protein Stability:	
Hsp 27	DCIS>N
Hsp 90	DCIS>N
GRP94	DCIS>N

[1]N: normal; DCIS: ductal carcinoma in situ

HIGH THROUGHPUT MOLECULAR PROFILING OF CANCER

Proteomics is advancing from the discovery-based analysis of 2D-gels to higher throughput analyses involving proteomic pattern recognition in both tissue and body fluids and the characterization of information flow within a cell through signal pathway profiling. Determining the level of activation of key components in signaling circuits can highlight disease-related alterations in pathways that may provide the drug targets of the future.

Biomarker Discovery and Proteomic Pattern Diagnostics

A promising technique that yields large amounts of low molecular weight protein expression data and allows for rapid protein pattern analysis of tumors and body fluids is SELDI-TOF MS (24-26). SELDI-TOF technology utilizes solid supports or "chips" made of aluminum or stainless steel engineered with bait surfaces 1 to 2 mm in diameter. The bait surfaces can be hydrophobic, cationic, or anionic chromatographic supports or based on "affinity supports" comprised of biochemical molecules such as antibodies, purified proteins such as receptors or ligands, or DNA oligonucleotides. Small amounts of solublized tissue or body fluid (volumes as small as 0.5 μL) are directly applied to the bait surface. After washing to remove unbound proteins, the proteins specifically interacting with the bait surface are analyzed by MS TOF, similar to standard MALDI-TOF analysis. The low molecular weight ionized proteins and peptides are recorded as mass signature peaks as they strike a detector plate based on their differential time of flight, and the data are displayed as a standard chromatograph (see Figures 2, 3). SELDI analysis software allows data to be viewed as a standard mass chromatograph or a gel-like density graph, as shown in Figure 2. Protein profiles can be obtained within minutes, and hundreds of proteins can be analyzed simultaneously from small numbers of cells. However, it is not yet possible to perform routine MS sequencing from protein peaks identified by SELDI analysis. Figure 2 shows assay validation data for SELDI analysis of LCM-enriched infiltrating breast cancer cells. In this example, similar protein expression patterns were observed in three independent microdissections of a single infiltrating ductal breast carcinoma. This similarity is reflected both in the mass chromatograph as well as the gel-view density graph. However, a broad mass-to-charge ratio (m/z) range, as illustrated in Figure 2, often disguises the presence of lower abundance proteins.

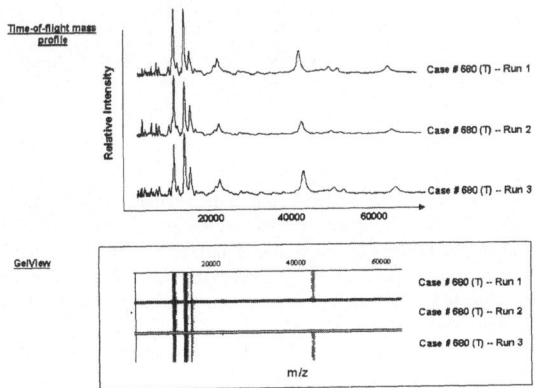

Figure 2. Reproducibility of protein profiles of microdissected breast invasive ductal carcinoma generated by SELDI-TOF analysis. Three independent microdissections of approximately 1500 cells each from a single breast tumor were subjected to SELDI-TOF analysis using a hydrophobic interaction bait surface. The top panel is the mass chromatogram generated for each dissection. Relative intensity is plotted on the y-axis and m/z ratio is plotted on the x-axis. The lower panel is the corresponding gel-view density graph of the data in the mass chromatograms.

Our own studies of several unmatched, microdissected populations of normal and tumor epithelial cells from frozen breast tissue show that, despite significant heterogeneity in protein expression between cases, potential tumor markers can be identified (Figure 3). Each density graph in Figure 3 represents approximately 3,000 normal or tumor epithelial cells isolated by LCM (500 laser pulses). Arrow A indicates a protein of m/z 12,000 that is preferentially expressed in all seven tumor cases compared to the normal cases. Paweletz et al.[27] have shown that reproducible and discriminatory protein biomarker profiles can be obtained from patient-matched normal, premalignant, malignant and metastatic cell populations from a variety of human tumors using LCM and SELDI-TOF analysis. Consistent protein changes were observed in eight matched sets of normal and malignant esophageal epithelium and three matched sets of microdissected prostate epithelial tissue, demonstrating that these combined technologies provide a means to rapidly generate protein expression profiles from microscopic lesions.

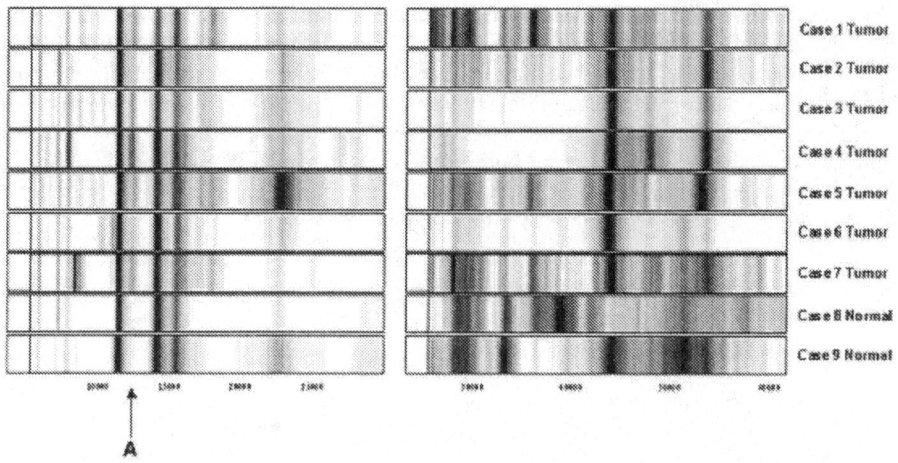

Figure 3. SELDI-TOF analysis of microdissected breast epithelium reveals a protein deregulated in a disease-specific manner. Approximately 3,000 cells were microdissected from seven different infiltrating ductal breast carcinomas and two unmatched normal breast tissue samples and subjected to SELDI-TOF analysis. The resulting gel-view density chromatograms (both panels, m/z 10,000-60,000) were aligned and compared and a protein of m/z 12,000, indicated by arrow A, was identified as overexpressed in the tumor samples compared to the unmatched normal tissue.

Despite the current limitations in deriving direct sequence information from protein peaks identified by SELDI-TOF, when combined with bioinformatics tools, this technology has the potential to revolutionize disease diagnosis, assessment of disease prognosis and toxicity screening. For example, a set of five biomarkers has been identified in urine that discriminates individuals with bladder transitional cell carcinoma from normal donors[28]. Also, a panel of serum biomarkers has also been identified to discriminate early stage breast cancers from non-cancer controls[29]. Our group has applied these technologies to the problem of ovarian cancer detection[30]. Currently, there are no effective screening tests available for the general population or women at high risk for the development of the disease. Ovarian cancer presents at advanced stages in more than 80% of patients and 5-year survival is 35% in this population. By contrast, more than 90% of stage I ovarian cancer patients survive 5 years[31]. These statistics strongly suggest that an effective diagnostic test for early stage ovarian cancer would have a significant impact on survival.

An iterative searching algorithm was designed and used to analyze SELDI spectra from a set of raw serum samples from women with ovarian cancer and unaffected control serums. The algorithm identified a "best-fit" pattern of peaks in the serum proteome that completely segregated ovarian cancer from non-cancer samples. This pattern correctly classified blinded serum samples from unaffected (n=69) and cancer (n=50) patients with 100% sensitivity and 95% specificity. Remarkably, this algorithm was able to correctly classify the serums from 18 Stage I ovarian carcinomas included in the blinded samples[30]. This study illustrates the power and general applicability of SELDI-TOF MS analysis of tumor cells and body fluids to the diagnosis and analysis of disease. Continuing improvements in the resolution and sensitivity of MS instruments should soon make it possible to obtain sequence from potential disease biomarkers and improve proteomic pattern diagnostics.

Multiplexed Protein Array Technologies

Protein microarrays represent a new technology that can profile the state of signaling pathway targets in small amounts of tissue such as those obtained during clinical biopsy procedures. These microarrays consist of an array of protein samples or baits such as antibodies, small molecules, small tissue samples or nucleic acids immobilized on a solid surface. The arrays can then be probed with mixtures of labeled proteins and those that are specifically captured by the bait surface can be detected by fluorescence, colorimetric or chemiluminescence means[32]. Our laboratory has developed an array, called the reverse phase protein array, that allows the assessment of the status of key signaling molecules in individual cell types from patient-matched, longitudinal study sets of normal, premalignant and cancerous lesions (Figure 4)[33]. In this approach, LCM-procured, pure cell populations are taken from human biopsy specimens, and a protein lysate is arrayed onto nitrocellulose slides. Several key technological components of this method offer unique advantages over tissue arrays[34] or antibody arrays[35, 36]. The reverse phase array can utilize denatured lysates so that antigen retrieval issues are not problematic, which is a large limitation for tissue arrays. These arrays can be comprised of non-denatured lysates derived directly from LCM-procured tissue cells so that protein-protein, protein-DNA, and/or protein-RNA complexes can be detected and characterized. Also, each patient sample is arrayed in a miniature dilution curve, providing an internal standard curve and allowing direct quantitative measurements to be made (Fig. 4A). Finally, reverse phase protein arrays do not require direct tagging of the protein as a read-out for the assay, thus yielding dramatic improvement in reproducibility, sensitivity and robustness of the assay over other techniques.

Reverse phase arrays can now be used to study key nodes in the cellular circuitry and to profile the functional state of protein pathways and signaling events within cells contained in biopsy samples. Recently, this platform was employed to address the basic but previously unanswered question of whether or not premalignant transformation is caused by an increase in the cell growth rate through the activation of the mitogenic growth pathways (e.g. phosphorylation of ERK) or whether early cancer is driven by a decrease in the cell death rate through the activation of apoptosis-inhibiting, pro-survival signaling pathways (e.g. phosphorylation of AKT). Reverse phase analysis of LCM-procured, patient-matched normal epithelial, premalignant, and invasive prostate carcinoma cells study sets revealed that phosphorylation and activation of AKT occurred as a critical early step in the progression of cancer (Figure 4B,C)[33]. Thus, the increase in the build-up of cells seen during early stage prostate cancer (prostatic intraepithelial neoplasia) is caused by an alteration of the cellular turnover by a decrease in the death rate, not induction of the growth rate. Consequently, inhibition of AKT activity through molecular targeted therapeutics may have profound impact in treating and prevention of prostate cancer progression.

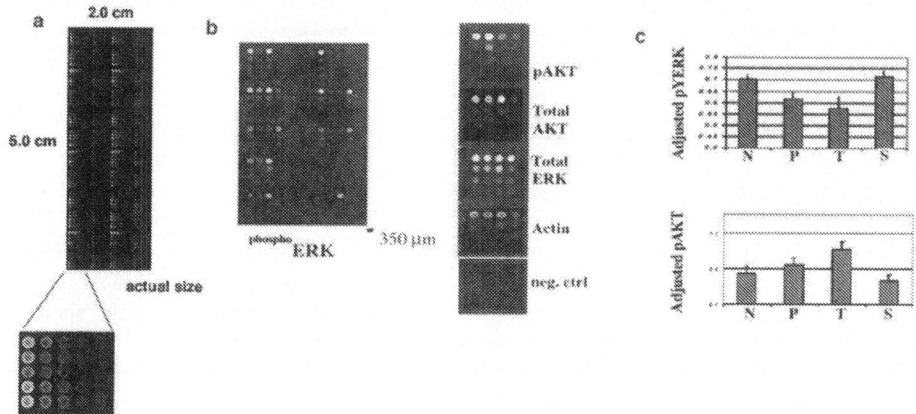

Figure 4. Signal pathway profiling using reverse-phase arrays. A) Arrays comprising miniature dilution curves of hundreds of patient specimens can be placed on one array. B) LCM-procured, patient-matched normal, premalignant, invasive cancer and stromal cells from prostate cancer patients were analyzed for ERK and AKT signaling using phosphospecific antibody reactivity. Normalization to the total cognate protein allows detailed molecular analysis. C) Adjusted levels of phosphorylated ERK (pERK) and AKT (pAKT) reveal an increasing activation of AKT and a concomitant decrease in the activation of ERK as the cancer cell progresses. N=normal; P=premalignant; T=tumor; S=stroma.

CONCLUSION

Evidence is emerging that every individual's cancer has a unique molecular signature, comprised of specific pathogenic molecular derangements. Thus, any given molecular targeted therapy will be effective for only the subset of patients that harbor a specific deregulated or defective protein. Discovery of new biomarkers for disease, proteomic pathway profiling and pattern diagnostics offer significant benefits in the areas of disease classification and survival outcome as well as in patient-tailored treatment selection and therapeutic efficacy and toxicity monitoring. In fact, we envision a time when molecular pathway profiling will be used to target multiple nodes in a pathogenic pathway, hopefully resulting in increased treatment efficacy and reduced toxicities.

References

1. Steiner, S. and Witsmann, F. Proteomics: Applications and opportunities in preclinical drug development., Electrophoresis. *21:* 2099-2104, 2000.
2. Celis, J., Kruhoffer, M., Gromova, I., Frederiksen, C., Ostergaard, M., Thykjaer, T., Gromov, P., Yu, J., Palsdottir, H., Magnusson, N., and Orntoft, T. Gene expression profiling: Monitoring transcription and translation products using DNA microarrays and proteomics., FEBS Lett. *480:* 2-16, 2000.
3. Oda, Y., Nagasu, T., and Chait, B. Enrichment analysis of phosphorylated proteins as a tool for probing the phosphoproteome., Nat. Biotech. *19:* 379-382, 2001.
4. Ducret, A., Desponts, C., Desmarais, S., Gresser, M., and Ramachandran, C. A general method for the rapid characterization of tyrosine-phosphorylated proteins by mini two-dimensional gel electrophoresis., Electrophoresis. *21:* 2196-2208, 2000.
5. Larsson, T., Bergstrom, J., Nilsson, J., and Karlsson, K. Use of an affinity proteomics approach for the identification of low-abundant bacterial adherins as applied on the Lewis(b) binding adhesin of Helicobacter pylori., FEBS Lett. *469:* 155-158, 2000.
6. Charlwood, J., Skehel, J., and Camilleri, P. Analysis of N-linked oligosaccharides released from glycoproteins separated by two-dimensional gel electrophoresis., Anal. Biochem. *284:* 49-59, 2000.
7. Fivaz, M., Vilbois, F., Pasquali, C., and vanderGoot, F. Analysis of glycosyl phosphatidylinositol-anchored proteins by two-dimensional gel electrophoresis., Electrophoresis. *21:* 3351-3356, 2000.
8. Lopez, M., Kristal, B., Chernokalskaya, E., Lazarev, A., Shestopalov, A., Bogdanove, A., and Robinson, M. High-throughput profiling of the mitochondrial proteome using affinity fractionation and automation., Electrophoresis. *21:* 3427-3440, 2000.
9. Koe, E., Burkhart, W., Blackburn, K., Koc, H., Moseley, A., and Spremulli, L. Identification of four proteins from the small subunit of the mammalian mitochondrial ribosome using a proteomics approach., Protein Sci. *10:* 471-481, 2001.
10. Godovac-Zimmerman, J., Sockic, V., Poznanovic, S., and Brianza, F. Functional proteomics of signal transduction by membrane receptors., Electorphoresis. *20:* 952-961, 1999.
11. Kidd, D., Liu, Y., and Cravatt, B. Profiling serine hydrolase activities in complex proteomes., Biochem. *40:* 4005-4015, 2001.
12. Adam, G., Cravatt, B., and Sorensen, E. Profiling the specific reactivity of the proteome with non-directed activity-based probes., Chemistry and Biol. *8:* 81-95, 2001.
13. Lewis, T., Hunt, J., Aveline, L., Jonscher, K., Louie, D., Yeh, J., Nahreini, T., Resing, K., and Ahn, N. Identification of novel MAP kinase pathway signaling targets by functional proteomics and mass spectroscopy., Mol. Cell. *6:* 1343-1354, 2000.
14. Ilag, L., Ng, J., and Jay, D. Chromophore-assisted laser inactivation (CALI) to validate drug targets and pharmacogenomic markers., Drug Dev't. Res. *49:* 65-73, 2000.
15. Chambers, G., Lawrie, L., Cash, P., and Murray, G. Proteomics: A new approach to the study of disease., J. Pathol. *192:* 280-288, 2000.
16. Rudert, F. Genomics and proteomics tools for the clinic., Curr. Opinion in Mol. Therapeutics. *2:* 633-642, 2000.
17. Hanash, S. Opermics: Molecular analysis of tissues from DNA to RNA to protein., Clin. Chem. and Lab. Med. *38:* 805-813, 2000.
18. Emmert-Buck, M., Bonner, R., Smith, P., Chuaqui, R., Zhuang, Z., Goldstein, S., Weiss, R., and Liotta, L. Laser capture microdissection., Science. *274:* 998-1001., 1996.
19. Wulfkuhle, J., Sgroi, D., Krutzsch, H., McLean, K., McGarvey, K., Knowlton, M., Chen, S., Shu, H., Sahin, A., Kurek, R., Wallwiener, D., Merino, M., Petricoin, E., Zhao, Y., and Steeg, P. Proteomics of human breast ductal carcinoma in situ (DCIS). In press., 2002.
20. Ornstein, D., Gillespie, J., Paweletz, C., Duray, P., Herring, J., Vocke, C., Topalian, S., Bostwick, D., Linehan, W., III, E. P., and Emmert-Buck, M. Proteomic analysis of laser capture microdissected human prostate cancer and in vitro prostate cell lines., Electrophoresis. *21:* 2235-2242, 2000.
21. Banks, R., Dunn, M., Forbes, M., Stanley, A., Pappin, D., naven, T., Gough, M., Harnden, P., and Selby, P. The potential use of laser capture microdissection to selectively obtain distinct populations of cells for

proteomic analysis - Preliminary findings., Electrophoresis. *20:* 689-700, 1999.

22. Eggling, F. v., Davies, H., Loms, L., Fiedler, W., Junker, K., Claussen, U., and Ernst, G. Tissue specific microdissection coupled with ProteinChip[R] array technologies: Applications in cancer research., Biotechniques. *29:* 1066-1070, 2000.

23. Gillespie, J., Ahram, M., Best, C., Swalwell, J., Krizman, D., Petricoin, E., Liotta, L., and Emmert-Buck, M. The role of tissue microdissection in cancer research, Cancer J. *7:* 32-39, 2001.

24. Hutchens, T. and Yip, T. New desorption strategies for the mass spectrometric analysis of macromolecules., Rapid Commun. Mass Spectrom. *7:* 576-580, 1993.

25. Merchant, M. and Weinberger, S. Recent advancements in surface-enhanced laser desorption/ionization time-of-flight mass spectometry., Electrophoresis. *21:* 1164-1167, 2000.

26. Isaaq, H., Veenstra, T., Conrads, T. and Felschow, D. The SELDI-TOF MS approach to proteomics: Protein profiling and biomarker identification., Biochem. Biophys. Res. Commun. *292:* 587-592, 2002.

27. Paweletz, C., Gillespie, J., Ornstein, D., Simone, N., Brown, M., Cole, K., Kohn, E., Linehan, W., Weber, T., Taylor, P., Emmert-Buck, M., Liotta, L., and Petricoin III, E. Rapid protein display profiling of cancer progression directly from human tissue using a protein biochip., Drug Dev't. Res. *49:* 34-42, 2000.

28. Vlahou, A., Schellhammer, P., Mendrinos, S., Patel, K., Kondlyis, F., Gong, L., Nasim, S. and Wright, Jr., G. Development of a novel proteomic approach for the detection of transitional cell carcinoma of the bladder in urine., Amer. J. Pathol. *158:* 1491-1502, 2001.

29. Li, J., Zhang, Z., Rosenzweig, J., Wang, Y., and Chan, D. Proteomics and bioinformatics approaches for identification of serum biomarkers to detect breast cancer., Clin. Chem. *48:* 1296-1304, 2002.

30. Petricoin III, E., Ardekani, A., Hitt, B., Levine, P., Fusaro, V., Steinberg, S., Mills, G., Simone, C., Fishman, D., Kohn, E. and Liotta, L. Use of proteomic patterns inserum to identify ovarian cancer., Lancet. *359:* 572-577, 2002.

31. Ozols, R., Rubin, S., Thomas, G. and Robboy, S. Epithelial ovarian cancer. In: Principles and practice of gynecologic oncology. Hoskins, W., Perez, C. and Young, R., eds. Philadelphia: Lippincott Williams and Wilkins. 981-1058, 2000.

32. Petricoin III, E., Zoon, K., Kohn, E., Barrett, C. and Liotta, L. Clinical proteomics: Translating benchside promise into bedside reality. Nat. Drug Disc. *1:* 683-695, 2002.

33. Paweletz, C., Charboneau, L., Bichsel, V., Simone, N., Chen, T., Gillespie, J., Emmert-Buck, M., Roth, M., III, E. P., and Liotta, L. Reverse phase protein microarrays which capture disease progression show activation of pro-survival pathways at the cancer invasion front., Oncogene. *20:* 1981-1989, 2001.

34. Torhorst, J., Bucher, C., Kononen, J., Haas, P., Zuber, M., Kochli, O., Mross, F., Dieterich, H., Moch, H., Mihatsch, M., Kallioneimi, O. and Sauter, G. Tissue microarrays for rapid linking of molecular changes to clinical endpoints., Amer. J. Pathol. *159:* 2249-2256, 2001.

35. Knezevic, V., Leethanakul, C., Bichsel, Vl, Worth, J., Prabhu, V., Gutkind, J., Liotta, L., Munson, P., Petricoin III, E. and Krizman, D. Proteomic profiling of the cancer micorenvironment by antibody arrays., Proteomics. *1:*1271-1278, 2001.

36. Sreekumar, A., Nyati, M., Varambally, S., Barrette, T., Ghosh, D., Lawrence, T. and Chinniyan, A. Profiling of cancer cells using protein microarrays: Discovery of novel radiation-regulated proteins., Cancer Res. *61:* 7585-93, 2001.

STRUCTURAL BASIS OF TUMORAL ANGIOGENESIS

Antonio Llombart-Bosch, José A. López-Guerrero, Carmen Carda Batalla, Amparo Ruíz Suarí, Amando Peydró-Olaya

Department of Pathology, University of Valencia, Avda. Blasco Ibañez, 17, 46010 Valencia, SPAIN

This work has been supported by grants FIS 01/ 0673 and FIS 01/702 from the Ministry of Health, Madrid, Spain.

INTRODUCTION

Mammalian cells require oxygen and nutrients for metabolism and growth. In all cases tissues possess a vascular and lymphatic network assuring the supply of these needs within 200 to 250μm. Multicellular organisms that grow beyond this size require the recruitment of new blood vessels, although some normal tissues are devoid of specific vascularization (cartilage, cornea, epidermis), obtaining their oxygen and metabolic supply through perfusion (Fig. 1).

Figure 1. Tumors require the constant formation of new blood vessels. Example of an ES/pPNET tumor.

The essential role of vascularization in solid tumors has been increasingly recognized in both primary tumor growth and in metastatic spread[1,2]. The observation that angiogenesis occurs in tumors is already 100 years old[3]. In 1971 Folkman proposed that both tumor growth and metastasis are angiogenic dependent[1]. More recently in 1976, Gullino proposed that pre-cancerous cells acquire angiogenic capacity on their way to final malignant transformation[4]. Shubik (1982) - based on three transplant methods for the study of tumoral neovascularization (chorioallantoic membrane, hamster cheek pouch chamber and the cornea) - described the existence of a considerable heterogeneity in vasculogenesis and angiogenesis, between carcinomas, sarcomas and melanomas as well as occasional formation of pseudovessels, lined with tumoral cells in malignant melanomas[5].

The creation of the concept of an **"angiogenic switch"**[6,7] serves to express the balance between pro-angiogenic and anti-angiogenic molecules: It is "on" when the balance favors the angiogenesis and is considered "off" when pro-angiogenic molecules are balanced by that of anti-angiogenic ones. Both pro and anti-angiogenic molecules

New Trends in Cancer for the 21st Century, edited by
Llombart-Bosch and Felipo, Kluwer Academic/Plenum Publishers, 2003

69

may arise from cancer cells, endothelial cells, stromal cells, blood and the extracellular matrix. In addition, this may change from tumor to tumor, or within the same tumor (original neoplasm, relapse, regression or metastasis).

Tumoral new vessel formation mimics vascular embryogenesis promoting the following processes (Fig.2):

Angiogenesis: The mechanism by which new vessels grow by branching from pre-existing vessels (mainly capillaries). The process may occur through *vascular sprouting* or by *intussusceptions* in which interstitial columns of tissue are incorporated into the lumen of newly formed or pre-existing vessels.

Vasculogenesis: De novo production of vessels originating from undifferentiated precursors (mesenchymal pluripotential cells with angioblastic capacity) forming an initial tubular network. At this stage the endothelial cells mature and integrate closely with smooth muscle cells, pericytes and the surrounding matrix.

Angiogenic Remodeling: The process by which the initial network is modified by pruning and vessel enlargement to form interconnecting branching figures characteristic of mature vasculature.

Lymphangiogenesis: The system by which endothelial vessels proliferate, producing new lymphatic, either by angiogenesis or vasculogenesis-like mechanism, induced by lymphatic endothelial growth factors and their receptors.

Arteriogenesis: The transformation of pre-existing arterioles to larger arterioles and arteries (collateral vessel formation after obstruction of a major artery).

Vascular co-option: Groups of avascular tumoral cells may co-opt pre-existing host vessels and start off as well vascularized small tumors.

Mosaic vessels: Tumoral cells in contact with the lumen, together with neoformed endothelial cells, interface, forming mosaics on the surface of the intratumoral capillaries.

Vascular mimicry: Tumoral cells of particular tumors transform themselves into a pseudoendothelium, mimicking new vessels that are incorporated into the vascular network.

Capillary drop-out: Regression induced in recently developed microvessels by anti-angiogenenic drugs.

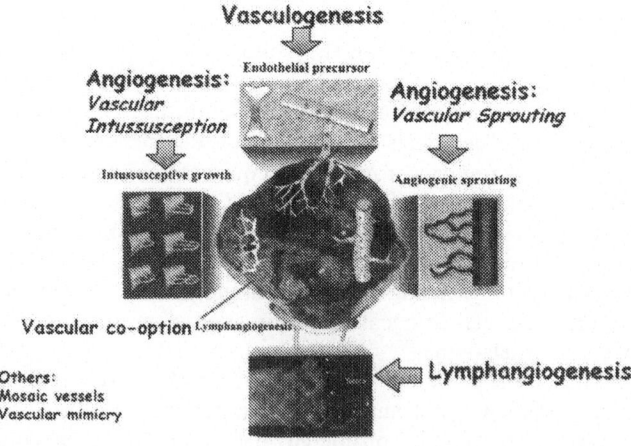

Figure 2. Major processes in new vessel formation in malignant tumors. Illustration adapted from Carmeliet P and Jain RK[8].

Therefore, within the complexity of a malignant tumor (mainly epithelial types of carcinoma), several vascular compartments and new growth shall be considered:

Vascular system pertaining to the host tissue including local capillaries and lymphatic network, peripheral to the tumor or in the major stromal component.

Vascular complex, associated to the neoformed stroma surrounding the tumor, or intermingled within the tumoral nests, in close contact to each other, but supported by an extracellular matrix that limits both compartments.

Neoformed capillary network induced by the tumoral cells through vasculogenesis or angiogenesis.

Tumor cell-to-tissue endothelial cell co-option in which mosaics of both tumoral cells and local endothelial cells are lined together, with no extracellular matrix (Mosaic blood vessels).

Tumoral cells mimicking functional endothelial cells supported only by an incomplete basal membrane (Tumoral mimicry).

All these structures may vary from tumor to tumor, particularly when considering epithelial, mesenchymal or lymphoid neoplasms, and also depend on the tissue in which the tumor arises or metastasizes. Occasionally up to 50% of neoplastic tissue may be composed of blood vessels. For instance, the density and distribution pattern of the vessels within mammary carcinomas adopts a sinusoidal irregular network, with dilated vessels that vary considerably in size and shape, and presenting focal aneurismal bulges, while melanomas show leashes and a radial distribution resembling the spokes of a wheel.

In consequence, the tumor architecture is rich, but heterogeneous and extremely variable, therefore somehow chaotic, leading to fields within the same tumor of hypoxic foci or hemorrhagic areas and well-preserved cell nests.

CELLS INVOLVED IN VASCULAR NEOGENESIS

Table 1. Cell components involved in the angiogenic process

Mesenchymal pluripotential cells with angioblastic capacity.
Endothelial cells.
Pericytes (smooth muscle like cells).
Adventicial fibroblasts.
Lymphocytes.
Platelets.
Monocytes and macrophages.
Inflammatory cells involved in tissue repair.
Myofibroblasts.
Neoplastic cells.

MAJOR VASCULAR SPECIFIC GROWTH FACTORS

A) Vascular endothelial growth factors (VEGF) and their receptors.

Comprise a family of 5 ligands PIGF / VEGF-A / VEGF-B / VEGF-C / VEGF-D and their respective receptors. VEGFR-1 (Fit-1) / VEGFR-2 (KDR/Flk-1) / VEGFR-3 (Fit-4). In addition, a number of accessory receptors occur such as NEUROPHILINS.

VEGF promotes endothelial cell proliferation and induces vascular leakage and permeability. The other various members of the family interact with a set of tyrosine kinase cell receptors that mediate the major growth and permeability actions of VEGF.

This is a potent and critical vascular regulator on post-natal life and early organ development[9].

Early tumoral growth together with Ang2 contributes to tumor vasculogenic co-option in avasculogenic neoplasms (small tumors or metastasis) favoring secondary tumoral vascular sprouting.

B) *The angiopoietins and their receptors.*

There are 4 members of the family: *Ang1 / Ang2 / Ang3 / Ang4*, ligands to the Ties family (Tie1 and Tie2) of tyrosine kinase cell receptors that are selectively expressed in the vascular endothelium. They participate in angiogenic remodeling and the stabilization of mature vessels in so far as they maximize interactions between the endothelial cells with their surrounding support cells and the interstitial matrix.

Ang1 may counteract the effect of VEGF on endothelial permeability, preventing leaks caused by the former.

Ang2 displays a similarly high affinity to Tie2. Biologically, it acts as an inhibitor of *Ang1*, allowing endothelial cells to revert to a more plastic stage, reminiscent of developing vessels. In tumoral growth, *Ang2,* together with VEGF, destabilizes the co-opted vessels causing endothelial apoptosis but later induces new angiogenic sprouting within the same neoplasm[9].

C) *The ephrins and their receptors.*

The Eph ligands and their receptors constitute the largest family of growth factor receptors. Exclusively related to vascular growth are: EPHRIN-A1 / EPHRIN-B1 / EPHRIN-B2 and their receptors, respectively: EphA2 / EphB2 / EphB3 / EphB4.

EPHRIN-B2 and its receptor EphB4 play key roles during vascular neogenesis. Moreover, EPHRIN-B2 marks the endothelium of the primordial arteries and EphB4 marks the endothelium of primordial venous vessels. In adult vessels, the EPHRIN-B2 continues detecting the arterial endothelium and their surrounding muscle cells, as well as the pericytes. This demonstrates the continuous role played by the ligand in adult arteries, perhaps regulating the relation between endothelium and muscle wall cells.

The maintenance of new vessels depends on the survival of endothelial cells. Normal adult endothelial cells can survive for years due to the activity of: VEGF, VE-cadherin and Ang1. The maturation of normal new vessels depends on the formation of a new basement membrane as well as smooth muscle cells and pericyte proliferation. PDGF-BB recruits new smooth muscle cells while TGF-b1 and Ang1/Tie2 stabilizes endothelial cells and smooth muscle cells.

In tumoral angiogenesis, EPHRIN-B2 is intensively re-expressed in sprouting vessels together with Ang2, a fact which indicates that venous or other uncommitted vessels do not exclusively condition this tumoral sprouting[9].

D) *Cyclooxigenases (COX-1 and COX-2).*

COX catalyzes the initial step in the biosynthesis of prostaglandins from arachidonic acid, being encoded by two genes, COX-1 and COX-2, that participate in the formation of several icosanoids such as PDG2, PGE2, PGI2, PGF2α and tromboxane A. COX-1 is expressed constitutionally in almost all tissues and has been considered as a housekeeper gene. In contrast, COX-2 is an inducible immediate early gene that is up-regulated by various stimuli. COX-2 regulates cancer-induced angiogenesis through the production of angiogenic factors such as VEGF and has been seen aberrantly increased in several epithelial cancers of the colon, gastric, esophagus, lung, bladder and endometrium[10-13]. Moreover, selective COX-2 inhibitors block angiogenesis in various cell systems[13].

Table 2. Major angiogenesis activators and their functional activity[8,9]

Activators	Functions
VEGF and family members	Stimulate angiogenesis, vasculogenesis, lymphangiogenesis, increased permeability and leukocyte adhesion.
VERGFR, NRP1	Integrate angiogenic and survival signals.
Ang1 and Tie2	Stabilize vessels; inhibit permeability.
PDGFR-BB and receptors	Recruit smooth muscle cells.
TGF-b1, Endoglin, TGF-b Receptors	Stimulate extracellular matrix production.
FGF, HGF, MCP-1	Stimulate angio and arteriogensis.
VE-Cadherin, PECAM (CD31)	Endothelial junctional proteins.
Ephrins	Regulate the arterial/venous specification.
PAI-1	Stabilizes nascent vessels.
NOS, COX-2	Stimulate angiogenesis and vasodilatation.
AC133	Regulates angioblastic capacity.
Chemokines	Pleiotropic role in angiogenesis.
Id1/Id3	Determine endothelial plasticity.
Integrins	Receptors for matrix molecules and proteinases.

HYPOXIA: ANGIOGENESIS AND VASCULAR REMODELING IN INFLAMMATION

In normal adult tissues vasculature is quiescent and only 0.01% of endothelial cells undergo mitosis. In non-malignant tissues, hypoxia and inflammation contribute to angiogenesis.

Hypoxia is a strong stimulus of angiogenesis through Hypoxia Inducible Transcription Factors (HIFs), which induce the expression of several angiogenic factors such as VEGF, NOS, PDGF, Ang2 and others. Moreover, it can induce vascular remodeling due to an imbalance between vasodilators (NO) and vasoconstrictors (endothelin-1).

Inflammation is associated with excessive angiogenesis.

These cells and other leukocytes release a number of angiogenic factors. Some of them are as follows: VEGF, Ang1, b-FIG, PDGF, TGF-b1, TNF-a, HGF, IGF-1, MCP-1 (monocyte chemotactic protein 1).

Inflammatory cells are also involved in vascular remodeling and negative control of angiogenesis.

Moreover, inflammatory cells have been implicated in the so-called "*adaptative angiogenesis*" that consists of the growth of pre-existing collateral arterioles after occlusion of a supply artery in the myocardium or in peripheral limbs. This adaptative angiogenesis results in functional and structurally normal arteries that are able to sustain their proper circulation and become adapted to physiological demands.

In granulation tissue and wound healing[14,15], vasculogenesis also takes place by activated cell division and endothelial sprouting of isolated cells or solid cell bundles. Several types of endothelial cells have been recognized with the support of immunohistochemistry and electron microscopy: undifferentiated perivascular cells, mesenchymal angioblasts, reactive endothelial cells, high-epithelioid endothelium, histiocytic endothelial cells, and mature endothelium.

It has not yet been confirmed if there are different cell varieties or diverse maturation stages of the same cell lineage.

MAJOR MECHANISMS OF VESSEL FORMATION IN THE EMBRYO

The first blood vessels develop from mesechymal cells that differentiate into endothelial cells and endothelial tubes, interconnecting with each other in order to organize a primitive blood vessel network. In addition, new blood vessels proliferate from this vascular plexus by angiogenesis, which is comprised of endothelial sprouting, splitting and cell fusion[16]. As soon as the first primordial vessels are formed, mural cells with smooth muscle cell lineages proliferate and become attached to the wall as pericytes[17]. The origin of the pericytes is less clear as they may be induced de novo from the mesenchyme surrounding the neoformed vessel[18]. Here, TGF-beta, Ang1 and its receptor Tie-2 seem to play a major role[8,9,19].

Continuous recruitment of endothelial cells and progenitor stem cells from the bone marrow environment and their subsequent mobilization into the peripheral blood contributes to a continuous tissue vascularization, promoting normal organogenesis. Despite major advances in their phenotypic identification, the molecular pathways involved in the angiogenic factor mediated recruitment remain poorly understood[20]. Hattori et al.,[21] have reported that VEGFR-1 is expressed in human CD34 cells, conveying signals for recruitment of hematopoyetic stem cells, and stimulating angiogenesis. Moreover, VEGFR-1 deficient mice die as embryos, presenting an excess of endothelial cells and vascularization[22]. Gerber et al.[23] have shown that VEGF regulates hematopoietic stem cell survival by an autocrine mechanism. Mice with VEGF deleted hematopoietic stem cells failed to survive or differentiate in vitro and failed to repopulate when lethally irradiated, while ligands to VEGFR-1 and VEGFR-2 will restore the gene-deleted hematopoiesis and the colony formation in vitro[24].

From the structural point of view, the embryonic angiogenesis discloses a sycitial origin of the angioblastic cell. The endothelial cells are identified in living embryos as mesenchymal or mesothelial coelomic cells that progressively produce lumina. This process of luminization may occur in several ways[25,26], including:
- Cell dissociation with subsequent rounding-up of mesenchymal angioblastic cells.
- Development of intercellular channels by confluence of several immature solid endothelial cells.
- Intracellular lumen formation initiated by the confluence of cytoplasm vacuoles and caveolae.
- Progressive maturation of these cells leads to the presence of cytoplasmic bundles of filaments and Weibel-Palade bodies as well as thigh intercellular junctions associated to clefts and gap-contacts.

MICROVESSEL DENSITY (MVD) FOR THE HISTOLOGICAL GRADING OF TUMOR ANGIOGENESIS.

Since 1972 several quantitative methods of grading tumor angiogenesis have been developed, measuring the amounts of neovascularization in the tumor and correlating it with the histological grade and clinical outcome[27-30]. The number of publications regarding MVD and the prognosis of tumors is extremely high[31] covering almost all types of neoplasms. At present, it is accepted that a high MVD count is a useful marker of poor prognosis and higher metastatic risk in a number of carcinomas, sarcomas and lymphomas, demonstrating that angiogenesis is a crucial event in the growth and metastasis of solid tumors[32]. Immunohistochemistry with several antibodies, such as human factor VIII - related antigen, CD31 and CD34 are accepted as being reliable for estimating angiogenesis[33-36], but not good indicators of therapeutic effectiveness or tumor regression with anti-angiogenic therapy[37]. Thus other parameters related to angiogenesis have been studied, such as the expression of VEGF[38] and TGF-b1[39] among others.

Carcinoma of the breast, both in situ and invasive, with and without lymph node metastasis, is a good model for the study of angiogenesis and related prognostic factors. In the development of a solid tumor two different stages occur, the first is a prevascular phase that may be present for long periods (preneoplasic phase and in situ carcinoma) being followed by a vascular phase that usually produces a rapid invasive growth. Most authors confirm that most vascularized carcinomas are associated with an increased risk of metastasis[30,40,41].

Studies by our own group[42] confirm that MVD is lower in DCIS than in invasive carcinoma. In addition, DCIS grade III (comedo carcinoma in situ) shows a greater MVD than DCIS grade I/II, confirming that this type of DCIS has a higher risk of progression (Fig. 3).

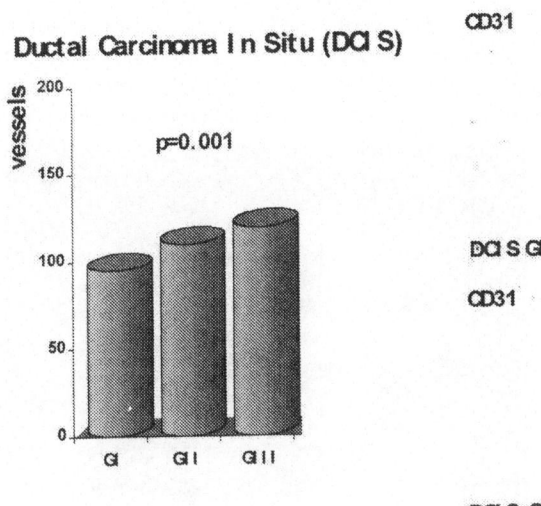

Figure 3. Angiogenesis in human tumors. A model in breast cancer. MVD is directly associated with the histological grade in DCIS of the breast. Microvessels are visualized after immunostaining with CD31.

In recent studies (non-published) we also confirm that local tumor relapse in invasive breast carcinomas is associated with a higher MVD than in the original tumor (Figure 4). Moreover, breast tumors that have caused bone marrow metastasis also present a higher MVD when compared to non- metastasizing carcinomas (Ruiz et al. 2003 in preparation).

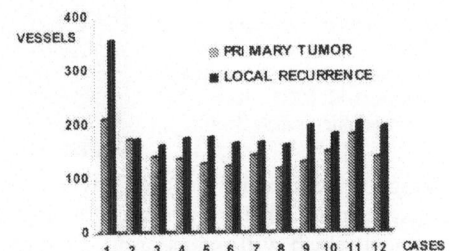

Figure 4. Angiogenesis in hbuman tumors. A model in breast cancer. MDV increases in recurrent tumors when compare with the primary neoplasm.

FINE STRUCTURE OF ENDOTHELIAL CELLS AND VESSELS IN TUMOR

Neoformed endothelia and vascular beds seen ultrastructurally are abnormal, presenting large irregularities. The number and size of endothelial cells varies. They are abnormal in size and shape and grow on top of each other, with microvilli or short digitations projecting into the lumen and presenting numerous endothelial fenestrate, intracytoplasmic vesicles and holes which cause numerous cell openings or widened inter-endothelial junctions. The endothelial cells can be highly attenuated[43,44]. Luminal microfolds are greatly enlarged at the endothelial surface. Caveolae have been defined as one of the major pathways for transcellular permeability[45] in endothelial cells. Tumor endothelia present abundant caveolae both near the luminal and in the abluminal compartment which may cause severe vascular leakage.

The basal laminae may be absent or reduplicated. In addition, smooth muscle cells and pericytes may be present, but irregularly distributed and do not function as normal contractile cells. The absence of pericytes and smooth muscle cells may lead to blood vessel dilatation, endothelial cell hyperplasia and microaneurism formation[46]. These defects cause the intratumoral vessels to become leaky.

Most of these alterations occur in the neoformed vessels located within the intratumoral vasculogenesis and to a lesser extent at the peripheral edges of the proliferation areas of the neoplasia, to which the extracellular matrix provides support and organizes the new vessel formation by angiogenesis (endothelial sprouting) (Fig.5).

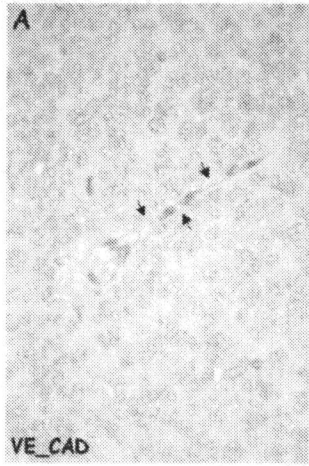
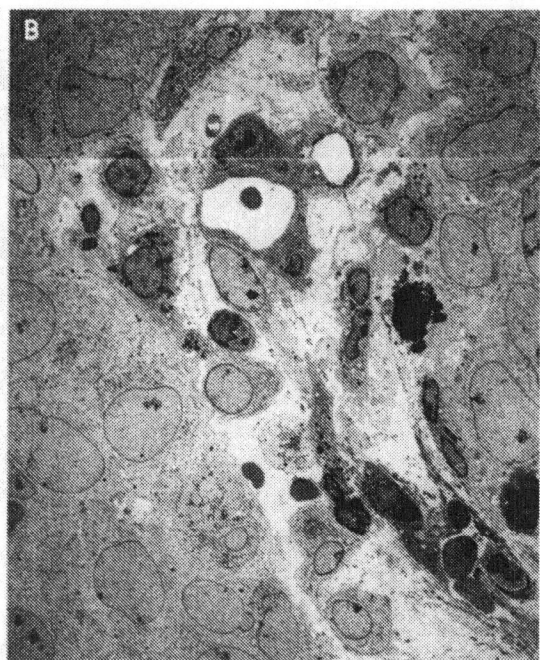

Figure 5. Neo-angiogenesis by vascular sprouting in a ES/pPNET tumor.
A, endothelial cells immuno-stained with VE-Cadherin; B, electron microscopy detail.

Vascular permeability and angiogenesis depends also on the type of tumor and the host tissue in which the cells are growing, because each organ has a diverse stromal component which will induce a different angiogenic switch due to a variable presence of pro and anti angiogenic molecules.

In order to evaluate the changes related mainly to edema present in the Central Nervous System, microvessels in peritumoral tissue have been studied comparatively with normal capillaries by morphometry and electron microscopy[47]. No statistical difference could be determined between normal and peritumoral capillaries as regards to diameter, endothelial thickness and wall thickness, but a number of structural changes were found regarding endothelial ultrastructure: the endothelial cells presented a three times vesicle density with surface connected caveolae. In addition, a thicker basal lamina and significantly reduced number of pericytes were found.

We have reviewed the vascular component in sarcomas particularly in Ewing's sarcoma (Es) of bone and soft tissue[48]. This small round cell sarcoma is a highly metastasizing tumor in children and young adults that presents a peculiar micro capillary network in which the tumoral cells group together in a perivascular irradiated pattern in continuity with necrotic fields and intermingled with apoptotic cells. The intratumoral capillaries seem to be close to the neoplastic cells and some continuity appears between them, being separated only by a tiny and discontinuous basal lamina. No pericytes are seen, while the reactive endothelial cells display a large, clear, watery cytoplasm with Weibel-Palade bodies, numerous pinocytic vesicles and filaments. The cell-to-cell contacts are irregular and leaky. Moreover, we have described an atypical Es, with angiogenic appearance[48-50], actually composed of malignant endothelial cells arranged in sheets or compact bands with a lobular pattern due to reticular septa and irregular clefts, reproducing luminization in early vascular stages and with occasional erythrocytes present.

MOSAIC BLOOD VESSELS IN TUMORS

Cancer cells can be located in the capillary walls of the tumor blood vessels, intermingled with normal endothelial cells. This event has been defended, with electron microscopical support, by several authors in the past[51]. The subject has been addressed by Maniotis et al.[52], considering this circumstance as "vascular mimicry" in which the actual tumoral cells acquire the capacity to build-up blood channels within the tumors (melanomas) thereby substituting the endothelial cells.

More recently, Chang et al.[53] have performed a number of elegant experiments in order to witness the presence of tumor cells covering the inner surface of the vessels, as endothelial cells do, in order to reveal what their functional significance may be. It is well known that tumor cells actively traverse the capillaries on their way to spreading metastatically into the blood stream.

Several questions are addressed by these authors on this subject, such as:

-Do the tumor cells actively participate in constituting the wall structure in a stable condition, or are they on their way to traversing the wall and shedding into the blood stream?

-How frequently does this process occur in human carcinomas such as colon cancer?

-Is the presence of mosaic blood vessels associated with an increase in the number of metastasis?

-What is the physiological behavior regarding the capacity to perfuse and be leaky compared to conventional intratumoral vessels?

Their findings were based on an animal model (tumor implants in immunodeficient mice) of the human colon carcinoma cell line LS140T, expressing a green fluorescent protein, while the tumoral endothelial cells were stained with CD31 and CD105 (endoglin) as well as a mixture of both antibodies. The observations were performed with confocal microscopy. In addition, 16 human colon carcinomas were quantified for the frequency of mosaic vessels with an analogous technique.

In the immunosuppressed mice, 13.7% of the tumor vessels were mosaic, a finding somewhat similar to that observed in the human carcinomas (13.6% mosaics). Based on the product of the mean proportion of mosaic vessels and the mean length of the studied perimeters of the vessels unstained with the endothelial markers, it was concluded that around 4% of the total luminal surface area is covered by tumor cells. Most of these tumor cells seem to be on their way to shedding and extravasating into the lumen. Basically, it has been previously demonstrated that nearly one million cells are shed per gram of tumor per day[54,55]. This finding is concordant with the data obtained by Chang et al., which could mean that about half of the tumor cells in contact with the lumen are in the process of shedding into the blood stream[53].

Numerous questions remain open about how these vessels are formed, and how stable they are while being sustained by only poorly developed attachments or imperfect cell to cell junctions and being submitted to numerous immunoreactive events. In addition, it is not clear what role circulating endothelial cell precursors may play in this type of mosaic formation, as well as the possible vascular co-option of endothelial cells that remain surrounded or displaced by the proliferation of tumoral cells (Fig. 6). Present findings differ from the proposed hypothesis of "vascular mimicry" in which the tumor cells are major participants in constructing the tumor vessels of the neoplasm[52].

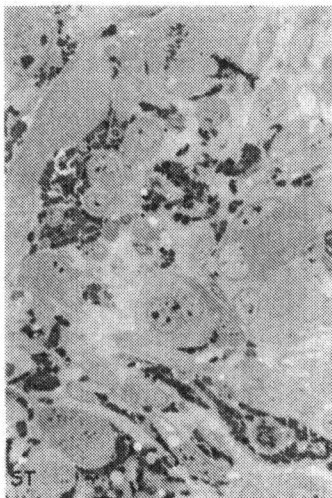 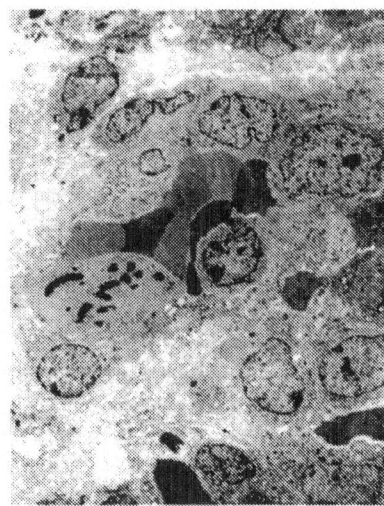

Figure 6. Semi-thin (ST) (left) and electron microscopic (right) sections illustrating the vascular mosaic in an osteosarcoma.

The finding of endothelial mosaics may have clinical significance since Mancuso et al.[56] have seen that resting and activated endothelial cells are significantly increased in the peripheral blood of cancer patients, while Browder et al.[57] have observed that the drug cyclophosphamide, widely used as an agent in high-dose chemotherapy, possesses a considerable antivascular activity which could imply the mobilization of neoplastic cells in patients receiving this agent together with autologous haemopoietic progenitor cells and G-CSF (granulocytic-colony stimulating factor).

LYMPHATIC VESSELS IN TUMORIGENSIS AND TUMORAL SPREAD

The importance of lymphatic vessels in tumor spread is beyond discussion. Most epithelial neoplasms and a large number of other tumors (sarcomas, melanomas, lymphomas) emigrate through the lymphatic system, colonizing the regional lymph nodes. This constitutes the first stage of cancer dissemination outside the initial infiltrative area. The presence of isolated cells in the cortical lymphatic sinus may be the first expression of a metastatic seeding in a neoplasm. The significance of the so-called "sentinel lymph node" has gained large clinical importance for the detection of early metastasis in breast and colon carcinoma, melanoma, etc.

A general belief was that within the malignant tumoral parenchyma there is no lymphatic vessel neoformation as seen in conventional angiogenesis. Thus, the tumoral cells reach the pre-existing lymphatic of the normal surrounding tissue by direct invasion in order to be transported to the regional lymph nodes[58]. Recent investigations into this question, based on the availability of specific lymphatic endothelial markers, indicate that this position is erroneous and that a tumoral lymphangiogenesis occurs, similar to that seen in conventional angiogenesis. What is still not clear is if vasculogenesis and lymphangiogenesis within a given neoplasm run along similar pathways, or constitute two different systems that may or may not be intermingled with each other.

A number of lymphatic endothelium markers have been discovered in recent years, but some of them express not only in the endothelial lymphatic, but also in blood vessels, making their distinction more difficult. The membrane protein LYVE1 is a transmembrane hyaluronic acid receptor, present in liver sinusoids[59] and PODOPLANIN is a membrane protein present in the glomerular podocytes of the kidney[60], both of which selectively stain the lymphatic. Another potential marker for this endothelium is VEGFR3 the receptor of the VEGFC and VEGFD[61]. Finally, the nuclear marker PROX1 is also expressed in the lymphatic, but not in blood vessels[62]. Based upon the detection of endothelial cells within several types of tumors with these new markers, there are now strong indications that confirm the major role played by the lymphatic, not only within the tumoral stroma, but also inside the neoplasm in close conjunction with the tumor cells, in a similar way as conventional blood endothelium does. Moreover, some heterogeneity seems to occur in the lymphatic that may display variable specialization depending on the type of tumor or its histological nature. Intratumoral connections between blood vessels and lymphatic vessels seem possible, becoming inter-connected as "vascular mimicry channels" in a common network of proliferating endothelial and tumoral cells in close continuity and supported by tiny ECM[63].

The clinical-pathological evidence of the frequent lymphatic metastatic spread of tumoral cells in carcinomas favors the hypothesis that a vigorous lynphangiogenesis occurs within a large number of epithelial neoplasms, independently of this second blood vessel component.

In the case of breast cancer it is well established that cancer cells spread mainly into the axillary lymph-nodes. Lymph-node positive cancer patients are associated with a shortened survival rate as compared with node-negative patients, this being one of the most important independent factors in breast cancer. Even small size neoplasms (2cm or smaller) show positive lymph-nodes (in over 20% of patients)[64].

Moreover, relatively little is known about the mechanism of metastatic spread in lymphatics. Lymphatics do not contain tight junctions or continuous basal laminae[65].

For intravasation the tumoral cells may only require cell adhesion to the endothelium and transmigration through intracellular gaps that occurs between lymphatic endothelial cells[66].

VEGFR-3 is a tyrosine-kinase receptor that binds to VEGF-C, playing an important role in angiogenesis and particularly as a lymphangiogenic marker in normal and tumoral tissues such as lymphangiomas, Kaposi sarcoma and other skin tumors[67-70]. In "in situ ductal carcinomas" of the breast VEGFR-3 expression has been detected in the proximal located "necklace vessels" surrounding the transformed ducts, while VEGF-C was located in the cytoplasms of the tumor cells. A large number of VEGFR-3 positive vessels were also found in invasive ductal carcinoma when compared to normal breast. VEGF-C stained intensively both in situ carcinoma and invasive cancer cells, which act as an angiogenic growth factor for local tumoral vessels that probably possess a lymphatic nature, as they were devoid of perycites or muscle cells. VEGF-C and VEGFR-3 seem to be components of a paracrine signaling network between cancer cells and lymphatic endothelium, modifying the permeability and inducing vasculogensis in breast cancer[71].

More recently, Skobe et al.[72], using an experimental model of orthoptic transplantation of human breast carcinomas into nude mice, have confirmed the occurrence of a vigourous lymphangiogenesis within the carcinoma stained with the endothelial marker LYVE-1, that was associated with a strong overexpression of VEGF-C present in the breast cancer cells, resulting in a significant increase in lymph-node and lung metastasis; this finding identifies tumoral lynphangiogenesis in breast carcinoma with VEGF-C. In addition, VEGF-D, also a member of the family of VEGF, is a ligand to VEGFR-3 that acts as a lymphatic endothelial receptor. Staker et al.[73], with an experimental mouse model, have demonstrated the capacity of this ligand for producing lymphangiogenesis within tumoral cell lines transplanted into nude mice overexpressing this molecule leading to the production of a high number of metastases into the lymph nodes.

TUMORS WITHOUT ANGIOGENIC SWITCH

Another question is if a solid tumoral growth can survive exclusively from the pre-existing vascular bed of the non-malignantly transformed tissue, without the angiogenic switch.

It seems clear that most epithelial tumors initially arise separated from the underlying vessels by a basement membrane that must be destroyed before the malignant cells have access to the vessels. Thus, it seems evident that the initial steps of tumor growth is in many cases avascular, with the tumor cells initially homing in on co-opted pre-existing vessels from the host. There are various ways in which tumoral cells induce angiogenesis[9]:

-Vascular co-opting of pre-existing host vessels (+Ang2).

-Angiogenic sprouting into the tumor (+VEGF, +Ang2 and +EPHRIN-B2).

- New intratumoral angiogenesis secondary to primary vessel regression of the co-opted vasculature induced after apoptosis (+Ang2) and secondary local hypoxia (+++VEGF).

Pezzella et al. have confirmed the hypothesis that if a tumor obtains sufficient blood supply from the pre-existing vasculature that already exists in the local tissue, it can grow without the need for the production of a vascular switch[74,75]. In a group of non-small lung cancers it has been found that CD31 immunoassaying of tumor vessels displays four distinct patterns: basal, papillary, diffuse and alveolar. The last is non-angiogenic (present in 15% of lung tumors). The immunostaining of this pattern shows tumoral cells filling the alveolar spaces, but the vessels belong to the alveolar spaces and not to the tumor itself. A clinical-pathological correlation has shown that the tumors with this vascular variety are more aggressive than those bearing other types of neovascularization[76].

New experiences by the same authors have demonstrated on angiogenic breast carcinomas that their metastasis in the lung can be non-angiogenic[77].

VASCULAR MIMICRY

Several investigators have for many years been discussing the evidence that cancer cells can become vascular lining cells and contribute to the formation of an intratumoral microvascular network[78-80]. Several electron microscopical studies have provided support for this hypothesis[43,81]. Recently, Maniotis et al.[52] have proposed a new concept for this situation under the term of "vascular mimicry" based on previous studies of Folberg et al.,[82] analyzing uveal and cutaneous melanomas both in vivo and in vitro. This hypothesis, although attractive, has given rise a number of controversies[83] and seems to be limited only to highly aggressive melanomas and their metastasis.

The early studies of Foldberg et al.,[84,85] based on malignant uveal melanomas, demonstrated the existence of particular types of channels with a basal lamina structure, that were stained with periodic-acid-Schiff stain (PAS stain), highlighting the presence of several types of loops within the tumoral parenchyma. Up to nine different types of channels were identified that could be organized into two main hierarchical groups: (a) those tumors with isolated straight parallel channels, and (b) a second group that contains a rich network of channels with loops and branching or isolated arcs. This second type of uveal melanomas was associated with high aggressivity and significant mortality from metastasis. Other groups have confirmed this finding[86,87].

These channels were considered by Maniotis et al.[52], as a system of "de novo" generation of pseudovascular structures devoid of endothelium, and lined externally by the melanoma cells that could generate an extracellular matrix. This novel process of microcirculation should be considered as being different from a true vasculogenesis, because the latter results from the neogenesis of the endothelial cell-lined vessel. Therefore, the "name of vascular mimicry shall be restricted to the process by which aggressive tumor cells generate non-endothelial cell-line channels delimited by extracellular matrix"[82].

Support in favor of this hypothesis has been provided by the group based upon immunohistochemical techniques: the melanoma cells express both vimentin and cytokeratin, in addition a focal positivity for Ulex lectin, CD31 and CD34 exists within the channels. Moreover, a number of proteins involved in angiogenesis, such as EPHA2 and TIE1, are expressed in the cell cultures of the aggressive melanoma[88,89]. No cells or nuclei are seen on the luminal side of the basement membrane. Red blood cells in single line (rouleaux) are frequently detected within the channels. Their ultra structure confirms the presence of melanoma cells localized externally of the PAS positive lamina, but with the absence of endothelial cells lining the lumen of the channels.

Using hybridization with cDNA microarrays, Maniotis et al., have found differences between the gene expression occurring in poorly invasive and in highly aggressive uveal melanomas[52]. About 210 known genes were expressed differentially with overexpression of TIE1, epithelial cell kinase, keratin 8 intermediate filaments and

Collagen type IV, suggesting that a genetic reversion to a embryonic genotype occurs in aggressive melanoma cells.

The numerous arguments against the existence of vascular mimicry in tumors have been previously well debated by McDonald et al.[83]. The presence of PAS stained networks is accepted, but they do not represent blood vessels or define microvascular architecture in uveal melanomas. These three-dimensional back to back loops of PAS positive stained basal lamina, could contain interconnecting tubular openings. This provides a favorable substrate for the in-growth of angiogenic or lymphatic vessels, in so far as both layers of the PAS positive net could separate from each other and form channels or tubular structures, leading to capillary growth. Open ends of the channels could explain the presence of red blood cells within these structures.

ANGIOGENESIS AND VASCULOGENESIS OF HUMAN TUMORS TRANSPLANTED TO RODENTS

Several animal models have been used to study the vascular neogenesis of human tumors transplanted into mice, rats, hamsters or immunodeficient nude mice. In addition, intravital microscopy is an established technology that allows non invasive imaging of vessel formation, opening up new possibilities for the analysis of angiogenesis and vasculogensis, as well as their architecture and function in xenografts[8].

Warren and Shubick[51] studied the growth of blood supply to melanoma transplants in golden hamster cheek pouch by optical and electron microscopy. They described three key patterns: firstly, the development of capillary sprouts that enter the tumor (angiogenesis) with leakage of erytrocytes cells between the tumoral cells; secondly, the presence of micro thrombi formation within the neoformed vessels, and finally the production of a central necrotic focus. Abnormal forms of microvascularization have been described in melanoma and sarcoma xenoptransplants by Konerding et al[90].

In order to go deeply into these findings we have undertaken a number of experiments using nude mice xenografts of human sarcomas transplanted into the subcutaneous pad of the mice, and followed up for several days and weeks after the graft. Three different types of sarcomas were used: a fast growing sarcoma with a mean time between transplants of 30 days, a slower growing osteosarcoma (60 days between grafts) and a more slow proliferating fibrosarcoma (90 days between transplants). All animals received the implant of a tumor chunk of 0.3-0.4 cm in size located in the subcutaneous pad.

The main object of this study was the analysis of:
- The microvasculature pre-existing within the tumor chunk before being transplanted into the nude-mice and their follow-up in the new host.
- The early stages of angiogenesis and vasculogenesis in the tumor transplant, provided by the new host.
- The types of vascular connections established between the host vasculature and the tumor graft.

The study was followed successively for 24 hours, 48 hours, one, two, three and four weeks, and the three types of sarcomas compared. None of them caused distant metastasis in nude mice when transplanted subcutaneously. The histological techniques (HE, PAS, reticuline stain) were complemented with Immunohistochemistry (CD34, VEGF, VEGFR1, VEGFR2, VEGFR3, VE-CAD and PDGFR) as well as electron microscopy (EM). See Fig.7 for schematic representation.

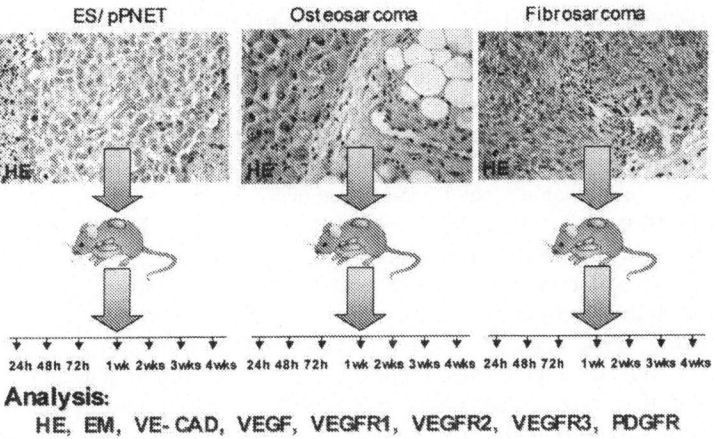

Figure 7. Schematic representation of our experience to study the phenomenon of angiogenesis in xenotransplanted tumors.

The vascular expression and neogenesis varies considerably from the fast growing ES/pPNET to the slow proliferating fibrosarcoma while the osteosarcoma reproduces patterns that are common in all three.

Original transplanted tumors posses their own vasculature provided by the host, being mainly composed of a fine network of capillaries in direct continuity with the tumor cells. This net is very rich in the osteosarcoma while the ES/pPNET presents a central co-opted vessel that is surrounded by a core of tumoral cells of a diameter of 300 microns in which a layer of 10 to 12 cells survives. Outside, these core cells are apoptotic or in lysis. The fibrosarcoma presents a vascularization coming from the peripheral capsule that provides micro-vessels invading the tumor and developing a poor intratumoral network.

Ultrastructurally we have seen numerous irregularities in the endothelial composition of the capillaries with the presence of poorly developed structures, the partial absence of basal laminae, the continuity of endothelial and tumoral cells as well as vascular mosaicism with sarcomatous cells directly in contact with the lumina that is filled with erythrocytes. These findings are particularly manifested in the osteosarcoma and to a lesser extent in the ES, but absent in the fibrosarcoma. The last of which always presents a continuous capillary endothelial lining with irregularities in size and diameter and with absence of pericytes.

24 to 48 hours after the implant, the tumors initiated an active angiogenic remodeling in the surrounding stroma that encircles the tumoral cells and is in continuity with the subcutaneous tissue of the mice. At first, intense capillary congestion and microhemorrhagies occurred. Endothelial sprouting with mitotic activity in the endothelial cells of the host capillaries of the host was seen. Activated angioblasts of mesenchymal origin, intermingled with numerous lymphocytes and macrophages, proliferated in these initial stages providing a neo-vasculogenesis through an in situ new vessel formation as seen in the embryo or in the early stages of cicatrization. Initial contacts occurred between the endothelial cells, these newly formed endothelial cells and the transplanted tumor cells, by co-option and sprouting forming tubular solid structures that later produce intracytoplasmic or intercellular caveolae and lumina, inside which erythrocytes appear. No clear basal lamina was seen.

At this stage a shell of 10 to 14 tumoral cells, up to 300 microns thick, remained morphologically well preserved while the more deeply located cells became isolated and suffered apoptosis, being transformed within the first week into a central necrotic mass. At this moment the tumor mass may shrink, diminishing in volume. Within the superficial rim of viable cells vasculogenesis and angiogenesis appeared simultaneously. Moreover, tumor-endothelial cell mosaics were detected in the two fast growing sarcomas (ES/pPNET and osteosarcoma) but not in the slow proliferating fibrosarcoma. Vascular mimicry was also detected at the end of the first week in the ES/pPNET and in the osteosarcoma using electron microscopy (Figure 8).

Between the first and the third week after transplant an intense neo-vasculogenesis and neo-angiogenesis appeared within the tumor parenquima in two different ways that were seen only in ES/pPNET and osteosarcoma. One, by intratumoral co-option of undifferentiated mesenchymal angioblasts that selectively proliferate, and two, by endothelial sprouting from the peripheral neoformed capillaries of the host (see Fig.5). The capillary network pre-existing from the original transplanted tumor mass may partially persist, providing a source for further intratumoral angiogenesis, but most of these endothelial cells suffer apoptosis.

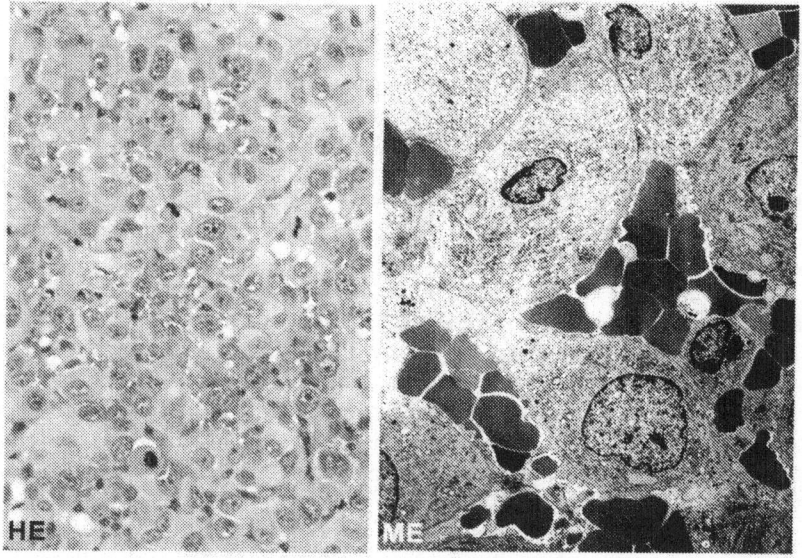

Figure 8. Vascular mimicry in a first week growing xenotransplanted human osteosarcoma.

At this stage the tumoral cells present an extremely intense metabolic activity with an overexpression of several vascular growth factors. We analyzed the expression of VEGF, VE-Cahderin, VEGFR1, VEGFR2, VEGFR3 and PDGFR. Figure 9 shows the evolution of the progressive increase in activity of all these factors, that start at 24 hours and continue during the first two weeks after the tumor transplantation. Only at the third week and after one month is the activity of the tumor cells, which produces vascular growth factors, stabilized and diminishes to a basal level similar to that prior to the transplantation.

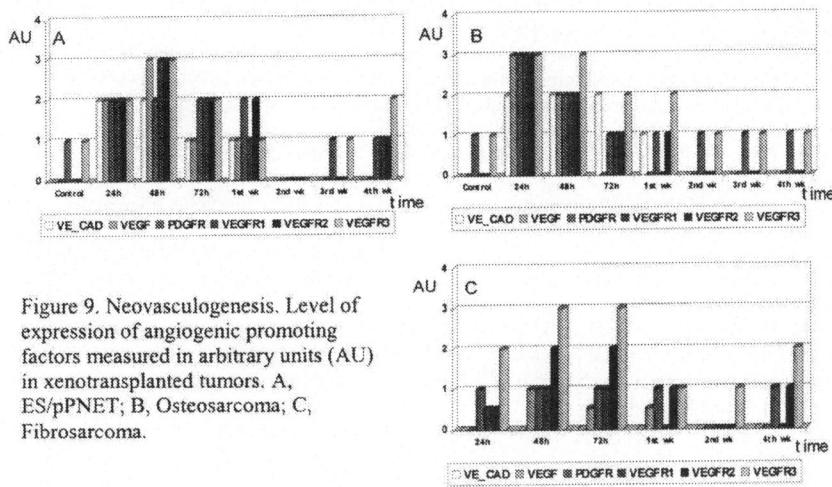

Figure 9. Neovasculogenesis. Level of expression of angiogenic promoting factors measured in arbitrary units (AU) in xenotransplanted tumors. A, ES/pPNET; B, Osteosarcoma; C, Fibrosarcoma.

Based upon present experience it seems evident that each tumor shows a different type of neovascularization. Fast growing sarcomas use all possibilities, including, not only vasculogenesis, angiogensis, vascular remodeling, vascular co-option, capillary drop-out, but also mosaic vessel formation and vascular mimicry. This circumstance is probably due, not only to the activation of vascular growth factors in the macrophages, but also to an autocrine stimulation of the tumor cells that initiates an active synthesis in the vascular growth factor within 24 hours of the transplant and lasting for several weeks. Therefore, these models provide excellent examples of all the systems that are involved in the recapillarization of a sarcoma.

References

1. Folkman J. Tumor angiogenesis, therapeutic implications. N Engl J Med 1971, 285:1182-1186.
2. Folkman J. Angiogenesis in cancer, vascular, rheumatoid and other diseases. Nat Med 1995, 1:27-31.
3. Goldman E. The growth of malignant disease in man and in the lower animals with special reference to the vascular system. Lancet 1907, 2:1236-1240.
4. Gullino FM. Angiogenesis and oncogenesis. J Nat Cancer Inst 1976, 6:111-124.
5. Shubik P. Vascularization of tumors: a review. J Cancer Res Clin Oncol 1982, 103:211-226.
6. Hanahan D, Folkman J. Patterns and emerging mechanims of the angiogenic switch during tumorogenesis. 1996 Cell, 86:363-364.
7. Hanahan D, Weinberg RA. The hallmarks of cancer. Cell 2000, 100:57-70.
8. Carmeliet P, Jain RK. Angiogenesis in cancer and other diseases. Nature Insight 2000, 407: 249-257.
9. Yancopoulos GD, Davis S, Gale NW, Rudge JS, Wiegand SJ, Holash J. Vascular-specific growth factors and blood vessel formation. Nature Insight 2000, 407:242-248.
10. Wilson KT, Fu S, Ramanujam KS, Meltzer SJ. Increased expression of inducible nitric oxide synthase and cyclooxygenase-2 in Barrett's esophagus and associated adenocarcinomas. Cancer Res 1998, 58:2929-2934.
11. Daniel TO, Liu H, Morrow JD, Crews BC, Marnett LJ. Thromboxane A2 is a mediator of cyclooxygenase-2-dependent endothelial migration and angiogenesis. Cancer Res 1999, 59:4574-4577.
12. Fujiwaki R, Iida K, Kanasaki H, Ozaki T, Hata K, Miyazaki K. Cyclooxygenase-2 expression in endometrial cancer: correlation with microvessel count and expression of vascular endothelial growth factor and thymidine phosphorylase. Hum Pathol 2002, 33:213-219.

13. Masferrer JL, Leahy KM, Koki AT, Zweifel BS, Settle SL, Woerner BM, Edwards DA, Flickinger AG, Moore RJ, Seibert K. Antiangiogenic and antitumor activities of cyclooxygenase-2 inhibitors. Cancer Res 2000, 60:1306-1311.
14. Bahr Th Wolff JR The formation of capillaries basement membrane during internal vascularization of the rat's cerebral cortex. Z.Zellforsch, 1972 133; 157-168.
15. Welt K Shippel K, Schippel G, Scheller W . Zu Ultrastruktur von Kapillarfeld im Skeletmuskel der weissen Ratte von 19 Fetaltag bis zum post-partum. Z. Mikr-Anat Forsch., 1974 88; 465-478.
16. Risau W. Mechanisms of angiogenesis. Nature 1997, 386:671-674.
17. Sims DE. The pericyte: a review. Tissue Cell 1986, 18:153-174.
18. Beck L Jr, D'Amore PA. Vascular development: cellular and molecular regulation. FASEB J 1997, 11:365-73.
19. Patan S. TIE1 and TIE2 receptor tyrosine kinases inversely regulate embryonic angiogenesis by the mechanism of intussusceptive microvascular growth. Microvasc Res 1998, 56:1-21.
20. Krause DS, Theise ND, Collector MI, Henegariu O, Hwang S, Gardner R, Neutzel S, Sharkis SJ. Multi-organ, multi-lineage engraftment by single bone marrow derived stem cell. Cell 2001, 105:639-677.
21. Hattori K, Heissig B, Wu Y, Dias S, Tejada R, Ferris B, Hicklin DJ, Zhu Z, Bohlen P, Witte L, Hendrikx J, Hackett NR, Crystal RG, Moore MA, Werb Z, Lyden D, Rafii S. Placental growth factor reconstitutes hematopoiesis by recruiting VEGFR1+ stem cells from bone-marrow microenviroment Nature Medicine 2002, 8:841-849.
22. Epstein SE, Kornowski R, Fuchs S, Dvorak HF. Angiogenesis therapy. Amides the type, the neglected potential for serius side effects. Circulation 2001, 1104:115-119.
23. Gerber HP, Malik AK, Solar GP, Sherman D, Liang XH, Meng G, Hong K, Marsters JC, Ferrara N. VEGF regulates hematopoietic stem cell survival by internal autocrine loop mechanism. Nature 2002, 417: 954-958.
24. Eriksson U, Alitalo K. VEGF receptor .1 stimulates stem-cell recruitment and new hope for angiogenesis therapies. Nature Medicine 2002, 8: 775-777.
25. Gonzalez Crussi, F. Vasculogenesis in the chick embryo. An ultrastructural study. Amer J Anat 1970, 130:441-460.
26. Rosai J, Gold J, Landy R. The hysticytoid hemangiomas. A unifying concept embracing several previously described entities of skin, soft tissue, large vessels bone and heart. Human Pathol 1979, 10:707-730.
27. Brem S, Cotran R, Folkman J. Tumor angiogenesis: a quantitative method for histologic grading. J Natl Cancer Inst 1972, 48:347-356.
28. Mlynek ML, van Beunigen D, Leder LD, Streffer C. Measurement of the grade of vascularisation in histological tumour tissue sections. Br J Cancer 1985, 52:945-948.
29. Srivastava A, Laidler P, Davies RP, Horgan K, Hughes LE. The prognostic significance of tumor vascularity in intermediate-thickness (0.76-4.0 mm thick) skin melanoma. A quantitative histologic study. Am J Pathol 1988, 133:419-423.
30. Weidner N, Semple JP, Welch WR, Folkman J. Tumor angiogenesis and metastasis--correlation in invasive breast carcinoma. N Engl J Med 1991, 324:1-8.
31. Hlatky L, Hahnfeldt P, Folkman J. Clinical application of antiangiogenic therapy: microvessel density, what it does and doesn't tell us. J Natl Cancer Inst 2002, 94:883-893.
32. Folkman J. Endothelial cells and angiogenic growth factors in cancer growth and metastasis. Introduction. Cancer Metastasis Rev 1990, 9:171-174.
33. Albonico G, Querzoli P, Ferretti S, Rinaldi R, Nenci I. Biological heterogeneity of breast carcinoma in situ. Ann N Y Acad Sci 1996, 784:458-461.
34. Bosari S, Lee AK, DeLellis RA, Wiley BD, Heatley GJ, Silverman ML. Microvessel quantitation and prognosis in invasive breast carcinoma. Hum Pathol 1992, 23:755-761.
35. Charpin C, Devictor B, Bergeret D, Andrac L, Boulat J, Horschowski N, Lavaut MN, Piana L. CD31 quantitative immunocytochemical assays in breast carcinomas. Correlation with current prognostic factors. Am J Clin Pathol 1995, 103:443-448.
36. Fox SB. Tumour angiogenesis and prognosis. Histopathology 1997, 30:294-301.
37. Kerbel R, Folkman J. Clinical translation of angiogenesis inhibitors. Nat Rev Cancer 2002, 2:727-739.
38. Guidi AJ, Schnitt SJ, Fischer L, Tognazzi K, Harris JR, Dvorak HF, Brown LF. Vascular permeability factor (vascular endothelial growth factor) expression and angiogenesis in patients with ductal carcinoma in situ of the breast. Cancer 1997, 80:1945-1953.

39. Harris AL, Zhang H, Moghaddam A, Fox S, Scott P, Pattison A, Gatter K, Stratford I, Bicknell R. Breast cancer angiogenesis--new approaches to therapy via antiangiogenesis, hypoxic activated drugs, and vascular targeting. Breast Cancer Res Treat 1996, 38:97-108.
40. Miliaras D, Kamas A, Kalekou H. Angiogenesis in invasive breast carcinoma: is it associated with parameters of prognostic significance?. Histopathology 1995, 26:165-169.
41. Santinelli A, Baccarini M, Colanzi P, Fabris G. Microvessel quantitation in intraductal and early invasive breast carcinomas. Anal Quant Cytol Histol 2000, 22:277-284.
42. Ruiz A, Almenar S, Cerda M, Hidalgo JJ, Puchades A, Llombart-Bosch A. Ductal carcinoma in situ of the breast: a comparative analysis of histology, nuclear area, ploidy, and neovascularization provides differentiation between low- and high-grade tumors. Breast J 2002, 8:139-144.
43. Hammersen F, Endrich B, Messmer K. The fine structure of tumor blood vessels. I. Participation of non-endothelial cells in tumor angiogenesis. Int J Microcirc Clin Exp 1985, 4:31-43.
44. Hashizume H, Baluk P, Morikawa S, McLean JW, Thurston G, Roberge S, Jain RK, McDonald DM. Openings between defective endothelial cells explain tumor vessel leakiness. Am J Pathol 2000, 156:1363-80.
45. Feng Y, Venema VJ, Venema RC, Tsai N, Behzadian MA, Caldwell RB. VEGF-induced permeability increase is mediated by caveolae. Invest Ophthalmol Vis Sci 1999, 40:157-67.
46. Hellstrom M, Gerhardt H, Kalen M, Li X, Eriksson U, Wolburg H, Betsholtz C. Lack of pericytes leads to endothelial hyperplasic and abnormal vascular morphogenesis. J Cell Biol 2001, 153:543-563.
47. Bertossi M, Virgintino D, Maiorano E, Occhiogrosso M, Roncali L. Ultrastructural and mophometric investigation of human brain capillaries in normal and peritumoral tissues. Ultrastruct Pathol 1997, 21:41-49.
48. Llombart-Bosch A, Peydro-Olaya A, Gomar F. Ultrastructure of one Ewing's sarcoma of bone with endothelial character and comparative review of the vessels in 27 cases of typical Ewing's sarcoma. Path Res Pract 1980, 167:71-87.
49. Llombart-Bosch A, Peydro-Olaya A, Lopez-Fernandez A, Zuzuarregui C. Sur le sarcomes reticulaires de la moelle osseuse type Ewing. Etude optique, histochimique and electronique de deux cas. Ann Anat Path 1970, 15:431-452.
50. Llombart-Bosch A, Pellin A, Carda C, Noguera R, Navarro S, Peydro-Olaya A. Soft tissue Ewing sarcoma--peripheral primitive neuroectodermal tumor with atypical clear cell pattern shows a new type of EWS-FEV fusion transcript. Diagn Mol Pathol 2000, 9:137-144.
51. Warren BA, Shubik P. The growth of the blood supply to melanoma transplants in the hamster cheek pouch. Lab Invest 1966, 15:464-478.
52. Maniotis AJ, Folberg R, Hess A, Seltor EA, Gardner LMG, Peér J, Trent JM, Meltzer PS, Hendrix MJC. Vascular channel formation by human melanoma cells in vivo and in vitro: vasculogenic mimicry. Am J Pathol 1999, 155:739-752.
53. Chang YS, Di Tomaso E, McDonald DM, Jones RS, Jain RK, Munn LL. Mosaic blood vessels in tumors: frequency of cancer cells in contact with flowing blood. Porc Nat Acad Sci USA 2000, 97:14608-14613.
54. Liotta LA, Kleinerman J, Saidel GM. Quantitative relationships of intravascular tumor cells, tumor vessels, and pulmonary metastases following tumor implantation. Cancer Res 1974, 34:997-1004.
55. Butler TP, Gullino PM. Quantitation of cell shedding into efferent blood of mammary adenocarcinoma. Cancer Res 1975, 35:512-516.
56. Mancuso P, Burlini A, Pruneri G, Goldhirsch A, Martinelli G, Bertolini F. Resting and activated endothelial cells are increased in the peripheral blood of cancer patients. Blood 2001, 97;3658-3661.
57. Browder T, Butterfield CE, Kraling BM, Shi B, Marshall B, O'Reilly MS, Folkman J. Antiangiogenic scheduling of chemotherapy improves efficacy against experimental drug-resistant cancer. Cancer Res 2000, 60;1878-1886.
58. Leu AJ, Berk DA, Lymboussaki A, Alitalo K, Jain RK. Absence of functional lymphatics within a murine sarcoma: a molecular and functional evaluation. Cancer Res 2000, 60:4324-4327.
59. Jackson DG, Prevo R, Clasper S, Banerji S. LYVE-1, the lymphatic system and tumor lymphangiogenesis. Trends Immunol 2001, 22:317-321.
60. Breitender-Geleff S, Soleiman A, Kowalski H, Horvat R, Amann G, Kriehuber E, Diem K, Weninger W, Tschachler E, Alitalo K, Kerjaschki D. Angiosarcomas express mixed endothelial phenotypes of blood and lymphatic capillaries: podoplanin as a specific marker for lymphatic endothelium. Am J Pathol 1999, 154:385-394.
61. Mandriota SJ, Jussila L, Jeltsch M, Compagni A, Baetens D, Prevo R, Banerji S, Huarte J, Montesano R, Jackson DG, Orci L, Alitalo K, Christofori G, Pepper MS. Vascular endothelial growth factor-C-mediated lymphangiogenesis promotes tumour metastasis. EMBO J 2001, 20:672-682.

62. Mouta-Carreira C, Nasser SM, di Tomaso E, Padera TP, Boucher Y, Tomarev SI, Jain RK. LYVE-1 is not restricted to the lymph vessels: expression in normal liver blood sinusoids and down-regulation in human liver cancer and cirrhosis. Cancer Res 2001, 61:8079-8084.

63. Ruoslahti E. Spezialization of tumour vasculature. Nature Reviews 2002, 2: 83-90.

64. Barth A, Craig PH, Silverstein MJ. Predictors of axillary lymph node metastases in patients with T1 breast carcinoma. Cancer 1997, 79:1918-19.

65. Leak LV. Electron microscopic observations on lymphatic capillaries and the structural components of the connective tissue-lymph interface. Microvasc Res 1970, 2:361-391.

66. O'Morchoe CC, O'Morchoe PJ. Differences in lymphatic and blood capillary permeability: ultrastructural-functional correlations. Lymphology 1987, 20:205-209.

67. Kaipainen A, Korhonen J, Mustonen T, van Hinsbergh VW, Fang GH, Dumont D, Breitman M, Alitalo K. Expression of the fms-like tyrosine kynase 4 gene becomes restricted to lymphatic endothelium during development. Proc Natl Acad Sci USA 1995, 92:3566-3570.

68. Jussila L, Valtola R, Partanen TA, Salven P, Heikkila P, Matikainen MT, Renkonen R, Kaipainen A, Detmar M, Tschachler E, Alitalo R, Alitalo K.Lymphatic endothelium and Kaposi sarcoma spindle cells detected by antibodies against the vascular endothelial growth factor receptor-3. Cancer Res 1998, 58:1599-1604.

69. Lymboussaki A, Partanen TA, Olofsson B, Thomas-Crusells J, Fletcher CD, de Waal RM, Kaipainen A, Alitalo K. Expression of the vascular endothelial growth factor C receptor VEGFR-3 in lymphatic endothelium of the skin and in vascular tumors. Am J Pathol 1998, 153:395-403.

70. Plate KH. From angiogenesis to lymphangiogensis. Nature Med 2001, 7:151-152.

71. Valtola R, Salven P, Heikkila P, Taipale J, Joensuu H, Rehn M, Pihlajaniemi T, Weich H, deWaal R, Alitalo K. VEGFR-3 and its ligand VEGF-C are associated with angiogenesis in breast cancer. Am J Pathol 1999, 154:1381-1390.

72. Skobe M, Hawighorst T, Jackson DG, Prevo R, Janes L, Velasco P, Riccardi L, Alitalo K, Claffey K, Detmar M. Induction of tumor lymphangiogenesis by VEGF-C promotes breast cancer metastasis. Nat Med 2001, 7:192-198.

73. Stacker SA, Caesar C, Badwin ME, Thormton GE, Williams RA, Prevo R, Jackson DG, Nishikawa S, Kubo H, Achen MG. VEGF-D promotes the metastatic spread of tumor cells via lymphatics. Nature Med 2001;7:186-191.

74. Pezzella F, Pastorino U, Tagliabue E, Andreola S, Sozzi G, Gasparini G, Menard S, Gatter KC, Harris AL, Fox S, Buyse M, Pilotti S, Pierotti M, Rilke F. Non-small-cell lung carcinoma tumor growth without morphological evidence of neoangiogenesis. Am J Pathol 1997, 151:1417-1423.

75. Pezzella F, Harris AL, Gatter KC. Ways of escape: are all tumors angiogenic? Histopathology 2001, 39:551-553.

76. Pastorino U, Andreola S, Tagliabue E, Pezzella F, Incarbone M, Sozzi G, Buyse M, Menard S, Pierotti M, Rilke F. Immunoghistochemical markers in stage I lung cancer: relevance to prognosis. J Clin Oncol 1997, 15:2858-2865.

77. Pezzella F. Evidence for novel non-angiogenic pathways in breast cancer metatasis. Breast Cancer Progression. Working Party. Lancet 2000, 355:1787-1788.

78. Willis RA. Pathology of tumors. London. Butterworth & Co.,Ltd 1948; pp136.

79. Vaupel P, Kallinowki F, Okunieff P. Blood flow, oxygen, and nutrients supply and metabolic microenvironment of human tumors. Cancer Res 1989, 49:6449-6465.

80. Majno G, Joris I. Cells Tissue and Disease.Principles of General Pathology. Cambridge. MA Blackwell Science, 1996 pp783.

81. Warren BA. The vascular morphology of tumors in Tumor Blood and Circulation: Angiogenesis, vascular morphology and blood flow of experimental and human tumors. Ed. Peterson H.I., Boca Raton, CRC Press Inc 1979. pp.1-48.

82. Folberg R, Hendrix MJC, Maniotis AJ. Vasculogenic mimicry and tumor angiogenesis. Am J Pathol 2000, 156:361-381.

83. McDonald DM, Munn L, Jain RK. Vasculogenic mimicry: How convincing, how novel, and how significant? Am J Pathol 2000, 156:383-388.

84. Foldberg R, Pe'er J, Gruman LM, Wooolson RF, Jeng G, Montangue PR, Moninger TO, YI H, Moore KC. The morphologic characteristics of tumor blood vessels as a marker of tumor progression in primary uveal melanoma: a matched case-control study. Human Pathol 1992, 23:1298-1305.

85. Foldberg R, Rummelt V, Parys-Van Ginderdeuren R, Hwang T, Woolson RF, Pe'er J, Gruman LM. The prognostic value of tumor blood vessel morphology in primary uveal melanoma. Ophtalmology 1993, 100:1369-1398.

86. Sakamoto T, Sakamoto M, Yoshikawa H, Hatta Y, Ishibashi T, Ohnishi Y, Inomata H. Histologic finding and prognosis of uveal malignant melanoma in Japanese patients. Am J Ophtalmology 1996, 12:276-283.
87. McLean IW, Keele KS, Burnier MN. Uveal melanoma: comparison of the prognostic value of fibrovascular lops, mean of the ten largest nucleoli, cell type and tumor size. Ophtalmology 1997, 104:777-780.
88. Pandey A, Shao H, Marks RM, Polverini PJ, Dixit VM. Role of B61 the ligand for the Eck receptor tyrosine kinase in TNF-alpha induced angiogenesis. Science 1995, 268:567-569.
89. Veilkola T, Karkainen M, Claesson-Welsh L, Alitalo K. Regulation of angiogenesis via vascular endothelial growth factor receptor. Cancer Res 2000, 60:203-212.
90. Konerding MA, Fait E, Dimitropoulou C, Malkusch W, Ferri C, Giavazzi R, Coltrini D, Presta M. Impact of fibroblast growth factor-2 on tumor microvascular architecture. A tridimensional morphometric study. Am J Pathol 1998, 152:1607-1616.

MATRIX METALLOPROTEINASES AND TUMOR PROGRESSION

José M.P. Freije, Milagros Balbín, Alberto M. Pendás, Luis M. Sánchez,

Xose S. Puente, and Carlos López-Otín*

Departamento de Bioquímica, Instituto Universitario de Oncología, Universidad de

Oviedo, 33006-Oviedo, Spain

ABSTRACT

The matrix metalloproteinases (MMPs) are a family of more than 20 distinct enzymes that are frequently overexpressed in human tumors. Functional studies have shown that MMPs play an important role in the proteolytic destruction of extracellular matrix and basement membranes, thereby facilitating tumor invasion and metastasis. In addition, these enzymes may also be important in other steps of tumor evolution including neoplastic cell proliferation and angiogenesis stimulation. On the basis of the relevance of MMPs in tumor progression, a number of different strategies aimed to block the unwanted activity of these enzymes in cancer have been developed. Unfortunately, most clinical trials with the first series of MMP inhibitors have failed to show clear benefit in patients with advanced cancer. Explanations for this lack of success include the failure to recognize the role of these enzymes in early stages of the disease as well as inadequacy of either the employed inhibitors or the proteases to be targeted.

The introduction of novel concepts such as tumor degradome, and global approaches to protease analysis, may facilitate the identification of the relevant MMPs that must be targeted in each individual cancer patient. On the other hand, the finding that MMPs are enzymes whose effects on biologically active substrates can have profound consequences on cell behaviour, suggests that selective inhibition of a limited set of MMPs at early stages of tumor evolution might be much more effective than using wide-spectrum inhibitors active against most family members, and administered to patients at late stages of the disease. Further studies directed to elucidate these questions

---

* Send correspondence to: Carlos López-Otín, Departamento de Bioquímica y Biología Molecular, Facultad de Medicina/Edificio S. Gascón, Universidad de Oviedo, 33006 Oviedo- SPAIN, Tel. 34-985-104201; Fax: 34-985-103564, E-mail:CLO@correo.uniovi.es

New Trends in Cancer for the 21ˢᵗ Century, edited by
Llombart-Bosch and Felipo, Kluwer Academic/Plenum Publishers, 2003

will be necessary to clarify whether any of the multiple strategies of MMP inhibition may be part of future therapeutic approaches to control tumor progression.

INTRODUCTION

A fundamental and distinctive feature of malignant tumors derives from their ability to invade other tissues and generate metastases at distant sites in the body. It is intuitively attractive to assume that proteolytic enzymes, through their capacity to degrade extracellular matrix components, may play a central role in cancer progression by allowing access of tumor cells to the vascular and lymphatic systems, thereby facilitating cancer dissemination[1]. Among the multiple proteases encoded in the human genome[2], members of the MMP family have raised enormous interest in cancer research due to their overexpression in multiple tumors as well as to their ability to degrade virtually all components of extracellular matrix and basement membranes[3]. In addition, recent studies have demonstrated that these enzymes also target a variety of substrates distinct from extracellular matrix components and influence basic processes essential in cancer including cell growth, differentiation, angiogenesis or apoptosis[4]. Furthermore, the generation of animal models of gain or loss of MMP functions has allowed the establishment of causal relationships between disregulated activity of these enzymes and tumor progression and have confirmed the essential roles of MMPs in early stages of tumor processes[4]. Taken together, these observations have prompted multiple studies aimed at evaluating MMPs as therapeutic targets in cancer[5]. This chapter will review the structure, function and regulation of MMPs and will discuss the different strategies for the development and use of new MMP inhibitors (MMPIs) designed to target selected MMPs at different cancer stages.

STRUCTURAL DESIGN OF MMPs

A prerequisite to therapeutically control a perturbed biological system is to understand the structure, function, and regulation of all its components in the physiological context. Recent advances have placed us in an optimal situation to improve our understanding of the association of MMPs with cancer. Thus, the availability of the human genome sequence has allowed us to confirm the presence of 24 distinct genes encoding MMP family members (Fig. 1). The structural design of most of these human MMPs is organized around a catalytic domain linked to a propeptide with an unpaired cysteine residue, which coordinates with the active site Zn^{2+} ion and is involved in maintaining enzyme latency. A signal peptide directs secretion from the cell, and a hemopexin carboxy-terminal domain contributes to establish substrate specificity and interactions with TIMPs. This is the basic organization of human collagenases and stromelysins. Gelatinases incorporate three fibronectin repeats within the catalytic domain. MT-MMPs show a C-terminal hydrophobic extension mediating its localization at the cell surface directly or via glycosylphosphatidylinositol-mechanisms. MT-MMPs also have a short insertion between the propeptide and the catalytic domain which comprises the consensus sequence RXK/RR involved in activation of these membrane enzymes by furin-like proteases. The evolution of some human MMPs has also progressed in the reverse direction leading to the loss of domains. This is the case of the two identified matrilysins, which lack the hemopexin domain and only exhibit the minimal domain organization required for secretion, latency and activity[6]. Finally, the increase in the number and diversity of MMPs has generated some classification problems, making necessary the introduction of a heterogeneous group named "other MMPs", and

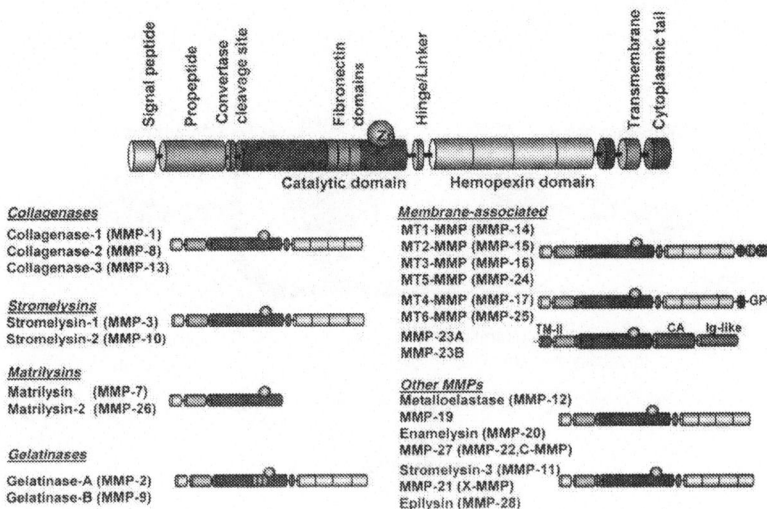

Figure 1. The MMPs: a family portrait. Domain structure of the 24 human MMP proteases, classified into different groups on the basis of domain organization. GPI, glycosylphosphatidylinositol. TM, type II transmembrane domain. CA, cysteine array. Ig, immunoglobulin domain.

FUNCTIONAL DIVERSITY OF MMPs

Closely parallel to the structural diversity of the MMP family members, recent studies including those derived from analysis of animal models of gain or loss of MMP function, have revealed that these enzymes are involved in multiple biological processes[3, 4]. Thus, MMPs participate in the tissue morphogenesis, maintenance and repair processes that occur in a variety of physiological conditions such as embryonic growth and development, reproductive processes, bone growth and resorption, angiogenesis or wound healing. Many of these events may also involve bioactive molecule processing by MMPs that regulate cell function during extracellular matrix remodeling.

Likewise, MMPs perform multiple functions in cancer beyond those derived from their ability to degrade extracellular matrix and basement membrane components during intravasation and extravasation of tumor cells[4] (Fig. 2). These additional functions include their participation during the very early stages of cancer in the creation of a pericellular microenvironment which ultimately leads to the genetic instability inherent to cancer development[8]. Furthermore, MMPs may favor the initiation and sustained growth of both primary tumors and metastases, by activating growth factors precursors, by inactivating growth factor binding proteins, or by releasing mitogenic molecules sequestered in the extracellular matrix surrounding cancer cells[10, 11]. MMPs may also participate in the processing of cell adhesion molecules, modifying cell-cell adhesion[12], and promoting cancer progression[13, 14]. Other actions of MMPs may lead to the destruction of chemokine gradients and alter the natural host defense system critical for host protection[15]. In addition, by cleavage of proapoptotic factors, MMPs may generate a more aggressive phenotype via generation of apoptotic resistant cells[16]. Finally, MMPs may regulate angiogenesis in cancer, both positively through their ability to mobilize or activate proangiogenic factors (17,18), or negatively via generation of angiogenesis inhibitors, such as angiostatin and endostatin, cleaved from large protein precursors[19-21].

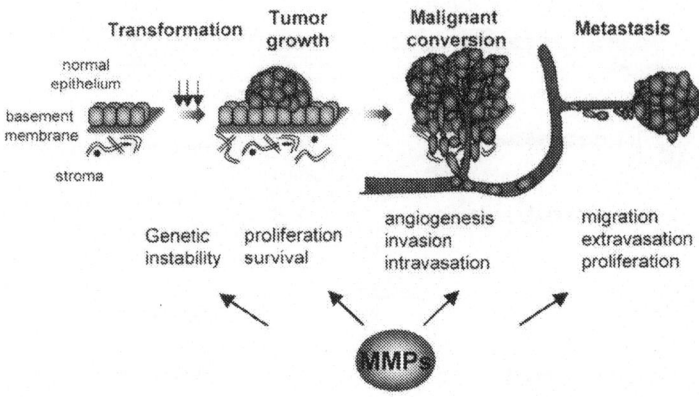

Figure 2. MMP functions in tumor development and progression. MMPs may perform classical roles in extracellular matrix degradation during intravasation and extravasation of tumor cells, but may target other substrates and influence basic processes in cancer such as regulation of cell proliferation, angiogenesis and apoptosis

Thus, the pattern that emerges in this protease family is one of diversity and complexity, in both structural and functional terms. Consequently, to develop MMP inhibition strategies for cancer therapy, we must consider that there are more than 20 distinct enzymes potentially important for the disease, and whose relevance may vary depending on the tumor type and the stage of tumor evolution in which the specific MMPs are produced or recruited from the stroma and immune cells. Moreover, the growing knowledge of the expanded roles for MMPs including those associated with early stages of tumor evolution, has rendered necessary a substantial change in the rationale for antiMMP-based therapies. Indeed, since a significant number of patients have micrometastases at the time of diagnosis, the possibility that MMP inhibition could be also of benefit in early stages of the disease has prompted the development of novel therapeutic approaches to try to block the MMP functions.

ENDOGENOUS CONTROL OF MMP EXPRESSION AND ACTIVITY

Because MMPs exhibit significant degradative potential against multiple substrates and influence many biological functions, their expression and activity in human tissues is strictly controlled both temporally and spatially. There are three major mechanisms for the endogenous regulation of MMP proteolytic functions: gene transcription, proenzyme activation, and inhibition of their enzymatic activity, although there are many other control points, from mRNA stabilization to protease autolysis, that can be very relevant in specific cases (Fig. 3). Collectively, these mechanisms function coordinately to assure that MMP expression and activity are circumscribed to those sites in which these enzymes are necessary. Unfortunately, malignant tumors use multiple strategies to avoid these stringent control mechanisms and generate the abnormal proteolytic activity associated with cancer progression.

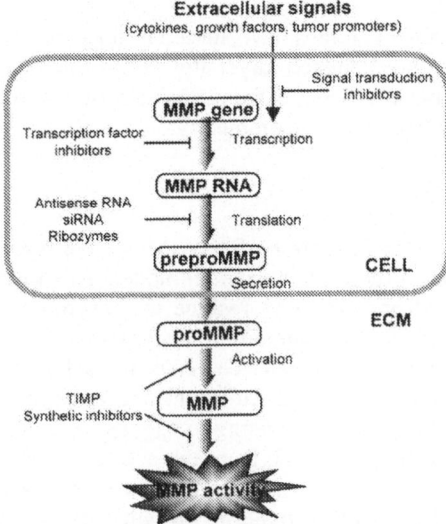

Figure 3. Levels of regulation of MMP expression and activity. Soluble factors, extracellular matrix-cell interactions or cell-cell contacts interact with cell surface receptors and initiate a cascade of events that lead to the generation of functional MMPs. The main levels of regulation and therapeutic intervention are shown.

Transcriptional regulation of MMPs

In contrast to the frequent lack of expression of these proteases under physiological conditions, MMP transcription is usually induced in tumor cells or in the surrounding stromal cells by a wide variety of agents including cytokines, growth factors, and oncogene products. In addition to soluble factors, extracellular matrix signals, changes in cell shape and other events such as mechanical stress that are physical in nature rather than chemical signals, may also result in MMP induction[22]. To date, no single factors have been identified that can be exclusively responsible for overexpression of the different MMPs in specific tumors, although TNF-α and IL-1 are regularly implicated in MMP overexpression. Likewise, the same MMP gene can be transcriptionally induced or repressed by different factors, such as TGF-β or retinoids, depending on the tumor cell type[23-25]. Hence, diverse factors and influences impact MMP expression in tumors in a complex manner. The signal transduction pathways mediating MMP transcriptional activation are also diverse, although the p38 MAPK pathway may be relevant in a number of cases[26-28]. In contrast to this variability, many extracellular signals and signal transduction pathways converge toward an AP-1 binding site present in the promoter region of most MMP genes[29]. The presence of this element, which binds members of the Fos and Jun families of oncoproteins, provides a general mechanism to account for MMP expression in malignant tumors. Nevertheless, there are additional nuclear factors, such as NFκB, Cbfa1, STATs and ETS family members, that contribute to the fine-tuning of MMP expression and account for the variable inducibility of MMP gene transcription in different tumors[30, 31]. Finally, the complexity of MMP transcriptional regulation is also increased due to the presence of single nucleotide polymorphisms (SNPs) in the promoter region of these genes that modify their transcriptional activity[32, 33].

In summary, although recent studies have started to uncover some common features underlying the apparent mechanistic diversity controlling MMP transcriptional activation, the emerging pattern derived from analysis of the regulatory factors and mechanisms is also one of diversity and complexity.

Activation of proMMPs

The mechanisms of *in vitro* activation of proMMPs have been extensively studied, leading to the development of the cysteine-switch model. This mechanism involves the participation of a conserved unpaired Cys residue in the prodomain of MMPs, as an essential molecular determinant for maintaining enzyme latency[34]. Once the shielding effect of the propeptide is withdrawn, water can enter the active site, become polarized by the active site glutamate residue and Zn^{+2} ion, and then function as the catalytic nucleophile. Other mechanisms such as binding to a ligand or to a substrate *in vivo*, may lead to a disengagement of the propeptide from the active center of the MMP, causing its activation[35]. Recent work has also clarified some partial aspects of the *in vivo* mechanisms responsible for MMP activation. In virtually all cases, the activation process requires the participation of other proteases from different classes, acting in proteolytic cascades. Once activated, these MMPs may also activate other proMMPs, thereby contributing to the amplification of the activation cascade[36].

An additional principle in the activation of MMPs is that it usually occurs in the immediate pericellular space, at sites with high-affinity for the respective enzyme precursors. The finding of MT-MMPs, a subfamily of membrane-bound MMPs with ability to activate proMMPs at the cell surface, and the identification of cell surface receptors for some proMMPs have provided strong support to the relevance of the focalization of activating mechanisms at the pericellular space. The proMMP-2 activation mechanism mediated by MT-MMPs is very complex and involves the formation of a multi-protein cell surface cluster that includes the presence of TIMP-2, which tethers proMMP-2 at its hemopexin C domain to a MT1-MMP molecule[37-39]. In contrast to these extracellular or pericellular mechanisms of proMMP activation, there are other family members such as MT-MMPs, MMP-11, MMP-23, and MMP-28 that are activated intracellularly through the action of furin-like proprotein convertases[40-42]. Remarkably, many proMMP activating enzymes are also deregulated during tumor progression, and different tumors overproduce a variety of activating enzymes[43].

Inhibition of mature MMPs

The activity of MMPs may also be regulated by a series of endogenous inhibitors that can be of wide-protease spectrum or specific for these enzymes. Thus, MMPs, like many other proteases, are inhibited by general inhibitors such as α2-macroglobulin[44]. In addition, they are also targeted by more specific inhibitors, including the TIMPs, the membrane-anchored glycoprotein RECK, and the tissue factor pathway inhibitor-2 (TFPI-2). Finally, it has been suggested that MMPs may be blocked by proteins containing TIMP-like domains in their structure.

The four human TIMPs are secreted extracellularly or anchored to the extracellular matrix, and inhibit the activity of MMPs by tight binding to form non-covalent complexes[45]. Despite TIMPs having been largely considered as specific inhibitors against MMPs, TIMP-3 also efficiently blocks the activity of ADAMs and ADAMTSs[46, 47]. It has long been suggested that the connective-tissue degrading activity of tumor cells may not only result from an increase in MMP levels but also from a decrease in TIMP production[48]. Consequently, the net balance between active proteases and inhibitors will be the final determinant of the tissue-degrading and bioactive molecular processing potential of tumors. However, not all the data are univocal in this regard. Thus, it has been reported that TIMPs levels are also increased during tumor progression and there are intriguing reports demonstrating paradoxical effects of these inhibitors in cancer such as growth promoting activities on tumor cells through nonproteolytic dependent mechanisms[49, 50]. In addition to TIMPs, RECK has been recently described as a regulator of extracellular matrix integrity and angiogenesis with an ability to inhibit the activity of several MMPs, but the molecular basis of this inhibition is still unclear[51]. Likewise, TFPI-2, a serine proteinase inhibitor, can also function as an inhibitor of MMPs through poorly understood mechanisms[52]. Another class of recently described endogenous MMP inhibitors is those containing TIMP-like domains, such as those present in PCPE (procollagen C-terminal proteinase enhancer)[53], NC1 domains of type IV collagen[54] or agrin[55]. Nevertheless, the targets of these putative MMP inhibitory activities in physiological and pathological conditions including cancer, remain unclear.

STRATEGIES FOR TARGETING MMPs IN CANCER

As deduced from the information discussed in the previous sections, our knowledge of MMPs has increased enormously over the past 20 years when the design of the first MMPIs was considered. However, the clinical efficacy of the first generation of MMPIs has been disappointing in most cases. For the next generation of MMPIs to control the unwanted activity of these enzymes during cancer development and progression, we need to introduce innovative strategies of MMP inhibition based on the utilization of the increased knowledge in this proteolytic system. In principle, inhibition can be targeted at any of the three major regulatory mechanisms that control the production and activity of MMPs: transcription, activation, and inhibition (Fig. 3). Nevertheless, we must consider that some of the mechanisms that fine-tune MMP activity—from mRNA stabilization to protease autolysis—may also be targeted for intervention in cancer therapy.

Strategies for targeting MMP gene transcription

There are three general approaches to inhibit MMP gene transcription: strategies based on either blocking extracellular factors mediating up-regulation of MMPs or enhancing the down-regulatory signals, interruption of signal transduction pathways, and targeting of nuclear factors responsible for inducing MMP gene expression[56]. In addition, gene-selective strategies for directly blocking or affecting efficiency of MMP synthesis, such as those based on ribozymes or on antisense-gene transfer constructs, are also of potential interest for cancer therapy[57-59].

The strategies aimed at blocking extracellular factors involved in synthesis of MMPs or at using suppressor factors for MMP expression are difficult to adopt for general applicability. This is because of the wide number of factors able to induce the production of these enzymes in each particular lesion and also because of the opposing effects of certain factors on the expression of distinct family members. However, recent studies have shown that factors such as interferons α, β, and γ may be useful to inhibit transcription of several MMP genes in different human cancer cells[60-62]. Another possibility is based on blocking those cytokines and cytokine receptors, such as TNF-α, IL-1, TNFR, or IL-1R with the ability to up-regulate MMP genes. This approach has already been translated into clinical applications for the treatment of arthritic processes that also involve a marked deregulation of MMP gene expression[63].

A second general strategy to block the production of MMPs in malignant tumors is aimed at targeting the signal transduction pathways that mediate their transcriptional induction. Thus, inhibition of p38 MAPK activity with SB203580 abolishes the expression of several MMPs in transformed keratinocytes and squamous cell carcinoma cells[27, 28]. Likewise, malolactomycin D suppresses the expression of several MMPs through blocking the activation of p38 MAPK[64]. Compounds such as manumycin A or halofuginone also block different signal transduction pathways that mediate MMP expression by tumor cells[65-67]. Therefore, it appears that inhibition of signaling pathways controlling MMP induction may be useful to suppress the functions mediated by these enzymes during tumor progression. In any case, it will be critical to demonstrate the absence of toxic effects derived from inhibition of signal transduction pathways operating in multiple physiological processes beyond their roles in cancer.

The third general approach to block the cascade of events leading to the inappropriate synthesis of MMPs by human tumors is to target the nuclear factors responsible for the transcriptional regulation of these genes. These strategies may focus on general factors such as AP-1 and NFκB that affect many MMP genes, or on more specific factors like Cbfa1 that selectively affects the expression of only some family members. The AP-1 site is the target for repression of MMP transcription by drugs such as glucocorticoids[68]. Nevertheless, these compounds affect so many genes distinct from MMPs that their potential usefulness for inhibiting the production of these enzymes is counteracted by their multiple side effects. This renders necessary the introduction of more specific compounds to block MMP synthesis. Very recently, it has been reported that natural products such as nobiletin or curcuminoids inhibit expression of MMPs in an AP-1-blocking dependent process[69, 70]. The NFκB nuclear factor also provides a general target for the blockade of MMP production. The importance of NFκB targeting in cancer has recently been reinforced with the finding that PS-341, a proteasome inhibitor that blocks the degradation of IκB and thereby maintains NFκB in an inactive status, may be effective for treatment of diverse tumor types[71, 72]. Hence, it will be interesting to examine the possibility that MMPs overexpressed in multiple myeloma[73] may be effectively down-regulated by PS-341 with commensurate beneficial effects for the patient. In addition to strategies focused on general factors, it should be possible to target nuclear factors like Cbfa1 that affect specific MMPs[74]. Such a strategy has potential for targeting different stages of tumor progression mediated by these enzymes, including formation of bone metastases[75]. The discovery of factors that affect only a small number of MMPs may be a powerful way to generate specificity in anti-MMP therapies, specificity that might otherwise be difficult to achieve at the level of inhibitors against the active forms of these enzymes. Finally, it may be interesting to restore the activity of transcription factors such as p53, MMAC/PTEN, and TEL that negatively regulate MMP expression, and whose activity may be lost during tumor progression[76-78]. Nevertheless, as in the case of the signal transduction blocking strategies, MMP inhibition must be seen as a desired but not sole target of these approaches that might have broad anti-tumor effects.

Strategies for targeting proMMP activation

Another possibility to target tumor MMPs is to focus on zymogen activation, the second major regulatory step in the control of MMP proteolysis. There are two general approaches in this regard based on either inhibiting the proMMP activating proteases or blocking the upstream activators of the proMMP activating enzymes. As mentioned above, essential MMP-activating enzymes such as the MT-MMPs, are also overexpressed in malignant tumors of different types, thereby being targets for cancer therapy by themselves. Thus, anti-MT1-MMP monoclonal antibodies inhibit proteolytic activity and impair endothelial cell migration and invasion of collagen and fibrin gels, opening the possibility of using these reagents in clinical trials[79]. Likewise, natural products such as green tea catechins have the ability to block the MT1-MMP dependent activation step of proMMPs[80]. On the other hand, the observation that proMT-MMPs are in turn activated by furin and other pro-protein convertases, suggests novel approaches to block the proteolytic cascade that leads to the generation of active MMPs. The use of a selective furin inhibitor, alpha 1-PDX, has resulted in the attenuation or complete abrogation of invasiveness and tumorigenicity of human cancer cells[81]. Furin inhibition was accompanied by deficient activation of MT1-MMP and reduced processing of proMMP-2, especially in the most aggressive cancer cell lines, suggesting that alpha-1 PDX may be useful as anticancer agent. Finally, recent reports have described additional strategies of targeting proMMP activation for cancer therapy. These are based on the use of thrombospondins[82, 83], endostatin[84], proteoglycans[85], or protease inhibitors originally designed against other proteases but apparently showing an indirect blocking effect on proMMP activation[86].

Strategies based on utilization of inhibitors of active MMPs

Although the MMP control points discussed above afford new possibilities for sites of intervention with novel cancer therapeutics, most strategies for MMP targeting have attempted to use endogenous inhibitors or to design synthetic drugs to abolish the proteolytic function of the active proteases and their activators. The ability of TIMPs to inhibit tumor growth in transgenic models provided convincing preclinical evidence in successful tests of the concept that MMPs are potential therapeutic targets for cancer[87,88]. However, TIMPs, as other protein-based treatments, suffer from poor pharmacokinetics. Furthermore, these protease inhibitors exhibit paradoxical effects and may have growth-promoting activity on tumor cells[49, 50]. Finally, tumor MMPs may not be easily accessible to exogenously added macromolecules such as TIMPs. Therefore, there is a need for developing synthetic MMPIs with ability to selectively target specific MMPs and devoid of the limitations associated with endogenous inhibitors.

Over the last decade, synthetic MMPIs for cancer treatment have undergone rapid clinical development[89]. Most of them have been designed as peptidic mimics of the amino acid sequence of collagen around the cleavage site by collagenases, with specificity imparted by the collagen-like sequence, and with the Zn^{2+} ion being chelated through a Zn-binding hydroxymate moiety incorporated at the terminus of the inhibitor. This approach was tremendously successful in developing tight binding inhibitors, and with further substitutions to the side chains, solubility, pharmacokinetics, and binding affinities were further improved as reflected by the drop in K_is from 10^{-7} M to the low nM range. Other approaches have used data derived from 3D structures of MMPs or from large-scale screening of compounds with MMP inhibitory properties, to design or identify non-peptidic molecules that selectively bind to the Zn-binding site of these enzymes. Bisphosphonates and tetracyclins, that are based on distinct structures and were originally designed for other clinical purposes, have also been shown to inhibit MMPs[90-92].

CLINICAL TRIALS WITH MMP INHIBITORS

Most clinical studies using synthetic MMPIs have not demonstrated significant efficacy in patients with advanced cancer[93]. However, a recently concluded clinical trial of patients with gastric carcinoma, has revealed a significant survival improvement after treatment with the British Biotech inhibitor Marimastat[94]. This compound was also as effective as gemcitabine in treatment of pancreatic carcinoma patients[95], and in combination with temozolomide led to a significant improvement in patients with gliobastoma multiforme[96]. Hence, despite the negative results in initial trials with hydroxymate-based MMPIs, these recent results should stimulate the further work needed in order to introduce these compounds for cancer treatment. In light of recent advances in our knowledge of MMPs, we can retrospectively conclude that the lack of efficacy of most MMPIs used in the diverse clinical trials with cancer patients were not unexpected due to a number of reasons that have been excellently reviewed recently[93,97], but at the time could not have been reasonably anticipated. First, we have learnt that MMPs play important roles in the early stages of cancer progression, and their contribution may be less in late phases of the disease[4]. Animal models of cancer development have also provided strong support for the increased efficacy of MMPIs in early stages of the disease[98]. Thus, MMPI-treatment of mice with pancreatic islet cancer led to a significant reduction in tumor burden only if the inhibitor was administered before the emergence of invasive carcinomas, but no effect was observed on the regression of these tumors. Likewise, MMPIs have been effective in the early stages of intestinal tumor formation, preventing further progression to malignancy[99]. As exemplified in the recent and encouraging clinical trial of glioblastoma treatment with Marimastat plus temozolomide[96], it is very important to design new clinical trials of MMPIs in selected early stage cancer and in combination with other drugs as an additional means to further validate this drug class. The failure of other clinical trials with MMPIs may have also been derived from the fact that most inhibitors are broad-spectrum agents with ability to target all MMPs, even those that can have paradoxical effects on tumor progression and favor the host instead of the tumor[93]. Therefore, MMPIs will interfere with bioactive molecule processing by MMPs in cancer, including those substrates that form part of the natural host defense mechanisms against tumor progression[100, 101]. Likewise, MMPIs can also inhibit other metalloproteases such as the ADAMTSs with ability to slow tumor evolution through their antiangiogenic activities[102, 103].

Taken together, these findings may explain some of the failures of anti-MMP therapy in cancer treatment, and emphasize the need for a detailed characterization of the adverse effects associated with the use of broad-spectrum inhibitors. Similarly, the finding that some MMPs and other metalloproteinases targeted by MMPIs may be beneficial for the host, implies that we need to know before and during treatment the molecular diagnosis of the proteases to be targeted in each particular tumor. At present, this problem is difficult to address because there are many MMPs potentially relevant to cancer, and different tumors exhibit unique MMP expression profiles. However, DNA microarrays have only recently been employed to define the MMP mRNA transcriptomes in different tumors and so the data to date have generally provided only an incomplete picture of the tumor MMP profiles. In addition, there are other proteases distinct from MMPs that are up-regulated during tumor progression. These enzymes may compensate for some of the MMP activities, in the case that these are blocked by MMPIs, thus making necessary the development of inhibitory strategies for these putative MMP-compensatory proteases.

THE APPLICATION OF DEGRADOMICS FOR THE RATIONAL USE OF MMPIs

As a theoretical approach to the global analysis of proteases associated with normal and pathological processes, we have recently introduced the new concepts of degradomics and degradomes, as complements of proteomics and proteomes[2]. Degradomics includes all genomic and proteomic studies focused on the identification and characterization of all proteases present in an organism, the substrates targeted by these proteases and their endogenous inhibitors. Extrapolating these ideas to cancer research, the degradome of a tumor would be the complete set of proteases produced by that specific tumor at a certain stage of development. We have also proposed that systematic comparisons between different tumors and analysis of different stages of tumor development by wide-scale degradomic approaches, including the use of protease chips[2], will be necessary to target the most appropriate MMPs in the different stages of tumor evolution. Furthermore, the definition of the differences in MMP expression patterns between the reactive stroma and the tumor tissue by degradomic techniques will identify the site where therapeutic levels of drug need to be achieved. This will further rationalize the achievable pharmacokinetic endpoints necessary for the appropriate delivery of MMPIs to the most appropriate tissue sites. Thus, degradomic analyses will greatly assist in the development of new MMPIs by defining the critical targets in oncology and thereby set the spectral breadth required for effective cancer treatment.

NEW AREAS FOR IMPROVEMENT OF MMP INHIBITORS

Another fundamental aspect in future attempts to improve the clinical efficacy of MMPIs derives from the need to design more selective inhibitors that should be devoid of some adverse reactions detected with broad-spectrum inhibitors. For this purpose it is essential to increase the number of 3D structures available for these enzymes[104-106]. New classes of MMPIs, such as small cyclic peptides selected in high-throughput screening approaches or mechanism-based synthetic inhibitors, may offer additional therapeutic possibilities[107, 108]. MMPIs extracted from different natural products, such as soy or green tea, are also being increasingly explored as antitumor agents[109]. Likewise, Neovastat, derived from extracts of shark cartilage and possessing potent MMP-inhibitory properties, is currently in clinical trials for the treatment of different malignancies[110].

The rational attempts to develop improved MMPIs must be complemented with significant advances from the clinical side of the problem. Thus, identification of the best surrogate markers of MMPI activity[93], or the development of novel procedures to assess the *in vivo* inhibition of MMPs remains as fundamental problems. Finally, it is also important to emphasize that MMPIs are only cytostatic drugs, hence necessitating combined administration with other anticancer cytotoxic therapies to achieve their maximum efficacy.

CONCLUSIONS AND OUTLOOK

MMPs are overexpressed in virtually all human malignant tumors and play essential roles in multiple stages of cancer development and progression. Therefore, inhibition of these enzymes continues to be an important therapeutic approach for this complex disease. The failure of some cancer clinical trials with MMPIs has raised doubts over the benefit of these compounds, but has also provided interesting information for their future improvement. These trials were carried out when the knowledge on this family was still very fragmentary, and in retrospect we can conclude that some of these MMPI trials could have been better designed. The recently published trial successes for MMPIs are encouraging, however, these promising results should be confirmed and extended. It will also be necessary to address the regulatory mechanisms resulting in MMP overexpression, with special emphasis in the identification of signals responsible for the interaction between stromal and tumor cells. This aspect is important to evaluate the possibility of targeting MMPs produced by stromal cells, whose genetic stability is higher that that of tumor cells[111, 112]. Likewise, more effective procedures for the delivery of MMP inhibitory drugs to cancer or stromal tissue, will be required.

From the clinical viewpoint, MMPs may spearhead the introduction of the tumor degradome concept to precisely define those proteases that should be targeted in each particular tumor. Also, the issue of broad-spectrum *vs* selective MMPIs must be addressed. Selective inhibition of a limited set of MMPs at early stages of the disease might be more effective than using wide-spectrum inhibitors active against most family members. It will also be necessary to delineate the precise roles of the diverse MMPs in tumor progression as well as to elucidate their multiple connections with other proteolytic systems, especially with ADAMs and ADAMTSs. Here, it will be essential to identify the *in vivo* substrates for these enzymes, other than extracellular matrix components, and whose processing by MMPs is responsible for much of the novel functions ascribed to MMPs in tumor development and evolution. Large-scale degradomic approaches to identify novel protein substrates of MMPs are being initiated to achieve this goal. It will also be important to explore the clinical relevance of new classes of MMPIs that block substrate-binding exosites or mask MMP substrate cleavage sites[113, 114], as well as the potential of MMP-activatable cytotoxics[115]. These studies will contribute to clarify whether any of the multiple strategies of MMP inhibition may be part of future therapeutic approaches to control tumor progression.

Acknowledgements

Our work is supported by grants from Comision Interministerial de Ciencia y Tecnologia-Spain, Gobierno del Principado de Asturias, and European Union.

References

1.   Chambers, A. F., Groom, A.C., and MacDonald, I.C. Dissemination and growth of cancer cells in metastatic sites. *Nature Rev Cancer* **2**, 563-572 (2002)

2. López-Otín, C. and Overall, C. M. Protease degradomics, a challenge for proteomics. *Nature Rev. Mol. Cell Biol.* **3**, 509-519 (2002)

3. Brinckerhoff, C. E. and Matrisian, L. M. Matrix metalloproteinases: a tail of a frog that became a prince. *Nature Rev. Mol. Cell Biol.* **3**, 207-214 (2002).

4. Egeblad, M. and Werb, Z. New functions for the matrix metalloproteinases in cancer progression. *Nature Rev. Cancer* **2**, 163-175 (2002).

5. Overall, C. M. and López-Otín, C Strategies for MMP inhibition in cancer: innovations for the posttrial era. *Nature Rev. Cancer.* **2**, 657-672 (2002)

6. Uría, J. A. and López-Otín, C. Matrilysin-2, a new matrix metalloproteinase expressed in human tumors and showing the minimal domain organization required for secretion, latency, and activity. *Cancer Res.* **60**, 4745-4751 (2000).

7. Velasco, G. *et al.* Cloning and characterization of human MMP-23, a new matrix metalloproteinase predominantly expressed in reproductive tissues and lacking conserved domains in other family members. *J. Biol. Chem.* **274**, 4570-4576 (1999).

8. Sternlicht, M. D. *et al.* The stromal proteinase MMP3/stromelysin-1 promotes mammary carcinogenesis. *Cell* **98**, 137-146 (1999).

9. Sternlicht, M. D. and Werb, Z. How matrix metalloproteinases regulate cell behavior. *Annu. Rev. Cell Dev. Biol.* **17**, 463-516 (2001)

10. Rifkin, D. B., Mazzieri, R., Munger, J. S., Noguera, I. and Sung, J. Proteolytic control of growth factor availability. *APMIS* **107**, 80-85 (1999).

11. Mañes, S. *et al.* The matrix metalloproteinase-9 regulates the insulin-like growth factor-triggered autocrine response in DU-145 carcinoma cells. *J. Biol. Chem.* **274**, 6935-6945 (1999).

12. Noe, V. *et al.* Release of an invasion promoter E-cadherin fragment by matrilysin and stromelysin-1. *J. Cell Sci.* **114**, 111-118 (2001).

13. Lochter, A. *et al.* Matrix metalloproteinase stromelysin-1 triggers a cascade of molecular alterations that leads to stable epithelial-to-mesenchymal conversion and a premalignant phenotype in mammary epithelial cells. *J. Cell Biol.* **139**, 1861-1872 (1997).

14. Ho, A. T., Voura, E. B., Soloway, P. D., Watson, K. L. and Khokha, R. MMP inhibitors augment fibroblast adhesion through stabilization of focal adhesion contacts and up-regulation of cadherin function. *J. Biol.Chem.* **276**, 40215-40224 (2001).

15. McQuibban, G. A. *et al.* Inflammation dampened by gelatinase A cleavage of monocyte chemoattractant protein-3. *Science* **289**, 1202-1206 (2000).

16. Fingleton, B., Vargo-Gogola, T., Crawford, H. C. and Matrisian, L. M. Matrilysin (MMP-7) expression selects for cells with reduced sensitivity to apoptosis. *Neoplasia* **3**, 459-468 (2001).

17. Yu, Q. and Stamenkovic, I. Cell surface-localized matrix metalloproteinase-9 proteolytically activates TGF-β and promotes tumor invasion and angiogenesis. *Genes Dev.* **14**, 163-176 (2000).

18. Stetler-Stevenson, W. G. Matrix metalloproteinases in angiogenesis: a moving target for therapeutic intervention. *J. Clin. Invest.* **103**, 1237-1241 (1999).

19. Dong, Z., Kumar, R., Yang, X. and Fidler, I. J. Macrophage-derived metalloelastase is responsible for the generation of angiostatin in Lewis lung carcinoma. *Cell* **88**, 801-810 (1997).

20. Cornelius, L. A. *et al.* Matrix metalloproteinases generate angiostatin: effects on neovascularization. *J. Immunol.* **161**, 6845-6852 (1998).

21. Ferreras, M., Felbor, U., Lenhard, T., Olsen, B. R. and Delaisse, J. Generation and degradation of human endostatin proteins by various proteinases. *FEBS Lett.* **486**, 247-251 (2000).

22. Kheradmand, F., Werner, E., Tremble, P., Symons, M. and Werb, Z. Role of Rac1 and oxygen radicals in collagenase-1 expression induced by cell shape change. *Science* **280**, 898-902 (1998).

23. Overall, C. M., Wrana, J. L. and Sodek, J. Independent regulation of collagenase, 72-kDa progelatinase, and metalloendoproteinase inhibitor expression in human fibroblasts by transforming growth factor-ß. *J. Biol. Chem.* **264**, 1860-1869 (1989).

24. Guérin, E., Ludwig, M. G., Basset, P. and Anglard, P. Stromelysin-3 induction and interstitial collagenase repression by retinoic acid: therapeutical implication of receptor-selective retinoids dissociating transactivation and AP-1-mediated transrepression. *J. Biol. Chem.* **272**, 11088-11095 (1997).

25. Uría, J. A., Jiménez, M. G., Balbín, M., Freije, J. M. P. and López-Otín, C. Differential effects of transforming growth factor-β on the expression of collagenase-1 and collagenase-3 in human fibroblasts. *J. Biol. Chem.* **273**, 9769-9777 (1998).

26. Jiménez, M. J. *et al.* A regulatory cascade involving retinoic acid, Cbfa1, and matrix metalloproteinases is coupled to the development of a process of perichondrial invasion and osteogenic differentiation during bone formation. *J. Cell Biol.* **155**, 1333-1344 (2001).

27. Simon, C., Goepfert, H. and Boyd, D. Inhibition of the p38 mitogen-activated protein kinase by SB 203580 blocks PMA-induced Mr 92,000 type IV collagenase secretion and in vitro invasion. *Cancer Res.* **58**, 1135-1139 (1998).

28. Johansson, N. *et al.* Expression of collagenase-3 (MMP-13) and collagenase-1 (MMP-1) by transformed keratinocytes is dependent on the activity of p38 mitogen-activated protein kinase. *J. Cell Sci.* **113**, 227-235 (2000).

29. Pendás, A. M., Balbin, M., Llano, E., Jimenez, M. G. and López-Otín, C. Structural analysis and promoter characterization of the human collagenase-3 gene (MMP13). *Genomics* **40**, 222-233 (1997).

30. Gutman, A. and Wasylyk, B. The collagenase gene promoter contains a TPA and oncogene-responsive unit encompassing the PEA3 and AP-1 binding sites. *EMBO J.* **9**, 2241-2246 (1990).

31. Bond, M., Fabunmi, R. P., Baker, A. H. and Newby, A. C. Synergistic upregulation of metalloproteinase-9 by growth factors and inflammatory cytokines: an absolute requirement for transcription factor NF-kappa B. *FEBS Lett.* **435**, 29-34 (1998).

32. Rutter, J. L. *et al.* A single nucleotide polymorphism in the matrix metalloproteinase-1 promoter creates an Ets binding site and augments transcription. *Cancer Res.* **58**, 5321-5325 (1998).

33. Biondi, M. L. *et al.* MMP1 and MMP3 polymorphisms in promoter regions and cancer. *Clin. Chem.* **46**, 2023-2024 (2000).

34. Springman, E. B., Angleton, E. L., Birkedal-Hansen, H. and Van Wart, H.E. Multiple modes of activation of latent human fibroblast collagenase: evidence for the role of a Cys73 active-site zinc complex in latency and a "cysteine switch" mechanism for activation. *Proc. Natl Acad. Sci. USA* **87**, 364-368 (1990).

35. Bannikov, G. A., Karelina, T. V., Collier, I. E., Marmer, B. L. and Goldberg, G. I. Substrate binding of gelatinase B induces its enzymatic activity in the presence of intact propeptide. *J. Biol. Chem.* **277**, 16022-16027 (2002).

36. Knauper, V. *et al.* Cellular mechanisms for human collagenase-3 (MMP-13) activation: evidence that MT1-MMP (MMP-14) and gelatinase A (MMP-2) are able to generate active enzyme. *J. Biol. Chem.* **271**, 17124-17131 (1996).

37. Sato, H. *et al.* A matrix metalloproteinase expressed on the surface of invasive tumour cells. *Nature* **370**, 61-65 (1994).

38. Strongin, A. Y. *et al.* Mechanism of cell surface activation of 72-kDa type IV collagenase. Isolation of the activated form of the membrane metalloprotease. *J. Biol. Chem.* **270**, 5331-5338 (1995).

39. Overall, C. M. *et al.* Identification of the tissue inhibitor of metalloproteinases-2 (TIMP-2) binding site on the hemopexin carboxyl domain of human gelatinase A by site-directed mutagenesis. The hierarchical role in binding TIMP-2 of the unique cationic clusters of hemopexin modules III and IV. *J. Biol. Chem.* **274**, 4421-4429 (1999).

40. Pei, D. and Weiss, S. J. Furin-dependent intracellular activation of the human stromelysin-3 zymogen. *Nature* **375**, 244-247 (1995).

41. Yana, I. and Weiss, S. J. Regulation of membrane type-1 matrix metalloproteinase activation by proprotein convertases. *Mol. Biol. Cell* **11**, 2387-2401 (2000).

42. Lohi, J., Wilson, C. L., Roby, J. D. and Parks, W. C. Epilysin, a novel human matrix metalloproteinase (MMP-28) expressed in testis and keratinocytes and in response to injury. *J. Biol. Chem.* **276**, 10134-10144 (2001).

43. Velasco, G. *et al.* Human MT6-matrix metalloproteinase: identification, progelatinase A activation, and expression in brain tumors. *Cancer Res.* **60**, 877-882 (2000).

44. Nagase, H., Itoh, Y. and Binner, S. Interaction of alpha 2-macroglobulin with matrix metalloproteinases and its use for identification of their active forms. *Ann. N. Y. Acad. Sci.* **732**, 294-302 (1994).

45. Brew, K., Dinakarpandian, D. and Nagase, H. Tissue inhibitors of metalloproteinases: evolution, structure and function. *Biochim Biophys Acta* **1477**, 267-283 (2000).

46. Amour, A. *et al.* The in vitro activity of ADAM-10 is inhibited by TIMP-1 and TIMP-3. *FEBS Lett.* **473**, 275-279 (2000).

47. Kashiwagi, M., Tortorella, M., Nagase, H. and Brew, K. TIMP-3 is a potent inhibitor of aggrecanase 1 (ADAM-TS4) and aggrecanase 2 (ADAM-TS5). *J. Biol. Chem.* **276**, 12501-12504 (2001).

48. Khokha, R. *et al.* Antisense RNA-induced reduction in murine TIMP levels confers oncogenicity on Swiss 3T3 cells. *Science* **243**, 947-950 (1989).

49. Corcoran, M. L. and Stetler-Stevenson, W. G. Tissue inhibitor of metalloproteinase-2 stimulates fibroblast proliferation via a cAMP-dependent mechanism. *J. Biol. Chem.* **270**, 13453-13459 (1995).

50. Jiang, Y., Goldberg, I. D. and Shi, Y. E. Complex roles of tissue inhibitors of metalloproteinases in cancer. *Oncogene* **21**, 2245-2252 (2002).

51. Oh, J. *et al.* The membrane-anchored MMP inhibitor RECK is a key regulator of extracellular matrix integrity and angiogenesis. *Cell* **107**, 789-800 (2001).
52. Herman, M. P. *et al.* Tissue factor pathway inhibitor-2 is a novel inhibitor of matrix metalloproteinases with implications for atherosclerosis. *J. Clin. Invest.* **107**, 1117-1126 (2001).
53. Mott, J. D. *et al.* Post-translational proteolytic processing of procollagen C-terminal proteinase enhancer releases a metalloproteinase inhibitor. *J. Biol. Chem.* **275**, 1384-1390 (2000).
54. Petitclerc, E. *et al.* New functions for non-collagenous domains of human collagen type IV. Novel integrin ligands inhibiting angiogenesis and tumor growth in vivo. *J. Biol. Chem.* **275**, 8051-8061 (2000).
55. Stetefeld, J. *et al.* The laminin-binding domain of agrin is structurally related to N-TIMP-1. *Nat. Struct. Biol.* **8**, 705-709 (2001).
56. Westermarck, J. and Kähäri, V. M. Regulation of matrix metalloproteinase expression in tumor invasion. *FASEB J.* **13**, 781-792 (1999).
57. Hua, J. and Muschel, R. J. Inhibition of matrix metalloproteinase 9 expression by a ribozyme blocks metastasis in a rat sarcoma model system. *Cancer Res.* **56**, 5279-5284 (1996).
58. Kondraganti, S. *et al.* Selective suppression of matrix metalloproteinase-9 in human glioblastoma cells by antisense gene transfer impairs glioblastoma cell invasion. *Cancer Res.* **60**, 6851-6855 (2000).
59. Nagavarapu, U., Relloma, K. and Herron, G. S. Membrane type 1 matrix metalloproteinase regulates cellular invasiveness and survival in cutaneous epidermal cells. *J. Invest. Dermatol.* **118**, 573-581 (2002).
60. Slaton, J. W. *et al.* Treatment with low-dose interferon-alpha restores the balance between matrix metalloproteinase-9 and E-cadherin expression in human transitional cell carcinoma of the bladder. *Clin. Cancer Res.* **7**, 2840-2853 (2001).
61. Ala-aho, R. *et al.* Inhibition of collagenase-3 (MMP-13) expression in transformed human keratinocytes by interferon-gamma is associated with activation of extracellular signal-regulated kinase-1,2 and STAT1. *Oncogene.* **19**, 248-257 (2000).
62. Ma, Z., Qin, H. and Benveniste, E. N. Transcriptional suppression of matrix metalloproteinase-9 gene expression by IFN-γ and IFN-β: critical role of STAT-1α. *J. Immunol.* **167**, 5150-5159 (2001).
63. Mengshol, J. A., Mix, K. S. and Brinckerhoff, C. E. Matrix metalloproteinases as therapeutic targets in arthritic diseases: bull's-eye or missing the mark? *Arthritis Rheum.* **46**, 13-20 (2002).
64. Futamura, M. *et al.* Malolactomycin D, a potent inhibitor of transcription controlled by the Ras responsive element, inhibit Ras-mediated transformation activity with suppression of MMP-1 and MMP-9 in NIH3T3 cells. *Oncogene* **20**, 6724-6730 (2001).
65. Zhang, Y. *et al.* Hyaluronan-CD44s signaling regulates matrix metalloproteinase-2 secretion in a human lung carcinoma cell line QG90. *Cancer Res.* **62**, 3962-3965 (2002).
66. McGaha, T. L., Phelps, R. G., Spiera, H. and Bona, C. Halofuginone, an inhibitor of type-I collagen synthesis and skin sclerosis, blocks transforming-growth-factor-beta-mediated Smad3 activation in fibroblasts. *J. Invest. Dermatol.* **118**, 461-470 (2002).
67. Elkin M, Reich R, Nagler A, Aingorn E, Pines M, de-Groot N, Hochberg A, Vlodavsky I. Inhibition of matrix metalloproteinase-2 expression and bladder carcinoma metastasis by halofuginone. *Clin. Cancer Res.* **5**, 1982-1988 (1999).
68. Karin, M. and Chang, L. AP-1-glucocorticoid receptor crosstalk taken to a higher level. *J. Endocrinol.* **169**, 447-451 (2001).
69. Sato, T. *et al.* Inhibition of activator protein-1 binding activity and phosphatidylinositol 3-kinase pathway by nobiletin, a polymethoxy flavonoid, results in augmentation of tissue inhibitor of metalloproteinases-1 production and suppression of production of matrix metalloproteinases-1 and –9 in human fibrosarcoma HT-1080 cells. *Cancer Res.* **62**, 1025-1029 (2002).
70. Mohan, R. *et al.* Curcuminoids inhibit the angiogenic response stimulated by fibroblast growth factor-2, including expression of matrix metalloproteinase gelatinase B. *J. Biol. Chem.* **275**, 10405-10412 (2000).
71. Adams, J. *et al.* Proteasome inhibitors: a novel class of potent and effective antitumor agents. *Cancer Res.* **59**, 2615-2622 (1999).
72. Tan, C. and Waldmann, T. A. Proteasome inhibitor PS-341, a potential therapeutic agent for adult T-cell leukemia. *Cancer Res.* **62**, 1083-1086 (2002).
73. Barille, S. *et al.* Metalloproteinases in multiple myeloma: production of matrix metalloproteinase-9 (MMP-9), activation of proMMP-2, and induction of MMP-1 by myeloma cells. *Blood* **90**, 1649-1655 (1997).
74. Jimenez, M. J. *et al.* Collagenase 3 is a target of Cbfa1, a transcription factor of the runt gene family involved in bone formation. *Mol. Cell Biol.* **19**, 4431-4442 (1999).

75. Yang, J. *et al.* Prostate cancer cells induce osteoblast differentiation through a Cbfa1-dependent pathway. *Cancer Res.* **61**, 5652-5659 (2001).

76. Sun, Y. *et al.* Wild type and mutant p53 differentially regulate the gene expression of human collagenase-3 (hMMP-13). *J. Biol. Chem.* **275**, 11327-11332 (2000).

77. Koul, D. *et al.* Suppression of matrix metalloproteinase-2 gene expression and invasion in human glioma cells by MMAC/PTEN. *Oncogene* **20**, 6669-6678 (2001).

78. Fenrick, R. *et al.* TEL, a putative tumor suppressor, modulates cell growth and cell morphology of ras-transformed cells while repressing the transcription of stromelysin-1. *Mol. Cell Biol.* **20**, 5828-5839 (2000).

79. Galvez, B. G., Matias-Roman, S., Albar, J. P., Sanchez-Madrid, F. and Arroyo, A. G. Membrane type 1-matrix metalloproteinase is activated during migration of human endothelial cells and modulates endothelial motility and matrix remodeling. *J. Biol. Chem.* **276**, 37491-37500 (2001).

80. Annabi, B. *et al.* Green tea polyphenol (-)-epigallocatechin 3-gallate inhibits MMP-2 secretion and MT1-MMP-driven migration in glioblastoma cells. *Biochim. Biophys. Acta.* **1542**, 209-220 (2002).

81. Bassi, D. E. *et al.* Furin inhibition results in absent or decreased invasiveness and tumorigenicity of human cancer cells. *Proc. Natl. Acad. Sci. USA* **98**, 10326-10331 (2001).

82. Rodriguez-Manzaneque, J. C. *et al.* Thrombospondin-1 suppresses spontaneous tumor growth and inhibits activation of matrix metalloproteinase-9 and mobilization of vascular endothelial growth factor. *Proc. Natl Acad. Sci. USA* **98**, 12485-12490 (2001).

83. Yang, Z., Strickland, D. K. and Bornstein, P. Extracellular matrix metalloproteinase 2 levels are regulated by the low density lipoprotein-related scavenger receptor and thrombospondin 2. *J. Biol.Chem.* **276**, 8403-8408 (2001).

84. Kim, Y. M. *et al.* Endostatin inhibits endothelial and tumor cellular invasion by blocking the activation and catalytic activity of matrix metalloproteinase. *Cancer Res.* **60**, 5410-5413 (2000).

85. Nakada, M. *et al.* Suppression of membrane-type 1 matrix metalloproteinase (MMP)-mediated MMP-2 activation and tumor invasion by testican 3 and its splicing variant gene product, N-tes. *Cancer Res.* **61**, 8896-8902 (2001).

86. Sgadari, C. *et al.* HIV protease inhibitors are potent anti-angiogenic molecules and promote regression of Kaposi sarcoma. *Nature Med.* **8**, 225-232 (2002).

87. Kruger, A., Fata, J. E. and Khokha, R. Altered tumor growth and metastasis of a T-cell lymphoma in Timp-1 transgenic mice. *Blood* **90**, 1993-2000 (1997).

88. Martin, D. C. *et al.* Transgenic TIMP-1 inhibits simian virus 40 T antigen-induced hepatocarcinogenesis by impairment of hepatocellular proliferation and tumor angiogenesis. *Lab. Invest.* **79**, 225-234 (1999).

89. Brown, P. D. Clinical studies with matrix metalloproteinase inhibitors. *APMIS* **107**, 174-180 (1999).

90. Duivenvoorden, W. C. *et al.* Doxycycline decreases tumor burden in a bone metastasis model of human breast cancer. *Cancer Res.* **62**, 1588-1591 (2002).

91. Cianfrocca, M. *et al.* Matrix metalloproteinase inhibitor COL-3 in the treatment of AIDS-related Kaposi's sarcoma: a phase I AIDS malignancy consortium study. *J. Clin. Oncol.* **20**, 153-159 (2002).

92. Boissier, S. *et al.* Bisphosphonates inhibit breast and prostate carcinoma cell invasion, an early event in the formation of bone metastases. *Cancer Res.* **60**, 2949-2954 (2000).

93. Coussens, L. M., Fingleton, B. and Matrisian, L. M. Matrix metalloproteinase inhibitors and cancer: trials and tribulations. *Science* **295**, 2387-2392 (2002).

94. Bramhall, S.R. *et al.* Marimastat as maintenance therapy for patients with advanced gastric cancer: a randomised trial. *Br. J. Cancer.* **86**, 1864-1870 (2002).

95. Bramhall, S. R., Rosemurgy, A., Brown, P. D., Bowry, C. and Buckels, J. A. Marimastat as first-line therapy for patients with unresectable pancreatic cancer: a randomized trial. *J. Clin. Oncol.* **19**, 3447-3455 (2001).

96. Groves, M. D. *et al.* Phase II trial of temozolomide plus the matrix metalloproteinase inhibitor, marimastat, in recurrent and progressive glioblastoma multiforme. *J Clin. Oncol* **20**, 1383-1388 (2002).

97. Zucker, S., Cao, J. and Chen, W. T. Critical appraisal of the use of matrix metalloproteinase inhibitors in cancer treatment. *Oncogene* **19**, 6642-6650 (2000).

98. Bergers, G., Javaherian, K., Lo, K. M., Folkman, J. and Hanahan, D. Effects of angiogenesis inhibitors on multistage carcinogenesis in mice. *Science* **284**, 808-812 (1999).

99. Fingleton, B. M., Heppner Goss, K. J., Crawford, H. C. and Matrisian, L. M. Matrilysin in early stage intestinal tumorigenesis. *APMIS* **107**, 102-110 (1999).

100. Pozzi, A. *et al.* Elevated matrix metalloprotease and angiostatin levels in integrin alpha 1 knockout mice cause reduced tumor vascularization. *Proc. Natl Acad. Sci. USA* **97**, 2202-2207 (2000).

101.Pozzi, A., LeVine, W. F. and Gardner, H. A. Low plasma levels of matrix metalloproteinase 9 permit increased tumor angiogenesis. *Oncogene* **22,** 272-281 (2002).

102.Vazquez, F. *et al.* METH-1, a human ortholog of ADAMTS-1, and METH-2 are members of a new family of proteins with angio-inhibitory activity. *J. Biol. Chem.* **274,** 23349-23357 (1999).

103.Cal, S. *et al.* Cloning, expression analysis, and structural characterization of seven novel human ADAMTSs, a family of metalloproteinases with disintegrin and thrombospondin-1 domains. *Gene* **283,** 49-62 (2002)

104.Gomis-Ruth, F. X. *et al.* Mechanism of inhibition of the human matrix metalloproteinase stromelysin-1 by TIMP-1. *Nature* **389,** 77-81 (1997).

105.Bode, W. *et al.* Structural properties of matrix metalloproteinases. *Cell Mol. Life Sci.* **55,** 639-652 (1999).

106.Morgunova, E., Tuuttila, A., Bergmann, U. and Tryggvason, K. Structural insight into the complex formation of latent matrix metalloproteinase 2 with tissue inhibitor of metalloproteinase 2. *Proc. Natl. Acad. Sci. USA.* **99,** 7414-7419 (2002).

107.Koivunen, E. *et al.* Tumor targeting with a selective gelatinase inhibitor. *Nat. Biotechnol.* **17,** 768-774 (1999).

108.Bernardo, M. M., Brown, S., Li, Z. H., Fridman, R. and Mobashery, S. Design, synthesis, and characterization of potent, slow-binding inhibitors that are selective for gelatinases. *J. Biol. Chem.* **277,** 11201-11207 (2002).

109.Garbisa, S. *et al.* Tumor gelatinases and invasion inhibited by the green tea flavanol epigallocatechin-3-gallate. *Cancer* **91,** 822-832 (2001).

110. Falardeau, P., Champagne, P., Poyet, P., Hariton, C. and Dupont, E. Neovastat, a naturally occurring multifunctional antiangiogenic drug, in phase III clinical trials. *Semin. Oncol.* **28,** 620-625 (2001).

111. Nielsen, B. S. *et al.* Collagenase-3 expression in breast myofibroblasts as a molecular marker of transition of ductal carcinoma in situ lesions to invasive ductal carcinomas. *Cancer Res.* 61, 7091-7100 (2001).

112. Bissell, M. J. and Radisky, D. Putting tumours in context. *Nature Rev.Cancer* 1, 46-54 (2001).

113. Silletti, S., Kessler, T., Goldberg, J., Boger, D. L. and Cheresh, D. A. Disruption of matrix metalloproteinase 2 binding to integrin αvβ3 by an organic molecule inhibits angiogenesis and tumor growth in vivo. *Proc. Natl Acad. Sci. USA* 98, 119-124 (2001).

114. Overall, C. M. Matrix metalloproteinase substrate binding domains, modules, and exosites: overview and experimental strategies. *Methods Mol. Biol.* 151, 73-114 (2001).

115. Liu, S., Netzel-Arnett, S., Birkedal-Hansen, H. and Leppla, S. H. Tumor cell-selective cytotoxicity of matrix metalloproteinase-activated anthrax toxin. *Cancer Res.* 60, 6061-6067 (2000).

ANGIOGENESIS INHIBITORS AND THEIR THERAPEUTIC POTENTIALS

Yihai Cao[*]

Microbiology and Tumor Biology Center, Karolinska Institutet, S-171 77
Stockholm, Sweden

INTRODUCTION

The observation that tumor growth is accompanied by increased vascularity was reported nearly a century ago[1]. The therapeutic potentials that target tumor blood vessels was suggested more than three decades ago[2]. Inspired by this hypothesis, many investigators have jointed to the field of antiangiogenesis with an obvious goal of finding angiogenesis inhibitors that block tumor growth and metastasis. Over the last decade, the field of antiangiogenesis has become one of the key focuses in development of new cancer therapeutic drugs. The simple reason that angiogenesis research has received tremendous surge is that other anti-cancer therapeutic strategies including chemotherapy and radiotherapy do not seem to effectively block tumor growth. On contrary, they often produce toxic side-effects and therapeutic resistance. Thus, the antiangiogenesis approach has raised a new hope for cancer patients.

Less than 10 years ago, only a few compounds, including several small chemical molecules and a couple of endogenous protein molecules have been described as angiogenesis inhibitors. These few angiogenesis inhibitors were barely enough to make a publishable table in a review article. Today, discovery of novel angiogenesis inhibitors has become a competitive business among many pharmaceutical companies with a hope to commercialize these compounds as therapeutic drugs against cancer and other angiogenesis dependent diseases. As a result, there is almost a new angiogenesis inhibitor being identified or reported every other week. Thus, it is almost impossible to give a complete overview of the entire field. According to their actions, angiogenesis inhibitors can be classified as: 1) Angiogenic factor antagonists; 2) Angiogenic factor receptor antagonists; 3) Protease inhibitors; 3) Anti-inflammatory compounds; 4) Matrix protein antagonists; 5) Cytokines; and 6) Direct endothelial cell inhibitors. Preclinical studies show that most of angiogenesis inhibitors effectively block tumor growth

Correspondence and reprint requests should be addressed to Yihai Cao, M.D., Ph.D. at the Microbiology and Tumor Biology Center, Karolinska Institute, S-171 77 Stockholm, Sweden. Tel: (+46)-8-728 7596, Fax: (+46)-8-31 94 70, E-mail: yihai.cao@mtc.ki.se

New Trends in Cancer for the 21st Century, edited by
Llombart-Bosch and Felipo, Kluwer Academic/Plenum Publishers, 2003

109

without causing toxicity. Excited by animal studies, many angiogenesis inhibitors are currently in various phases of human cancer trials even without knowing the underlying mechanisms of their actions. As a consequence, early clinical evaluations of their therapeutic potentials have generated some disappointments. These ongoing clinical studies have raised several important questions: 1) Can the antitumor effect of an angiogenesis inhibitor in animal models be directly translated into those in human patients? 2) What is a fundamental difference between a spontaneous human cancer and an experimental tumor in animals? 3) What are the differences of human tumor neovascularization and experimental animal tumor angiogenesis? 4) What are the underlying mechanisms of angiostatic actions of these inhibitors? 5) How does an angiogenesis inhibitor affect a well-established human tumor growth? The answers to these questions are unknown. Without knowing the functional mechanisms and the difference of vascular biology between human and animals, it is difficult to predict the consequence of clinical trials. In fact, several major angiogenesis inhibitors have suffered setbacks in early clinical trials[3]. In order to better understand their biological functions and mechanisms of actions, we have characterized several angiogenesis inhibitors at the molecular level.

FEATURES OF TUMOR VESSELS

Many elegant experiments in animal models have shown that tumor growth and metastasis are dependent on the newly formed blood vessels. It is still worthwhile to mention a simple experiment that provides conclusive evidence that angiogenesis is a prerequisite for tumor growth and antiangiogenesis can block tumor growth. In the rabbit cornea, when a tiny piece tumor tissue is implanted, the tumor implant changes its growth rate from linear to exponential once newly formed blood vessels reached to the tumor tissue[4]. At the prevascular stage, a tiny tumor tissue consisting of several millions of cells remains in its dormant stage for about 10 days without growth. Survival of these cells in an avascular tumor is dependent on free diffusion of nutrients, O_2 and growth factors. The tumor implant is unable to grow beyond volumes of 2-3 mm^3. However, these living tumor cells are able to produce potent angiogenic factors, such as vascular endothelial growth factor/vascular permeability factor (VEGF/VPF) and fibroblast growth factor-2 (FGF-2), which switch on an angiogenic phenotype of the tumor implant. Once newly formed blood vessels reach the tumor implant, the growth of the tumor is exponential. In fact, the tiny tumor implant grows beyond the size of the entire eye organ within a couple of days. In contrast, mechanical disruptions of tumor-induced vessels in the cornea can completely arrest tumor growth. From this simple experiment, we conclude: 1) tumor cells are able to recruit new blood vessels from the host; 2) tumor growth is dependent on angiogenesis; and 3) interference with tumor-induced blood vessel growth can stop tumor growth.

Although tumors are able to recruit new blood vessels from the host, there are fundamental differences between tumor vessels and host tissue vessels. Morphologically, tumor vessels are irregular, heterogeneous and leaky. These features are considered as hallmarks of destruction of normal blood vessel integrity[5]. The endothelial cells are disorganized and irregularly shaped, sometimes overlapped each other, and luminal projections, which lead to abluminal sprouts. It has been reported the blood vessels in tumors consist of mosaic cell types including tumor cells[6, 7]. Although mural cells have been found on tumor vessels, they have unusually loose association with endothelial cells[8]. In addition, tumor vessels contain the abnormal basement membrane including changes of matrix protein composition, assembly, and structures.

Unlike normal blood vessels in a healthy tissue, there is no clear distinction between arterioles and venules among tumor vessels. As a result of this abnormal vessel architecture, blood flows in tumor vessels are chaotic. For example, a single vessel transports blood to distal tumor cells and removes it from the tumor tissue. Thus, the tumor tissue is relatively hypoxic with poorly oxygenated blood.

VASCULAR ENDOTHELIAL GROWTH FACTOR AND OTHER TUMOR-PRODUCED ANGIOGENIC FACTORS

The abnormality of the tumor vessel architecture represents the imbalanced production of tumor angiogenic factors and inhibitors. It is believed that tumors overexpress angiogenic factors and decrease production of angiogenesis inhibitors, although the concept of down-regulation of inhibitors in tumor tissues needs to be further validated. More than a dozen of tumor angiogenic factors and cytokines have been isolated[9]. Among these angiogenic factors, the VEGF family has become a central focus in today´s tumor angiogenesis research, simply because most tumors, if not all, express VEGF at high levels. The VEGF family is comprised of five structurally related members including VEGF-A, placenta growth factor (PlGF), VEGF-B, VEGF-C, and VEGF-D. The biological functions of the VEGF family are mediated by activation of three structurally homologous tyrosine kinase receptors, VEGFR-1, VEGFR-2 and VEGFR-3[10]. VEGF and PlGF-2 also bind to a non-tyrosine kinase receptor, neuropilin-1[11, 12]. However, the biological signals mediated by neuropilin-1 in endothelial cells are not known. According to their receptor binding patterns and angiogenic features, the members of the VEGF family can be further divided into three subgroups: 1) VEGF, which binds to VEGFR-1 and VEGFR-2, and induces vasculogenesis, angiogenesis and vascular permeability; 2) PlGF and VEGF-B, which bind only to VEGFR-1, with unknown physiological and pathological functions; 3) VEGF-C and VEGF-D, which interact with both VEGFR-2 and VEGFR-3, and induce both blood angiogenesis and lymphangiogenesis[10, 13]. Accumulating evidence has pointed to that VEGFR-2, in response to VEGF, mediates angiogenic signals for blood vessel growth and VEGFR-3 transduces signals for lymphatic vessel growth[14]. The function of VEGFR-1 is poorly understood. Similar to VEGF, PlGF can be generated as at least three alternatively spliced isoforms of the same gene, PlGF-1, PlGF-2 and PlGF-3[15, 16, 17].

PlGF-1 ANTAGONIZES VEGF-INDUCED ANGIOGENESIS AND TUMOR GROWTH BY THE FORMATION OF FUNCTIONALLY INACTIVE HETERODIMERS

Formation purification of heterodimers

Similar to the platelet-derived growth factor (PDGF) family, all members in the VEGF family naturally exist as dimeric proteins in order to interact with their specific receptors. In addition to homodimers, PlGF and VEGF-B can form heterodimers with VEGF when these factors are produced in the same cell[18, 20]. We have previously reported that PlGF-1 preferentially forms heterodimers with VEGF intracellularly[18, 19]. PlGF-1/VEGF heterodimers are naturally present in tissues when both factors are synthesized in the same population of cell. To study the role of PlGF/VEGF heterodimers in regulation of angiogenesis, we expressed recombinant human PlGF-1 and VEGF$_{165}$ monomers with different molecular weights. Using an in vitro refolding method and two-affinity columns, we were able to purify the PlGF-1/VEGF heterodimers to homogeneity.

PlGF-1/VEGF heterodimers lacks angiogenic activity in vivo

To test their *in vivo* angiogenic features, we analyzed all three dimeric factors in the mouse corneal angiogenesis model[10]. As expected, VEGF homodimers induced a robust corneal angiogenic response with a high number of microvessels that forming a primitive vascular network at the leading edge. In contrast, the same amount of PlGF-1 homodimers or PlGF-1/VEGF heterodimers failed to stimulate corneal angiogenesis. PlGF-1 did not seem to interfere with VEGF-induced neovascularization when both PlGF and VEGF homodimers were co-implanted in mouse corneas. Quantification of corneal neovascularization showed that PlGF-1 and PlGF-1/VEGF lacked detectable angiogenic responses in this *in vivo* assay.

Formation of PlGF-1/VEGF heterodimers in tumor cells

Because PlGF-1 forms functionally defective heterodimers with VEGF *in vitro*, we hypothesized that overexpression of PlGF-1 could lead VEGF molecules to form PlGF-1/VEGF heterodimers in tumor cells and thus antagonize the angiogenic activity of VEGF produced by tumors. To test this hypothesis, we expressed hPlGF-1 to a high level using a retroviral vector in a well-characterized murine fibrosarcoma, with a VEGF-dependent *in vivo* growth. The presence of hPlGF-1 and hVEGF cDNAs was confirmed by Southern blot analysis. Overexpression of hVEGF in murine fibrosarcoma cells resulted in the formation of hVEGF/hVEGF homodimers and hVEGF/mVEGF heterodimers, that were co-precipitated by an antibody specific to hVEGF. The different forms of VEGF dimers were converted to monomers under reducing conditions. In addition to the $mVEGF_{164}$ isoform, $mVEGF_{120}$ also participated in the formation of heterodimers with $hVEGF_{165}$. Similarly, high levels of hPlGF-1 expression resulted in the formation of hPlGF-1/hPlGF-1 homodimers and hPlGF-1/mVEGF heterodimers as detected in complexes precipitated by a specific anti-hPlGF-1 antibody. These dimers were reduced to monomers in the presence of a reducing agent.

To quantify the amounts of various dimeric molecules secreted by tumor cells, we performed a sensitive sandwich ELISA assay using specific antibodies against each factor, either two antibodies against the same factor but raised in different species (homodimers) or two antibodies against different factors (heterodimers). As expected, a high level of mVEGF homodimers (2430 pg/ml) was detected in conditioned medium from *wt* T241 tumor cells. The majority of mPlGF produced by *wt* T241 were involved in heterodimerization with mVEGF, suggesting that mPlGF preferentially formed heterodimers with mVEGF, rather than mPlGF/mPlGF homodimers. Only low levels of mVEGF homodimers (770 pg/ml) were found in the conditioned media of hPlGF-T241-1 and hPlGF-T241-2 cells grown at the same conditions. In contrast, virtually all mVEGF molecules were present as hPlGF-1/mVEGF heterodimers in PlGF-1-overexpressing hPlGF-T241-1 (7,500 pg/ml) and hPlGF-T241-2 tumor cells (73,000 pg/ml). Although different levels of hPlGF were produced in hPlGF-T241-1 and hPlGF-T241-2 tumor cells, both these high levels efficiently depleted mVEGF homodimers.

Lack of stimulatory activity on endothelial cells by PlGF-1-overexpressing cells *in vitro*

To study the chemotactic activity, we tested the effect of conditioned media derived from various transduced and non-transduced cells in a modified Boyden chemotaxis assay. As expected, VEGF elicited a strong chemotactic response on VEGFR-2-expressing PAE cells. Similarly, conditioned medium from *wt* T241 cells significantly stimulated VEGFR-2/PAE cell migration. High expression levels of hVEGF enhanced the chemotactic activity produced by T241 cells. In contrast, both PlGF-1 homodimers and PlGF-1/VEGF heterodimers lacked such a chemotactic effect on these endothelial cells, and expression of hPlGF-1 completely abolished the chemotactic effect produced by T241 cells. None of these factors or conditioned media induced VEGFR-1/PAE cell motility. Similar results were obtained with primary HUVE cells. Addition of hVEGF homodimers at the concentration of 50 ng/ml to VEGFR-2/PAE cells induced a spindle-like cell shape with reorganization of actin fibers, a feature that both PlGF-1 homodimers and PlGF-1/VEGF heterodimers lack. Furthermore, VEGFR-1-expressing PAE cells did not respond to any of these three factor-treatments. Incubation with conditioned medium from *wt* T241 cells resulted in an elongated spindle-like cell shape in VEGFR-2/PAE cells, similar to that induced by hVEGF, confirming that T241 cells secrete high levels of mVEGF. This effect was completely abrogated after expression of hPlGF-1, indicating that a majority of the mVEGF molecules participated in formation of heterodimers with hPlGF-1. In contrast, overexpression of hVEGF in T241 cells led to remarkable cell shape changes and actin reorganization. Again, conditioned media from all cell lines failed to induce a similar change in endothelial morphology of VEGFR-1/PAE cells.

Overexpression of PlGF-1 in tumor cells suppresses of tumor growth

Overexpression of hPlGF-1 in T241 cells did not alter the growth rates of two independent tumor clones in culture. The *wt* T241 tumor cells grew rapidly *in vivo*, and visible tumors were readily detectable 6 days after implantation. Expression of hVEGF in these cells significantly accelerated tumor growth. Tumors expressing hVEGF grew invasively into surrounding tissues and resulted in early visible metastases in other organs such as spine and liver. In contrast, expression of hPlGF-1 remarkably delayed tumor growth and visible tumors were only detectable by day 12 after implantation. These tumors remained at a similar small average size of about 70 mm^3 by day 16 after implantation. At day 16 after tumor implantation, approximately 90% inhibition of tumor growth was scored in hPlGF-1-expressing tumors as compared with the *wt* T241 tumors. Similarly, highly significant reductions of primary tumor volumes were found in both PlGF-1-expressing tumor clones. Immunohistochemical studies showed that hPlGF-1-expressing tumors had significantly reduced neovascularization as compared with *wt* T241 tumors. In contrast, hVEGF-expressing tumors were highly vascularized with an average of more than 300 microvessels per optical field. In addition to high vessel counts, some of the microvessels were dilated with a thin endothelial layer. The invasive growth feature of hVEGF-expressing tumors led to early metastasis of tumor cells into other organs such as spine and liver. Biopsy examination revealed that 100% of hVEGF-T241 tumor bearing mice had hepatic metastases. Both liver volume and weight of hVEGF-T241 tumor bearing mice were significantly larger than those of control animals. Overproduction of VEGF by tumor cells not only resulted in hemorrhagic lesions in hepatic metastases, but also caused destruction of regular hepatocyte sinusoidal organization as compared to liver structures of wt T241- or hPlGF-1-T241-tumor bearing mice.

SWITCH ON MULTIPLE ANGIOGENIC FACTORS DURING TUMOR PROGRESSION AND POTENTIAL DEVELOPMENT OF DRUG RESISTANCE BY USING SINGLE ANGIOGENIC FACTOR ANTAGONISTS

As the genome of tumor cells is unstable, they constantly undergo genetic mutations, which lead to alternations of gene expression patterns. As a result of genetic mutations, tumors consist of heterogenous cell populations. Thus, expression patterns of pro-angiogenic factors can be altered along tumor progression and single angiogenic factor antagonists may encounter drug resistance problems. As most tumors produce VEGF at high levels, development of VEGF antagonists is an obvious approach to block tumor angiogenesis. These VEGF antagonists include VEGF mRNA antisense, neutralizing antibodies to VEGF and its receptors, soluble VEGF receptors, and VEGFR-2-siganlling inhibitor. In animal models, these VEGF antagonists have produced remarkable effects in suppression of tumor growth. For example, VEGF neutralizing antibodies and soluble VEGF receptors completely prevented tumor growth[21, 22]. However, if a tumor produces other angiogenic factors such as FGF-2, the tumor may become resistant to anti-VEGF treatment. In fact, an early tumor may only secrete one or two angiogenic factors whereas a large progressive tumor can produce many angiogenic factors[23]. For example as shown in Fig. 1, more than 50% newly diagnosed breast cancers produce only VEGF. In subsequent tumor progression, recurrences and metastases, production of other angiogenic factors including, FGF-2, TGF-β, PlGF, PD-ECGF and pleiotrophin is switched on. Anti-VEGF reagents might stress tumor cells to select for colonies producing other proangiogenic factors such as FGF-2. Thus, VEGF antagonists may not be effective in the treatment of all cancers. Such a principle may also apply to other anti-single factor approaches including anti-FGF-2 and anti-PDGFs. Thus, single angiogenic factor antagonists may encounter problems due to the development of drug resistance, as tumor cells may most likely alter their angiogenic stimulator expression profiles. However, a recent study has provided some exceptional evidence that VEGF plays an essential and non-replaceable role of tumor angiogenesis in a mouse pancreatic tumor model[24]. In contrast to antagonists for single angiogenic factors, general angiogenesis inhibitors that block common pathways of tumor angiogenesis could bypass drug resistance and thus prove therapeutically effective against all cancer types.

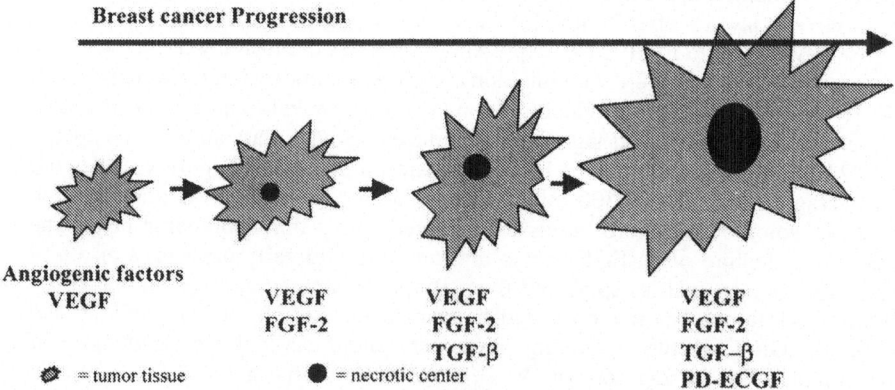

Figure 1. Switch on multiple angiogenic factors during tumor progression. An early lesion of breast cancer only expresses VEGF as an angiogenic stimulus. During tumor progression, expression of multiple other angiogenic factors is turned on.

DIRECT ANGIOGENESIS INHIBITORS

In contrast to single angiogenic factor antagonists, angiogenesis inhibitors that block a common angiogenic pathway would be more effective for cancer treatment. Alternatively, those angiogenesis inhibitors that directly inhibit endothelial cell proliferation, migration or differentiation would also overcome the drug resistant problem as the genome of endothelial cells is stable. Several angiogenesis inhibitors including angiostatin and endostatin have been reported to directly inhibit endothelial cell growth although the underlying mechanisms of their actions are not fully understood.

Angiostatin and its related fragments

The structure of angiostatin includes the first four kringle domains of plasminogen. A Kringle (*kringla* in Swedish) is a type of Scandinavian cookie folded into two rings. This term was originally adopted to describe a triple loop structure linked by three pairs of disulfide bonds present in prothrombin. Kringle structure exists in many proteins that can contain anything from one to several kringles. The primary amino acid sequence of each kringle domain is composed of approximate 80 amino acids. In addition to the six conserved cysteine residues in their predicted positions, amino acids flanking the third and fourth cysteines are also highly conserved. However, other amino acids in the primary structure are less conserved among various kringles. Amino acid sequence analysis of kringle domains of human angiostatin shows that K1, K2, K3 and K4 display considerable similarity (about 50% identity)[25]. Both NMR and X-ray crystallography demonstrate that the high degree of primary sequence homology translates into a remarkably uniform conformation. Among these individual kringles, K1 has been identified as the most potent inhibitor for endothelial cell growth. K3 exhibits higher inhibitory potency than K2. Surprisingly, K4 is virtually inactive in suppression of endothelial cell growth. Indeed, a short version of angiostatin that only contains the first three kringle domains without K4 (K1-3) seems to be more active than K1-4 in inhibition of endothelial cell growth[25]. It is this form of angiostatin that is in clinical trials in the treatment of human cancer. It should be cautiously emphasized that, due to its smaller size, K1-3 may have a relatively short half-life *in vivo*. Thus, *in vitro* activity should not be directly translated into the *in vivo* effects. Kringle 4 is a special segment that manifests high affinity for lysine binding. In addition, K1 has been reported to bind to lysine with relatively high affinity. Since K1, but not K4, is a potent endothelial inhibitor and both kringles bind to lysine, lysine binding does not seem to play critical role in suppression of angiogenesis. Another unique feature of K4 is that it contains two clusters of positively charged lysine residues, adjacent to cysteine 22 and cysteine 80. Inspection of the three dimensional structure reveals that these lysines, together with lysine 59 configure an exposed and positively charged area in K4, whereas other kringles lack such a cationic cluster[25]. Whether this lysine-enriched domain in K4 contributes to the loss of endothelial inhibitory activity is not known. However, one could speculate that a cationic domain may interact with a negatively charged domain in another protein, such as the heparan sulfate proteoglycans (HSPGs) in the extracellular matrix. This interaction could simply sequester K4 and prevent it from endothelial inhibition. The kringle structure is essential to maintain the anti-endothelial activity of angiostatin. Disruption of intrachain and interchain disulfide bonds by reducing reagents completely abolishes the anti-endothelial activity of angiostatin[25]. This information is important in manufacturing biologically active angiostatin and other kringle fragments for the use in antiangiogenesis. Similarly, unfolded or misfolded angiostatin or kringles expressed as cytosolic proteins should not be used in searching for angiostatin receptor(s) and studying molecular mechanisms. For example, angiostatin expressed in bacterial cells has to be appropriately refolded in order to inhibit endothelial cell growth and angiogenesis.

Like other individual kringle domains, the K5 domain of human plasminogen contains 80 amino acid residues. Primary structure alignment shows that K5 exhibits remarkable sequence identity (about 60%) with K1 although K2, K3 and K4 also share significant homologies with K5[26]. Similar to K1 and K4, K5 is a lysine-binding kringle of human plasminogen. Unlike K4, K5 lacks clusters of lysine residues in its primary structure. It was hypothesized that K5 might inhibit endothelial cell growth and angiogenesis. Surprisingly, both proteolytic and appropriately folded recombinant K5 displays remarkably more potent anti-endothelial effect than the other individual kringle domains. In fact, K5 alone exhibits several folds greater effect than the K1-4 of angiostatin[26]. This unexpected finding suggests that K5 might inhibit endothelial cell growth via a separate mechanism, or that K5 is a more potent inducer of inhibitory targets on endothelial cells. It is concluded from these *in vitro* studies that the ranking order of endothelial cell inhibition is K5>K1-3>K1-4>K1>K3>K2>K4. However, these *in vitro* data have not been directly translated into antiangiogenic activity *in vivo*. For example, K5 has been found to be less active than angiostatin in suppression of angiogenesis in the chick chorioallantoic membrane assay and the mouse corneal angiogenesis model. Insufficient suppression of *in vivo* angiogenesis by K5 is mainly due to its relatively short half-life *in vivo*. Thus, antiangiogenic effect of a given compound must be tested in *in vivo* angiogenesis models but not only in *in vitro* endothelial cell cultures.

Based on the findings that both angiostatin and K5 inhibit endothelial cell growth, it was speculated that a combination of these two fragments would produce greater effect. Indeed, *in vitro* studies show that a combination of K1-4 and K5 produce a remarkably synergistic activity on suppression of capillary endothelial cell growth[27]. These results suggest that angiostatin and K5 might inhibit endothelial cell proliferation via separate pathways. This initial study stimulated the effort of obtaining a fragment of the entire kringle domain (K1-5) of human plasminogen. Urokinase-activated plasmin has been used to proteolytically release a fragment containing the K1-4 plus the most part of K5 (K1-5) of human plasminogen. Similar to a combination of angiostatin and K5, K1-5 displays approximately 50-fold greater activity than angiostatin on inhibition of endothelial cell growth. Consistent with these *in vitro* results, K1-5 has been found to produce potent antiangiogenic and antitumor activities at low doses at which angiostatin is inactive. Like angiostatin and K5, the inhibitory activity of K1-5 is restricted to the endothelial lineage but does not affect other cell types. Recently it has been found that K1-5 is a naturally occurring angiogenesis inhibitor in the body[28]. This finding suggests that K1-5 plays a role in regulation of physiological and pathological angiogenesis.

Antiangiogenic mechanisms of angiostatin

The angiostatic mechanism of most endogenous angiogenesis inhibitors remains an enigma. Mechanistic studies of angiogenesis inhibitors have become a focus of many academies and pharmaceutical companies. Despite great efforts, little is known about endothelial cell components with which these inhibitors interact. The endothelial cell targets include endothelial cell surface receptors, signaling pathways, activation of gene expression and signals leading to quiescent endothelial phenotypes. As a consequence, lack of molecular mechanisms has become one of the most common criticisms of reviewers to exclude publications of most research articles in high impact journals.

Although several studies indicate that endothelial cell apoptosis, suppression of integrin signaling pathways, antagonistic effect of growth factor-induced signaling pathways, regulation of oncogenes and tumor suppressor genes and repression of endothelial cell cycles have been suggested to be involved in antiangiogenic activities of these inhibitors, none of the data provide compelling mechanistic evidence, especially in *in vivo* settings. However, these studies have pointed that the underlying mechanisms of endogenous angiogenesis inhibitors are complex and require many signaling players to coordinately suppress angiogenesis. As angiostatin is in clinical trials, it is essential to understand the underlying antiangiogenic mechanism. Although the answer to this question remains unknown, it is worthwhile to mention a couple of studies. Some have reported the isolation of possible receptors of angiostatin (ATPase, Angiomoietin)[29, 30, 31]. Another study suggests that angiostatin could prevent the G2/M transition of endothelial cell cycle[32]. Recently, it has been demonstrated that endothelial apoptosis may play a role in mediation of antiangiogenic activity of angiostatin[33]. It would be interesting to see if kringle domains of other proteins can also inhibit endothelial cell growth through the same pathways.

ORAL ANGIOGENESIS INHIBITORS

Although many antiangiogenic protein molecules have been shown to effectively block tumor growth and metastasis in mice, their therapeutic values in the treatment of human cancers are still questionable. Several dose and mechanistic related obstacles need to be resolved before a large number of cancer patients can be considered for therapy. According to animal studies, relatively large dosages (20-100 mg/kg) of these angiogenesis inhibitors have to be delivered in order to reach maximal effects. When these amounts are translated into human trials, it is unattractive to deliver huge amounts of biologically active recombinant proteins for long-term, if not life-span, treatments of a large number of cancer patients. In addition to high dosages, frequent injections of these angiogenesis inhibitors are also required. Therefore, discovery of small molecules in natural products as angiogenesis inhibitors is an important approach in improving or even replacing the current antiangiogenic therapy in the treatment of cancer and other diseases. Indeed, of the 20 best-selling non-protein drugs in 1999, 9 were derived or developed as the result of leads generated by natural products. Among these natural products, "functional food" has become increasingly appreciated by both medical professionals and the general public, due to its health benefits. These "daily" consumed natural products have shown beneficial effects correlated with lower risks of developing lethal diseases such as cancer and heart diseases, and they can be obtained without prescriptions. Polyphenols, especially flavonoids, that are rich in fruits, soybeans, vegetables, herbs, roots and leaves, act as active components in prevention of cancer, heart diseases and diabetes. For example, fresh green tea contains large amounts of catechin polyphenols, while resveratrol and quercetin are enriched in grapes, red wine and other food products. These compounds have been extensively studied for their effects in suppression of tumor growth and prevention of heart diseases in animal models. Several years ago, our laboratory reported that catechins in green tea suppress angiogenesis when they were given orally[34]. Excited by this initial finding, more than 20 other polyphenols molecules present in various plant extracts have been found to inhibit angiogenesis[35, 36]. Although their activities are non-specific for tumors and the underlying mechanisms are complex, these natural compounds have several great advantages over other anticancer therapeutic agents: 1) Many of these polyphenols are rich in our daily diets and can be easily obtained in grocery stores without prescriptions.

2) These polyphenol-enriched natural products are usually available at low costs. 3) Ingestion of these natural products does not require FDA approvals. 4) Polyphenol small molecules can usually be sufficiently absorbed after oral ingestion. 5) They rarely have any side-effects, as many have been used as food products for centuries. 6) The half-life of many polyphenols in the body is relatively long. 7) They are ideal therapeutic agents for long-term prevention and treatment of diseases such as angiogenesis dependent diseases. For example, antiangiogenesis compounds may have to be delivered for the rest of a cancer patient's life. As oral angiogenesis antagonists, we would like to emphasize that these compounds are non-specific angiogenesis inhibitors. They generally inhibit the growth of a wide spectrum of cell types. However, endothelial cells seem to be more sensitive to these polyphenols than other cell types, because relatively low concentrations of these polyphenols can result in endothelial cell inhibition. Thus, selective inhibition of angiogenesis can be achieved by using low dosages.

Based on the chemical structures of these natural antiangiogenic polyphenols, it most likely seems possible to identify more potent and specific angiogenesis inhibitors from their synthetic analogs. For example, flavopiridol is a synthetic flavone derivative with potent anti-endothelial, antiangiogenic and antitumor effect. Currently, flavopiridol is in phase II clinical trials for the treatment of various cancer forms in humans. We speculate that both natural and synthetic polyphenolic compounds will become important therapeutic agents in cancer and other angiogenesis dependent diseases. These compounds, either alone or in combinations with other current therapeutic strategies, will produce beneficial effects against most common human diseases including cancer and cardiovascular diseases.

CONCLUSIONS

Antiangiogenesis has become one of the most exciting approaches in the development of cancer drugs. There is no doubt that blockage of tumor blood supply will be beneficial for cancer patients. Indeed, many available angiogenesis inhibitors have produced remarkable antitumor effects in mice models. However, it is uncertain if these angiogenesis inhibitors will produce similar effects in human patients. According to cancer therapy history, translation of animal results into clinical therapy is a highly risky jump. The most frequently encountered problem in the past is why a molecule or a drug can block tumor growth in mice but fails in human trials. There is no satisfactory answer to this old question. There is a fundamental difference between experimental animal tumors and spontaneous human cancers. For example, in mouse transplantable tumor models, an implanted tumor grows into a relatively large size within a few weeks, whereas a spontaneous human cancer may take years to grow into a similar size. Thus, growth rates of blood vessels between a mouse tumor and a human tumor may be different. This difference may influence expression levels of angiogenic markers, which these drug target. In addition, a slow-growing spontaneous human tumor has a long history of gene mutations and contains many more heterogeneous cell populations than a mouse fast-growing tumor. Thus, a human cancer may produce multiple angiogenic factors and becomes resistant to the treatment with single angiogenic factor antagonists. Although numerous protein and chemical molecules are found to inhibit angiogenesis, the underlying mechanisms of their actions are poorly understood. Without knowing molecular mechanisms, the outcomes of their human trials are unpredictable. In fact, several ongoing antiangiogenic clinical trials including angiostatin, endostatin, avastin and matrix metalloproteinase inhibitors are all disappointing[3]. Sadly, the failure of these trials implies that we have a long way to go before finding a panacea to cure cancer.

References

1. Algire, G. H., Chalkley, H. W., Legallais, F. Y., and Park, H. D. (1945) Vascular reactions of normal and malignant tissues in vivo. *J. Natl Cancer Inst* 6, 73-85
2. Folkman, J. (1971) Tumor angiogenesis: therapeutic implications. *N Engl J Med* 285, 1182-1186.
3. Dembner, A. (2002) Tumor fighting drugs suffer setbacks. *Boston Globe* Teusday, C1-C2
4. Gimbrone, M. A., Jr., Cotran, R. S., Leapman, S. B., and Folkman, J. (1974) Tumor growth and neovascularization: an experimental model using the rabbit cornea. *J Natl Cancer Inst* 52, 413-427.
5. McDonald, D. M., and Baluk, P. (2002) Significance of blood vessel leakiness in cancer. *Cancer Res* 62, 5381-5385.
6. Folberg, R., Hendrix, M. J., and Maniotis, A. J. (2000) Vasculogenic mimicry and tumor angiogenesis. *Am J Pathol* 156, 361-381.
7. Maniotis, A. J., Folberg, R., Hess, A., Seftor, E. A., Gardner, L. M., Pe'er, J., Trent, J. M., Meltzer, P. S., and Hendrix, M. J. (1999) Vascular channel formation by human melanoma cells in vivo and in vitro: vasculogenic mimicry. *Am J Pathol* 155, 739-752.
8. Hashizume, H., Baluk, P., Morikawa, S., McLean, J. W., Thurston, G., Roberge, S., Jain, R. K., and McDonald, D. M. (2000) Openings between defective endothelial cells explain tumor vessel leakiness. *Am J Pathol* 156, 1363-1380.
9. Cao, Y. (1998) Endogenous angiogenesis inhibitors: angiostatin, endostatin, and other proteolytic fragments. *Prog Mol Subcell Biol* 20, 161-176.
10. Cao, Y., Linden, P., Farnebo, J., Cao, R., Eriksson, A., Kumar, V., Qi, J. H., Claesson-Welsh, L., and Alitalo, K. (1998) Vascular endothelial growth factor C induces angiogenesis in vivo. *Proc Natl Acad Sci U S A* 95, 14389-14394.
11. Migdal, M., Huppertz, B., Tessler, S., Comforti, A., Shibuya, M., Reich, R., Baumann, H., and Neufeld, G. (1998) Neuropilin-1 is a placenta growth factor-2 receptor. *J Biol Chem* 273, 22272-22278.
12. Soker, S., Takashima, S., Miao, H. Q., Neufeld, G., and Klagsbrun, M. (1998) Neuropilin-1 is expressed by endothelial and tumor cells as an isoform-specific receptor for vascular endothelial growth factor. *Cell* 92, 735-745.
13. Makinen, T., Jussila, L., Veikkola, T., Karpanen, T., Kettunen, M. I., Pulkkanen, K. J., Kauppinen, R., Jackson, D. G., Kubo, H., Nishikawa, S., Yla-Herttuala, S., and Alitalo, K. (2001) Inhibition of lymphangiogenesis with resulting lymphedema in transgenic mice expressing soluble VEGF receptor-3. *Nat Med* 7, 199-205.
14. Ferrara, N., and Alitalo, K. (1999) Clinical applications of angiogenic growth factors and their inhibitors. *Nat Med* 5, 1359-1364.
15. Cao, Y., Ji, W. R., Qi, P., and Rosin, A. (1997) Placenta growth factor: identification and characterization of a novel isoform generated by RNA alternative splicing. *Biochem Biophys Res Commun* 235, 493-498.
16. Maglione, D., Guerriero, V., Viglietto, G., Delli-Bovi, P., and Persico, M. G. (1991) Isolation of a human placenta cDNA coding for a protein related to the vascular permeability factor. *Proc Natl Acad Sci U S A* 88, 9267-9271.
17. Maglione, D., Guerriero, V., Viglietto, G., Ferraro, M. G., Aprelikova, O., Alitalo, K., Del Vecchio, S., Lei, K. J., Chou, J. Y., and Persico, M. G. (1993) Two alternative mRNAs coding for the angiogenic factor, placenta growth factor (PlGF), are transcribed from a single gene of chromosome 14. *Oncogene* 8, 925-931.
18. Cao, Y., Chen, H., Zhou, L., Chiang, M. K., Anand-Apte, B., Weatherbee, J. A., Wang, Y., Fang, F., Flanagan, J. G., and Tsang, M. L. (1996) Heterodimers of placenta growth factor/vascular endothelial growth factor. Endothelial activity, tumor cell expression, and high affinity binding to Flk-1/KDR. *J Biol Chem* 271, 3154-3162.
19. Cao, Y., Linden, P., Shima, D., Browne, F., and Folkman, J. (1996) In vivo angiogenic activity and hypoxia induction of heterodimers of placenta growth factor/vascular endothelial growth factor. *J Clin Invest* 98, 2507-2511.
20. Olofsson, B., Pajusola, K., Kaipainen, A., von Euler, G., Joukov, V., Saksela, O., Orpana, A., Pettersson, R. F., Alitalo, K., and Eriksson, U. (1996) Vascular endothelial growth factor B, a novel growth factor for endothelial cells. *Proc Natl Acad Sci U S A* 93, 2576-2581.

21. Kim, K. J., Li, B., Winer, J., Armanini, M., Gillett, N., Phillips, H. S., and Ferrara, N. (1993) Inhibition of vascular endothelial growth factor-induced angiogenesis suppresses tumour growth in vivo. *Nature* 362, 841-844.
22. Millauer, B., Shawver, L. K., Plate, K. H., Risau, W., and Ullrich, A. (1994) Glioblastoma growth inhibited in vivo by a dominant-negative Flk-1 mutant. *Nature* 367, 576-579.
23. Relf, M., LeJeune, S., Scott, P. A., Fox, S., Smith, K., Leek, R., Moghaddam, A., Whitehouse, R., Bicknell, R., and Harris, A. L. (1997) Expression of the angiogenic factors vascular endothelial cell growth factor, acidic and basic fibroblast growth factor, tumor growth factor beta-1, platelet-derived endothelial cell growth factor, placenta growth factor, and pleiotrophin in human primary breast cancer and its relation to angiogenesis. *Cancer Res* 57, 963-969.
24. Inoue, M., Hager, J. H., Ferrara, N., Gerber, H. P., and Hanahan, D. (2002) VEGF-A has a critical, nonredundant role in angiogenic switching and pancreatic beta cell carcinogenesis. *Cancer Cell* 1, 193-202.
25. Cao, Y., Ji, R. W., Davidson, D., Schaller, J., Marti, D., Sohndel, S., McCance, S. G., O'Reilly, M. S., Llinas, M., and Folkman, J. (1996) Kringle domains of human angiostatin. Characterization of the anti-proliferative activity on endothelial cells. *J Biol Chem* 271, 29461-29467.
26. Cao, Y., Chen, A., An, S. S., Ji, R. W., Davidson, D., and Llinas, M. (1997) Kringle 5 of plasminogen is a novel inhibitor of endothelial cell growth. *J Biol Chem* 272, 22924-22928.
27. Cao, R., Wu, H. L., Veitonmaki, N., Linden, P., Farnebo, J., Shi, G. Y., and Cao, Y. (1999) Suppression of angiogenesis and tumor growth by the inhibitor K1-5 generated by plasmin-mediated proteolysis. *Proc Natl Acad Sci U S A* 96, 5728-5733.
28. Li, T. S., Kaneda, Y., Ueda, K., Hamano, K., Zempo, N., and Esato, K. (2001) The influence of tumour resection on angiostatin levels and tumour growth--an experimental study in tumour-bearing mice. *Eur J Cancer* 37, 2283-2288.
29. Moser, T. L., Kenan, D. J., Ashley, T. A., Roy, J. A., Goodman, M. D., Misra, U. K., Cheek, D. J., and Pizzo, S. V. (2001) Endothelial cell surface F1-F0 ATP synthase is active in ATP synthesis and is inhibited by angiostatin. *Proc Natl Acad Sci U S A* 98, 6656-6661.
30. Moser, T. L., Stack, M. S., Asplin, I., Enghild, J. J., Hojrup, P., Everitt, L., Hubchak, S., Schnaper, H. W., and Pizzo, S. V. (1999) Angiostatin binds ATP synthase on the surface of human endothelial cells. *Proc Natl Acad Sci U S A* 96, 2811-2816.
31. Troyanovsky, B., Levchenko, T., Mansson, G., Matvijenko, O., and Holmgren, L. (2001) Angiomotin: an angiostatin binding protein that regulates endothelial cell migration and tube formation. *J Cell Biol* 152, 1247-1254.
32. Griscelli, F., Li, H., Bennaceur-Griscelli, A., Soria, J., Opolon, P., Soria, C., Perricaudet, M., Yeh, P., and Lu, H. (1998) Angiostatin gene transfer: inhibition of tumor growth in vivo by blockage of endothelial cell proliferation associated with a mitosis arrest. *Proc Natl Acad Sci U S A* 95, 6367-6372.
33. Claesson-Welsh, L., Welsh, M., Ito, N., Anand-Apte, B., Soker, S., Zetter, B., O'Reilly, M., and Folkman, J. (1998) Angiostatin induces endothelial cell apoptosis and activation of focal adhesion kinase independently of the integrin-binding motif RGD. *Proc Natl Acad Sci U S A* 95, 5579-5583.
34. Cao, Y., and Cao, R. (1999) Angiogenesis inhibited by drinking tea. *Nature* 398, 381.
35. Brakenhielm, E., Cao, R., and Cao, Y. (2001) Suppression of angiogenesis, tumor growth, and wound healing by resveratrol, a natural compound in red wine and grapes. *Faseb J* 15, 1798-1800.
36. Cao, Y., Cao, R., and Brakenhielm, E. (2002) Antiangiogenic mechanisms of diet-derived polyphenols. *J Nutr Biochem* 13, 380-390.

MUTATED TYROSINE KINASES AS THERAPEUTIC TARGETS IN MYELOID LEUKEMIAS

Martin Sattler, Blanca Scheijen, Ellen Weisberg, James D. Griffin [*]

Department of Medical Oncology, Dana-Farber Cancer Institute, and the Dept. of Medicine, Brigham and Women's Hospital and Harvard Medical School, Boston, MA USA

ABSTRACT

Tyrosine kinases are commonly mutated and activated in both acute and chronic myeloid leukemias. Here, we review the functions, signaling activities, mechanism of transformation, and therapeutic targeting of two prototypic tyrosine kinase oncogenes, BCR-ABL and FLT3, associated with chronic myeloid leukemia (CML) and acute myeloid leukemia (AML), respectively. BCR-ABL is generated by the Philadelphia chromosome translocation between chromosomes 9 and 22, creating a chimeric oncogene in which the *BCR* and c-*ABL* genes are fused. The product of this oncogene, BCR-ABL, has elevated ABL tyrosine kinase activity and transforms hematopoietic cells by exerting a wide variety of biological effects, including reduction in growth factor dependence, enhanced viability, and altered adhesion of chronic myelocytic leukemia (CML) cells. Elevated tyrosine kinase activity of BCR-ABL is critical for activating downstream signalling cascades and for all aspects of transformation, explaining the remarkable clinical efficacy of the tyrosine kinase inhibitor, imatinib mesylate (STI571). By comparison, FLT3 is mutated in about one third of all cases of AML, most often through a mechanism that involves an internal tandem duplication (ITD) of a small number of amino acid residues in the juxtamembrane domain of the receptor. As is the case for BCR-ABL, these mutations activate the kinase activity constitutively, activate multiple signaling pathways, and result in an augmentation of

[*] Corresponding author: James D. Griffin, Department of Medical Oncology, Dana-Farber Cancer Institute, 44 Binney Street, Boston, MA 02115, USA, E-mail: james_griffin@dfci. harvard.edu , Phone: 617-632-3360, Fax: 617-632-4388,

New Trends in Cancer for the 21st Century, edited by
Llombart-Bosch and Felipo, Kluwer Academic/Plenum Publishers, 2003

121

proliferation and viability. Transformation by FLT3-ITD can readily be observed in murine models, and FLT3 cooperates with other types of oncogenes to create a fully transformed acute leukemia. FLT3 tyrosine kinase inhibitors are currently being evaluated in clinical trials and may be very useful therapeutic agents in AML.

TYROSINE KINASE ONCOGENES IN LEUKEMIA

Activating mutations in tyrosine kinase oncogenes are the most common type of mutations detected in human myeloid leukemias. In "chronic" myeloid leukemias such as CML or chronic myelomonocytic leukemia, there is considerable evidence that an activated tyrosine kinase oncogene, by itself, is sufficient to cause the disease. However, in "acute" myeloid leukemias, other mutations are also required. This latter "two-hit" hypothesis for AML is validated in murine models of leukemia, and is very useful in designing novel therapeutic strategies.

More than 95% of patients with CML have translocations that activate the ABL kinase. Furthermore, although not discussed further here, patients with chronic myelomonocytic leukemia (CMML) often show activation of the PDGF receptor beta, and occasionally in other tyrosine kinases as well. In animal models, BCR-ABL appears to be sufficient to cause a myeloproliferative or lymphoproliferative syndrome without the requirement of mutations in other known oncogenes, although this remains a controversial topic.

In AML, transformation is likely to be associated with multiple oncogenic events. Tyrosine kinase mutations by themselves are probably sufficient to cause myeloproliferative disease, but must cooperate with a second oncogene to cause AML. For instance, FLT3-ITDs are sufficient to cause a myeloproliferative phenotype with normal differentiation in bone marrow transplant assay, but not AML. Gene rearrangements involving transcriptional regulators, like AML1/ETO, CBFβSMMHC, or PML/RARα fusion proteins, may impair hematopoietic differentiation, but when present alone are also not sufficient to cause AML. A unifying hypothesis is that two different classes of mutations are required for the AML phenotype characterized by an oncogene, such as a tyrosine kinase that confers a proliferative and/or survival advantage of hematopoietic progenitors, and secondly an oncogene that results in impaired differentiation. For example, *FLT3-ITDs* would exemplify Class I mutations that confer proliferative and/or survival advantage to cells through activation of the STAT, RAS/MAPK and PI3K/AKT pathways, and would be complemented by a Class II mutation exemplified by the *AML1/ETO* gene rearrangement that result in impaired differentiation and the AML phenotype[1, 2]. Besides support from animal models, this hypothesis is underscored by the observation that mutations in distinct Class I genes, rarely co-exist in the same patient. Similarly, the t(8;21), inv(16), t(15;17) and 11q23 gene rearrangements that are typical of Class II mutations are not present concurrently in the same blasts. Thus, in the vast majority of patients, only one mutation from each class is present in each patient.

BCR-ABL

BCR-ABL is the best studied tyrosine kinase oncogene in human leukemia. The incidence of CML is approximately 5 cases per 100,000 individuals per year, a rate that increases with patient age, and the disease accounts for 7% to 15% of all leukemias in adults[3]. There is no evidence that genetic predisposition plays a role in the development of CML, but evidence from studies of Hiroshima atomic bomb survivors and patients who underwent radiation therapy for ankylosing spondylitis shows that ionizing radiation can cause CML [3]. Using sensitive nested polymerase chain reaction (PCR), very low levels of BCR-ABL transcripts can sometimes be detected in the blood of healthy people, but there is no indication that such people will develop CML. The BCR-ABL oncogene, generated by the Philadelphia (Ph) chromosome translocation, t(9;22)(q34;q11), was first described by Nowell and Hungerford in 1960[4]. The fusion of the BCR and ABL genes results in the production of a constitutively active tyrosine kinase that enhances proliferation and viability of myeloid lineage cells. BCR-ABL is likely to be sufficient by itself to cause chronic myelogenous leukemia (CML), but over time other genetic events occur and acute leukemia develops. There are 3 different BCR/ ABL proteins that are generated by 3 different breakpoints in the BCR gene. p190BCR-ABL is associated with acute lymphocytic leukemia (ALL), p210BCR-ABL is associated with CML, and p230BCR-ABL is associated with chronic neutrophilic leukemia[5-14]. However, it is currently not known how these 3 forms of BCR-ABL differ from each other in signaling. The constitutive activation of the tyrosine kinase activity of ABL is the initial and most critical signaling event associated with the BCR-ABL oncogene, and is crucial for all transforming functions of the oncogenes. CML is typically diagnosed after patients present with fatigue, weight loss, or abdominal symptoms, and appear to have an elevated white blood cell count. The chronic or stable phase is characterized by a massive expansion of myeloid cells, a packed marrow, leukocytosis, and splenomegaly. Differentiation of myeloid cells is normal however, and it is usually easy to distinguish CML from other types of myeloid leukemia. The initial stable phase is followed in many cases by transformation to an acute leukemic phase, called blast crisis. The diagnosis of CML is confirmed by demonstration of the Ph chromosome or detection of BCR-ABL transcripts by PCR. In the blast crisis phase, new cytogenetic events are common, but the Ph chromosome is always retained. Approximately 50% of patients with CML have a predominance of myeloid blasts, 25% have lymphoid blasts, and 25% have undifferentiated or other blasts, but blasts from multiple lineages can co-exist as well. The prognosis of patients in blast phase treated with standard chemotherapy is quite poor, with a median survival of 3 to 9 months[15]. The therapy of both stable- and blast-phase CML has undergone a dramatic change with the introduction of the small molecule tyrosine kinase inhibitor, imatinib mesylate (Glivec, Gleevec, STI571; Novartis Pharma AG), which blocks the kinase activity of ABL and leads to reduced viability and proliferation of CML cells. Essentially all stable-phase patients have a complete hematologic response, and many become Ph-negative over a period of months. Patients in blast phase also respond well to STI571, although the majority relapse after a few months [16-18]. The drug is remarkably well tolerated, despite the fact that it is also an excellent inhibitor of the PDGFR and c-KIT[16,19-24]. Allogeneic bone marrow transplantation is the only known curative therapy for CML, and there are many studies currently focused on combining imatinib with other therapies, including BMT.

TRANSFORMATION BY BCR-ABL

Rowley[25] showed in 1973 that the Ph chromosome is the result of a reciprocal translocation involving the long arms of chromosomes 9 and 22. The Ph chromosome was found in cells of the myeloid, megakaryocytic, and erythroid lineages, suggesting that the disorder originates in a stem cell with pluripotent capabilities. The molecular genetics of the Ph chromosome were studied in detail in the early 1980s. In 1983 Heisterkamp et al.[7] showed c-*ABL* to be located on the segment of chromosome 9 that is translocated to chromosome 22. The breakpoints in chromosome 22 were found to occur over a very short stretch of DNA (5 to 6 kilobases), called the breakpoint cluster region (BCR). The breakpoints occurred in the middle of a gene, now called *BCR*, that is widely expressed and normally involved in regulating the oxidative burst in neutrophils. In CML, the classic fusion is b2a2 or b3a2 fusing exon 2 (b2) or exon 3 (b3) of c-*BCR* to exon 2 (a2) of c-*ABL*, leading to an oncoprotein of 210 kDa molecular weight[8-10]. In the case of Ph-positive ALL, there is fusion with the production of an oncoprotein of 190 kDa molecular weight[11-14]. A third translocation is associated with chronic neutrophilic leukemia, encoding a 230 kDa BCR-ABL protein[6]. Each of these oncoproteins contains the same segment of c-ABL, differing in the amount of BCR present in the oncogene.

The biological activities of BCR-ABL include the induction of proliferation, inhibition of apoptosis, altering adhesion, and supporting genomic instability. However, the propensity for CML to evolve into blast crisis over time, due to the accumulation of new mutations, is still not well understood. The alteration in adhesion, homing, and migration caused by *BCR-ABL* is of particular interest and may contribute substantially to the pathogenesis of CML. BCR-ABL has prominent effects on the function of integrins, which are important in hematopoietic cells for growth regulation, migration in and out of the marrow, and in numerous functions of mature myeloid cells. CML cells have a diminished capacity to adhere to stromal layers[26] and to fibronectin or its proteolytic fragments [27], all ascribed to altered functions of ß1 integrins.

FUNCTIONAL DOMAINS OF BCR-ABL AND THEIR ROLE IN TRANSFORMATION

c-BCR and c-ABL have multiple functional domains that contribute to different aspects of transformation by BCR-ABL.

BCR

Structurally, the c-BCR protein contains an oligomerization domain, a DBL-homology and a guanosine triphosphate (GTP)-ase activating protein (GAP)-homology domain[28]. The oligomerization domain of c-BCR is contained within the first 61 amino acids and mediates oligomerization of c-BCR. In BCR-ABL, this domain is required for activation of the ABL kinase and this activation is essential for transformation of target cells[29]. c-BCR can be substituted in other transforming *ABL* oncogenes by protein structures that cause oligomerization, such as TEL[30]. The kinase activity in BCR/ ABL also results in autophosphorylation including a tyrosine at position 177 in c-BCR, which has been identified as a major GRB2 SH2 binding site in BCR-ABL[31-33]. GRB2 is constitutively linked through SH3 domain interactions to SOS, resulting in activation of RAS. A BCR-ABL mutant with a phenylalanine (Phe) substitution (Tyr177Phe) reduced Ras activation in some assays[31-33]. In hematopoietic cells this BCR-ABL mutant can still activate Ras and can be transforming, suggesting that there are multiple pathways in *BCR/ ABL*-transformed hematopoietic cells that lead to activation of Ras. Ras belongs to a family of small GTPases that include Rac and Rho. There are a number of downstream effectors of Ras including serine and threonine kinases like RAF, extracellular signal-regulated kinase, or phosphatidylinositol 3–kinase (PI3K)[34]. Recent evidence suggests an unexpected role for Tyr177 in the induction of CML-like myeloproliferative disease by BCR-ABL in a murine leukemia model. Mutation of Tyr177 to Phe reduces the myeloproliferative disease induced by BCR-ABL, and leads to B- and T-lymphoid leukemias of prolonged latency in mice. This is consistent with the fact that the v-Abl oncoprotein, which lacks interaction with Grb2, does not induce a CML-like disease[35, 36].

In addition, we have recently found that phosphorylated Tyr177 recruits the scaffolding adapter Gab2 by means of a Grb2/Gab2 complex[37]. Compared to wild type BCR-ABL-expressing BaF3 cells, cells expressing BCR-ABL-Y177F exhibit markedly reduced Gab2 tyrosine phosphorylation and decreased association of phosphatidylinositol-3 kinase (PI3K) and Shp2 with both Gab2 and BCR-ABL. Activation of the PI3K/Akt and Ras/Erk pathways, cell proliferation and migration are decreased in BCR-ABL-Y177F cells. Most importantly, primary murine marrow cells from Gab2-/- mice are resistant to myeloid transformation by BCR-ABL. Our results identify Gab2 and its associated proteins as key mediators of leukemogenic signaling by BCR-ABL.

ABL KinaseDomain

As noted above, the transformation of cells by BCR-ABL is entirely dependent on an intact kinase domain of ABL. The tyrosine kinase c-Abl was identified as the cellular homolog of the transforming protein in the murine Abelson leukemia virus[38]. Mice with c-Abl gene disruption have perinatal mortality and display facial abnormalities and reduced osteoblast function. Also, the spleen is abnormal, and development of T-cell and especially B-cell progenitors in the bone marrow is reduced[39-41]. Although the exact function of c-ABL is unknown, it has been shown to be involved in transcriptional regulation and possibly is activated in response to certain types of DNA damage[42-44]. The kinase activity of c-ABL is regulated by the interaction of its SH3 domain with the activation loop of the tyrosine kinase domain. It has been suggested that autophosphorylation of c-ABL changes the conformation of this regulatory loop to stabilize the active conformation[45,46]. The ABL kinase inhibitor STI-571 takes advantage of these structural requirements by interacting with the conserved but rather less specific ATP binding sites, as well as the activation loop that has to be in an inactive conformation[47].

SH2 and SH3 Domains

The SH domains of c-ABL define its role as tyrosine kinase and are important in mediating and modulating the transforming activity in BCR-ABL. Mutation of the SH3 but not the SH2 domain of c-ABL has been demonstrated to generate a transforming protein in fibroblasts, but not in hematopoietic cells[48,49]. Thus, the ABL SH3 domain can potentially interact with an inhibitor of transformation. The role of the ABL SH2 domain in transformation by BCR-ABL is controversial. The ABL SH2 domain is not required for transformation in some assays but appears to be required for autocrine or paracrine growth factor independence in vitro[33, 50-53]. An interesting difference was found in the requirement of the SH2 domain for the induction of a CML-like disease in mice. Comparing p190BCR-

ABL and p210BCR-ABL, the SH2 domain was not required for induction of a B-lymphoid leukemia in mice. Under conditions in which BCR-ABL induced a CML-like myeloproliferative disease, p210 SH2 mutants were less efficient at this induction than p190 mutants[54].

CRKL Binding Site

*(X)*CRKL has been identified as a highly tyrosine phosphorylated protein in CML cells[55-57]. It is an adapter protein containing one SH2 followed by two SH3 domains and is closely related to v- Crk and c-Crk. *v-crk* is the oncogene in the avian retrovirus CT10 and has a deletion of the C-terminal SH3 domain[58]. Deletion of the CRKL-SH3 binding site, a proline rich domain in BCR-ABL, reduces the ability of the oncoprotein to transform fibroblasts[59]. However, this BCR/ ABL mutant transforms myeloid cells, causing growth factor independence[60]. CRKL has the potential function to link tyrosine-phosphorylated proteins to enzymes and lead to activation of pathways that could contribute to transformation.

Actin-Binding Domain

The BCR-ABL fusion protein is localized to the cytoskeleton through an actin-binding site in the C-terminus[61]. In myeloid cells transfected with the oncogene *BCR-ABL*, the actin cytoskeleton is rearranged with more F-actin than normal cells, and BCR-ABL colocalizes with the actin cytoskeleton. The actin-binding domain may also be important for transformation of fibroblasts[62] and the induction of a lethal leukemia by BCR-ABL. However, although the actin-binding domain of ABL enhances development of leukemia, it does not appear to be required[63].

CRITICAL SIGNALING PATHWAYS BY BCR-ABL

The *BCR-ABL* oncogene exerts several biologic effects on hematopoietic cells that are partly dependent on the model system being studied. In cell line models and in vivo studies in mice, *BCR-ABL* is mitogenic, induces factor independence, inhibits apoptosis, and alters integrin-mediated adhesion and motility. In primary CML cells, the major defects associated with BCR-ABL are aberrant regulation of adhesion and possibly enhanced motility and viability, although not all investigators agree on the latter. Studies have suggested, however, that very immature primary myeloid cells from patients in the stable phase of CML are more likely to show enhanced viability and growth-factor independence. BCR-ABL activates several different signaling pathways that enhance viability and proliferation.

In CML cell lines and cells from CML patients, the JAK/STAT pathway has been demonstrated to be constitutively activated. STAT1 and STAT5 were found to be the major tyrosine-phosphorylated STATs in p210BCR-ABL–containing cells[64, 65]. In cell lines transformed by p190BCR-ABL, there is also activation of STAT6[66]. Several oncogenes have been shown to be associated with constitutive phosphorylation of STAT5, and STAT5 has been reported to be phosphorylated in a variety of malignant disorders in addition to than CML[67, 68]. STAT5 has several important structural domains, including a DNA-binding sequence, an SH2 domain, and a transactivation domain. Phosphorylation of Tyr694 of STAT5A and Tyr699 of STAT5B creates a binding site for the SH2 domain of another STAT5 molecule[69-71, 72, 73]. The role of STAT5 in hematopoiesis of adult mice is not clear, because mice with a targeted disruption of the *STAT5A* and *STAT5B* genes have largely normal blood counts[74]. However, these mice had reduced myeloid progenitor counts, suggesting that STAT5 might be required to support immature hematopoiesis. Furthermore, STAT5 may also be required for normal fetal erythropoiesis[75]. This is consistent with the fact that BCR/ ABL produces leukemias in *STAT5A/B* double knockout mice, but with a reduced amount of pure myeloid leukemias[76]. We have shown that overexpression of a dominant negative form of STAT5B (STAT5; aminoacids 1-683) that lacks Tyr699 and the transcriptional activation domain in a BCR/ ABL-transformed hematopoietic cell line inhibited STAT5- dependent transcription and reduced growth and viability but did not cause cell cycle arrest[77]. A point mutation of the *STAT5* gene leading to a constitutively active form of STAT5 can support growth of the murine BaF3 cells line in the absence of murine IL-3[78]. Constitutive activation of STAT5, as described for CML cells, may therefore help to maintain viability in hemopoietic cells and thereby contribute to the myeloproliferative disease. Interestingly, disruption of the gene for interferon consensus sequence binding protein (ICSBP), a transcription factor of the interferon regulatory factor family, leads to abnormalities of hematopoiesis in mice. Mice that do not express ICSBP develop a blood disorder similar to CML, exhibiting a stable phase followed by a blast phase[79]. In CML cells, the expression levels of ICSBP are reduced or absent[80]. Overexpression of ICSBP negatively regulates normal hematopoiesis in mice and inhibits BCR-ABLinduced leukemia[81].

The PI3K family of enzymes regulates a variety of biological functions in different systems, such as apoptosis, mitogenesis, integrin activation, membrane trafficking, membrane ruffling, and chemotaxis. PI3K can phosphorylate PI at the D3 position and in vivo produces mainly PI-(3,4)-bisphosphate and PI-(3,4,5)-trisphosphate, which function as second messengers[82, 83]. The lipid products are thought to be involved in the membrane recruitment and activation of pleckstrin homology (PH) domain–containing proteins[84, 85] and may interact with FYVE motifs (Fab1p, YOTB, Vac1p, EEA1)[86, 87] or SH2 domains[88]. A role for PI3K as a pleiotropic regulator of signal transduction pathways and biological functions includes in part the functional regulation of AKT (survival, growth), Rac (motility, survival), S6kinase (protein synthesis), and others. PI3K can also be regulated by Ras and regulate Ras function itself [82, 83]. The p85 regulatory subunit of PI3K contains 2 SH2 domains (N- and C-terminal) and an SH3 domain. p85-PI3K can associate via its SH2 or SH3 domains to activated hematopoietic growth factor receptors (such as the c-KIT receptor[89]) and to signaling proteins (such as IRS-1[90], c-CBL[91], and GAB2[92, 93]). The p110 catalytic subunit functions to interact with protein tyrosine kinases and tyrosine-phosphorylated proteins, which results in the activation of PI-3 lipid kinase activity[94, 95]. BCR-ABL leads to constitutive activation of PI3K. In cell lines and mouse models, PI3K is important in transformation by BCR-ABL[91, 96, 97]. PI3K has been shown to have a regulatory function in apoptosis, and this may be of particular importance to CML because one of the biological effects of BCR-ABL in primary CML cells is a reduction in the sensitivity to certain inducers of cell death [98, 99]. Activation of AKT, the anti-apoptotic PH-domain containing serine/threonine kinase, by PI3K in BCR-ABL-transformed cells appears to play a major role in transformation[100]. AKT is the cellular homolog of v-Akt, which causes thymomas in mice[101, 102]. Activation of AKT requires both recruitment to the membrane and phosphorylation at threonine-308 and serine-473, likely by PDK1[103, 104]. There are many downstream antiapoptotic targets of AKT, for example, AKT can phosphorylate Bad and subsequently prevent cytochrome C release[105]. Bad is an inducer of apoptosis and it competes with Bax for binding to Bcl-2 and Bcl-xL. AKT can also regulate gene expression through direct phosphorylation of forkhead transcription factors [106]. Phosphorylation of the proapoptotic forkhead proteins on specific serine and threonine residues leads to export from the nucleus, binding to 14-3-3 proteins, and suppression of forkhead-induced gene transcription. BCR-ABL also inhibits the expression of p27Kip1 through the AKT pathway[107, 108]. p27Kip1 is a widely expressed inhibitor of cdk2, an essential cell cycle kinase regulating entry into the S phase. Suppression of the p27Kip1 protein level by BCR-ABL through PI3K/AKT is likely to lead to an accelerated entry into the S phase. AKT-independent mechanisms of PI3K include the activation of Rho, Rac, and Cdc42 proteins[109,110]. These small GTP-binding proteins signal towards the cytoskeleton and BCR-ABL causes cytoskeletal abnormalities. In BCR-ABL-transformed cells, Rac is downstream of PI3K and its activation is required for transformation[111]. Levels of bioactive inositol lipids generated by PI3K are regulated by polyinositol phosphatases. The most prominent members include the tumor suppressors PTEN and SHIP (SH2-domain containing inositol-5-phosphatase)[112,113]. The polyinositol-5-phosphatase SHIP1 is of special interest because its protein levels are dramatically downregulated by BCR-ABL[114]. Also, SHIP1 knockout mice develop a myeloproliferative syndrome characterized by a dramatic increase in numbers of GM progenitor cells in the marrow and spleen[115]. It is therefore possible that downregulation of SHIP1 contributes to the myeloproliferative phenotype in CML. Nevertheless, the mechanism whereby SHIP1 causes a myeloproliferative phenotype in mice is unknown.

Transformation of the hematopoietic cell lines with BCR-ABL results in an increase in reactive oxygen species compared with quiescent untransformed cells[116]. ROS contribute to several cellular functions and are known to be involved in the regulation of signal transduction, gene expression, and proliferation[117]. The biological effects of ROS vary widely in different cells and include modulation of signaling pathways by directly altering the activity of protein kinases and protein phosphatases (PTPases)[118, 119]. It is not known how BCR-ABL modulates the levels of ROS. We have demonstrated that inhibition of the mitochondrial respiratory chain by rotenone significantly decreases intracellular ROS levels[116]. This result suggests that mitochondria are an important source for ROS in BCR-ABL-transformed cells. In addition, it is also possible that BCR-ABL affects the protein levels or enzymatic activities of 1 or more enzymes that regulate ROS. Elevated levels of ROS have also been observed in cytokine signaling, such as in transforming growth factor-β[120], epidermal growth factor[121], PDGF[122], GM-CSF, IL-3, steel factor, and thrombopoietin[123]. Increased production of ROS is sufficient to cause a transforming phenotype itself. Overexpression of the superoxide-generating NADPH oxidase Mox1 in NIH3T3 fibroblasts increases cell growth and induces tumors in athymic mice[124]. Interestingly, the inhibition of SOD by the estrogen derivative 2-methoxy-estradiol kills leukemia cells but not normal lymphocytes[125]. SOD catalyzes the reduction of superoxide to H_2O_2. This finding suggests that SOD regulates a fine balance between cell survival and free-radical-mediated cell death. It has been suggested that ROS may act as second messengers to regulate activities of redox-sensitive enzymes, including protein kinases and protein phosphatases. Consistent with a potential role of ROS in BCR-ABL signaling, the PTPase activity in untransformed cells is decreased upon BCR-ABL transformation[116].

Furthermore, BCR-ABL-induced tyrosine phosphorylation can be inhibited by the addition of reducing agents, and the ABL kinase activity can be upregulated by ROS[116]. Overall, increased levels of ROS in BCR-ABL-transformed cells are consistent with a model in which increased ROS amplify BCR-ABL signaling, possibly by regulating redox-sensitive proteins such as cellular PTPases. The response of regulators of transcription to changes in the cellular redox status has been well described. Nuclear factor (NF)-kB; p53; and AP-1, the family of JUN/FOS transcription factors, can be regulated in response to redox signaling.

A SIGNALING MODEL FOR BCR-ABL

From the studies cited above, it is possible to derive a model explaining many of the mechanisms of transformation of the *BCR-ABL* oncogene. BCR activates the ABL tyrosine kinase, probably through oligomerization, promotes cytoplasmic localization, and activates at least 1 unique signaling pathway through the autophosphorylation site at Tyr177. The ABL tyrosine kinase phosophorylates itself, recruting signaling proteins with SH2 domains, phosphorylates neighboring proteins in the cytoskeleton and cytoplasm, and thereby activates signaling pathways normally controlled by hematopoietic growth factor receptors. When this oncogene is expressed in hematopoietic stem cells, proliferation and viability are enhanced. It is not clear if BCR-ABL increases self-renewal of hematopoietic stem cells, but it clearly does not block myeloid differentiation. The effects of p190BCR-ABL on immature B cells may be somewhat different in this regard. In CML, the myeloproliferative syndrome is a preleukemic disorder in many respects. Most importantly, mutations in other genes accumulate over time, resulting in progressive blocks in differentiation, and ultimately, acute leukemia. The signaling pathways discussed here, including Ras, PI3K, and JAK/STAT, have all been shown to play important roles in transformation, at least in some models. It seems unlikely that there is a single critical pathway activated by this oncogene that is uniquely responsible for transformation. Rather, there is likely to be substantial overlap in the biological effects resulting from each of these pathways and also substantial cross talk between them. From a clinical perspective, the ideal target for drug development is the tyrosine kinase itself, and the remarkable clinical activity of STI571, even in blast phase, has supported this concept completely. It is not currently known if the addition of other drugs blocking specific pathways downstream of BCR-ABL will have synergistic activity with imatinib mesylate, but such studies are underway. Overall, the success of STI571 is a testimony to the success of decades of scientific research on CML. The identification of the Philadelphia chromosome, demonstration of a translocation between chromosomes 9 and 22, identification of BCR and ABL as the translocated genes, and identification of the biochemical activities of BCR-ABL all played essential and critical roles in this story.

FLT3

The murine Flt3/Flk-2 receptor was cloned because of its structural relationship to c-fms, thus named fms-like tyrosine kinase 3[126], and simultaneously by degenerate PCR on a fetal liver cDNA library based on the conserved kinase domain of tyrosine kinase receptors (fetal liver kinase 2)[127]. The human homologue, originally termed stem cell tyrosine kinase-1 (STK-1), encodes a protein of 993 amino acids with 85% identity and 92% similarity with the corresponding mouse Flt3 protein[128, 129]. The Flt3 receptor has the same general structure as four other tyrosine kinase receptors that comprise the type III receptor tyrosine kinases (RTK) subfamily: c-Fms, the receptor for colony-stimulating factor-1 (CSF-1), c-Kit, and both of the receptors for platelet-derived growth factor (PDGFRα and PDGFRβ). Each of these receptor molecules has five immunoglobulin-like (Ig) domains in the extracellular region and a split catalytic domain in the intracellular part of the receptor.

The ligand for the Flt3 receptor (FL) encodes a type 1 transmembrane protein, but soluble and membrane-bound isoforms can be generated as a result of alternative splicing of mRNAs[130, 131]. FL mRNA transcripts are present in a wide variety of human and mouse tissues. The Flt3 receptor is preferentially expressed in primitive CD34$^+$ hematopoietic stem cells, pro-B cells and immature CD4$^-$CD8$^-$ thymocytes in addition to gonads, placenta and brain. In primary tumors, increased expression of Flt3 is detected on most leukemic samples of AML and B-ALL, but generally only at low levels on T-ALL[132,133]. Interestingly, Flt3 is the most differentially expressed gene that distinguishes a subset of human acute leukemias involving the mixed-lineage leukemia gene (*MLL*) (high expression) from conventional B-precursor ALL and AML[134]. FL stimulates proliferation and colony formation of the vast majority of adult and pediatric AML-leukemic cells and promotes their survival, although to a variable extent[135-137].

As predicted from the Flt3 expression pattern, FL potently enhances the colony-stimulating activity on hematopietic progenitor cells in synergy with G-CSF, GM-CSF, M-CSF, IL-3, IL-6, IL-11, IL-12 or KL. FL can also support proliferation of murine B cell progenitors alone or in combination with IL-7 or KL. In contrast, FL has no growth stimulating activity on progenitor cells committed to the erythrocyte, megakaryocyte, eosinophil, or mast cell lineages[138-140]. FL enhances the production of dendritic cells (DC) from CD34$^+$ (!) BM progenitor cells in combination with GM-CSF, TNF and IL-4. In vivo treatment of mice with FL results in dramatic increase of DC in all primary and secondary lymphoid tissues[141], and in humans it induces both CD11c$^+$ and CD11c$^-$ DC subsets[142, 143]. The phosphorylated cytoplasmic domain of murine Flt3 transduces activation signals through direct interaction with Grb2 and the p85 subunit of PI3K (Tyr-958), and phosphorylation of SHIP, Shc, Vav, RasGAP and PLCγ[144-146]. FLT3 also activates Stat5, but apparently only *Stat5a$^{-/-}$*, and not *Stat5b$^{-/-}$*, bone marrow progenitor cells are unresponsive to FL-mediated proliferative effects[147].

Detailed analysis in *flt3$^{-/-}$* mice has indicated that mainly primitive B lymphoid progenitor cells are affected in the absence of Flt3 expression. However, normal numbers of functional B cells are present in the periphery, and total composition and cell numbers of hematopoietic organs and peripheral blood are indistinguishable between *flt3$^{-/-}$* and wild-type mice. Although the Flt3 receptor is expressed on murine and human cell populations enriched for hematopoietic stem and progenitor cells, the population of multipotential and myeloid colony-forming progenitors is not affected in *flt3$^{-/-}$* mice. Only competitive repopulation experiments reveal a significant defect of Flt3-deficient stem cells, where reconstitution of the hematopoietic system is less efficient in comparison to wild-type stem cells, especially of the lymphoid lineage. In contrast, *flt3L$^{-/-}$* mice display an overt reduction in leukocyte counts of bone marrow, spleen, lymph nodes and peripheral blood, with additional defects in dendritic and NK cells[148].

Mutations in FLT3 have been commonly detected in primary samples from patients with AML. The most common mutation is an internal tandem duplication (ITD) in the juxtamembrane (JM) domain of *FLT3* in AML[149]. Subsequent studies have shown that FLT3 tandem duplications are present in 17-27% of *de novo* adult AML, 14-17% of childhood AML cases, in 3-5% of MDS, 20% of acute promyelocytic leukemia, and 3% of pediatric ALL, expressing myeloid antigens [150-153]. The presence of ITD in FLT3 correlates with a poor outcome in adult and pediatric AML. Disease-free and overall survival is even more inferior in FLT3-ITD cases lacking the wild type FLT3 allele[154]. The length of the ITD is variable, but the duplicated sequence is selected for in-frame fusions, and mostly involves the Tyr-rich stretch 587-NEYFYVDFREYEYD-560 located in exon 11. The FLT3-ITD receptor activates Stat5 and the MAP kinase pathway and promotes increased phosphorylation of AKT. Interestingly, in a murine BMT assay, FLT3-ITD, but not wild type FLT3, even with high expression levels, induces a myeloproliferative phenotype[155]. Remarkably, elongation of the JM portion rather than introduction of new tyrosine residues generates ligand-independent dimerized versions of Flt3., Several kinds of missense mutations at Asp-835 located in the activation loop of the second tyrosine kinase domain of FLT3 have been found in 7% of AML cases and 3% of MDS and ALL cases[156, 157]. All D835-mutant FLT3 variants induce constitutive tyrosine phosphorylation and confer IL-3-independence in 32D cells. D835 mutations occur independently of FLT3-ITD[157], arguing that each variant may contribute to the pathogenesis of acute leukemia.

FLT3 is the single most commonly mutated gene in AML, and confers a poor prognosis in most patients. As a consequence, there has been an intensive effort to develop FLT3-selective inhibitors as therapeutic reagents. This approach has been validated in part by activity of the STI571 ABL kinase inhibitor in CML blast crisis. Preclinical studies in cell culture and murine models of leukemia mediated by FLT3-ITD provide further support for this strategy[158-160]. For example, the tyrphostin AG1296, a selective inhibitor of FLT3, KIT and PDGFßR, inhibits the growth of BaF3 cells transformed by FLT3-ITD, as well as FLT3 autophosphorylation and activation of downstream targets such as STAT5A/B[158]. Although none of these compounds would be suitable for consideration in clinical trials in humans, these experiments provide evidence that FLT3 inhibition may be an effective approach to the subset of leukemias with activating mutations in FLT3, and perhaps for AML associated with overexpression of the wildtype FLT3.

FLT3 inhibitors with suitable pharmocokinetic and toxicity profiles for clinical testing have been reported in abstract form. For example, CT53518 (Millenium), a novel piperazinyl quinazoline, is a submicromolar inhibitor of FLT3, as well as PDGFßR and c-KIT. CT53518 has activity both in cell culture and in animal models of leukemia[161]. CEP-701 (Cepahlon), an orally bioavailable inhibitor of FLT3-ITD and activating loop mutants, has activity in a murine model based on injection of FLT3-ITD transfected BaF3 cells[162], as well as in primary AML cells in culture containing FLT3-ITD[163]. SU5614, SU5416 and SU11248 (SUGEN) mediate inhibition of FLT3-ITD transformed cells in vitro and in vivo[164, 165]. PKC412, a benzoylstaurosporine from Novartis Pharmaceuticals was developed as a VEGFR inhibitor, and had minimal toxicity in a Phase I trial in solid tumor patients. PKC412 is also a potent submicromolar inhibitor of FLT3-ITD in cell culture and murine models of leukemia[166], and is currently in clinical trials in AML. Each of these drugs has pharmacokinetic and toxicity profiles suitable for Phase I/II testing. It appears likely that several FLT3-selective inhibitors will be tested in clinical trials within the next year, with hope and promise for improving therapy in AML.

CONCLUSION

It is clear that tyrosine kinase oncogenes have emerged as major therapeutic targets in myeloid leukemias. In myeloproliferative syndromes such as CML or CMML, where a mutated kinase is likely to be the only oncogene present, therapy with a tyrosine kinase inhibitors can frequently induce dramatic and long-lasting remissions. In more advanced phases of CML, however, the remissions are partial and of shorter duration. This is due in many cases to the development (or emergence of preformed) drug resistance. In AML, where other oncogenes are present, it seems most likely that FLT3 inhibitors will be active, but not sufficient by themselves to cure the disease. Many questions remain. For example, is it possible to combine TK inhibitors in either CML or AML with standard chemotherapy and improve the remission rate and duration? Can signal transduction inhibitors be used in combination, and if so, is it more efficacious to target multiple points on a single, critical pathway, or is it better to target distinct pathways that are both important? What are the mechanisms of resistance to TK inhibitors, and how can they be circumvented, or prevented? Finally, activated tyrosine kinases are present in about 40% of patients with AML, but are there still other unidentified kinases that are mutated in the remaining 60%? Overall, it is clear that the concept of oncogene-targeted therapy has been validated, and it will be of great interest to determine the impact of this type of therapy for both hematologic and epithelial malignancies in the future.

REFERENCES

1. Dash A, Gilliland DG. Molecular genetics of acute myeloid leukaemia. Baillieres Best Pract Res Clin Haematol. 2001;14:49-64.
2. Gilliland DG. Hematologic malignancies. Curr Opin Hematol. 2001;8:189-191
3. Li FP. Epidemiology of chronic leukemia, in Wiernik P.H., Canellos G.P., Kyle R.A., et al (eds). Neoplastic Disease of the Blood. New York, Churchill Livingstone. 1991:7-14
4. Nowell PC, Hungerford DA. Chromosome studies on normal and leukemic human leukocytes. J Natl Cancer Inst. 1960;25:85-109
5. Kurzrock R, Shtalrid M, Romero P, Kloetzer WS, Talpas M, Trujillo JM, Blick M, Beran M, Gutterman JU. A novel c-abl protein product in Philadelphia-positive acute lymphoblastic leukaemia. Nature. 1987;325:631-635.
6. Pane F, Frigeri F, Sindona M, Luciano L, Ferrara F, Cimino R, Meloni G, Saglio G, Salvatore F, Rotoli B. Neutrophilic-chronic myeloid leukemia: a distinct disease with a specific molecular marker (BCR/ABL with C3/A2 junction). Blood. 1996;88:2410-2414.
7. Heisterkamp N, Stephenson JR, Groffen J, Hansen PF, de Klein A, Bartram CR, Grosveld G. Localization of the c-Abl oncogene adjacent to a translocation breakpoint in chronic myelocytic leukaemia. Nature. 1983;306:239-242
8. Heisterkamp N, Stam K, Groffen J, de Klein A, Grosveld G. Structural organization of the Bcr gene and its role in the Ph' translocation. Nature. 1985;315:758-760
9. Ben-Neriah Y, Daley GQ, Mes-Masson AM, Witte ON, Baltimore D. The chronic myelogenous leukemia-specific p210 protein is the product of the Bcr/Abl hybrid gene. Science. 1986;233:212-214
10. Shtivelman E, Lifshitz B, Gale RP, Canaani E. Fused transcript of abl and bcr genes in chronic myelogenous leukaemia. Nature. 1985;315:550-554
11. Fainstein E, Marcelle C, Rosner A, Canaani E, Gale RP, Dreazen O, Smith SD, Croce CM. A new fused transcript in Philadelphia chromosome positive acute lymphocytic leukaemia. Nature. 1987;330:386-388
12. Clark SS, McLaughlin J, Crist WM, Champlin R, Witte ON. Unique forms of the abl tyrosine kinase distinguish Ph'-positive CML from Ph'-positive ALL. Science. 1987;235:85-88

13. Walker LC, Ganesan TS, Dhut S, Gibbons B, Lister TA, Rothbard J, Young BD. Novel chimaeric protein expressed in Philadelphia positive acute lymphoblastic leukaemia. Nature. 1987;329:851-853

14. Chan LC, Karhi KK, Rayter SI, Heisterkamp N, Eridani S, Powles R, Lawler SD, Groffen J, Foulkes JG, Greaves MF, et a. A novel abl protein expressed in Philadelphia chromosome positive acute lymphoblastic leukaemia. Nature. 1987;325:635-637

15. Kantarjian H, Faderl S, Talpaz M. Chronic Myelogenous Leukemia, in DeVita VT Jr, Hellman S, Rosenberg SA (eds). Cancer: Priniples and Practice of Oncology. Philadelphia, Lippincott Williams and Williams. 2001:2433-2447

16. Druker BJ, Tamura S, Buchdunger E, Ohno S, Segal GM, Fanning S, Zimmermann J, Lydon NB. Effects of a selective inhibitor of the Abl tyrosine kinase on the growth of Bcr-Abl positive cells. Nat Med. 1996;2:561-566.

17. Donato NJ, Talpaz M. Clinical use of tyrosine kinase inhibitors: therapy for chronic myelogenous leukemia and other cancers. Clin Cancer Res. 2000;6:2965-2966.

18. Goldman JM. Tyrosine-kinase inhibition in treatment of chronic myeloid leukaemia. Lancet. 2000;355:1031-1032.

19. Deininger MW, Goldman JM, Lydon N, Melo JV. The tyrosine kinase inhibitor CGP57148B selectively inhibits the growth of BCR-ABL-positive cells. Blood. 1997;90:3691-3698.

20. Carroll M, Ohno-Jones S, Tamura S, Buchdunger E, Zimmermann J, Lydon NB, Gilliland DG, Druker BJ. CGP 57148, a tyrosine kinase inhibitor, inhibits the growth of cells expressing BCR-ABL, TEL-ABL, and TEL-PDGFR fusion proteins. Blood. 1997;90:4947-4952.

21. Wang WL, Healy ME, Sattler M, Verma S, Lin J, Maulik G, Stiles CD, Griffin JD, Johnson BE, Salgia R. Growth inhibition and modulation of kinase pathways of small cell lung cancer cell lines by the novel tyrosine kinase inhibitor STI 571. Oncogene. 2000;19:3521-3528.

22. Buchdunger E, Cioffi CL, Law N, Stover D, Ohno-Jones S, Druker BJ, Lydon NB. Abl protein-tyrosine kinase inhibitor STI571 inhibits In vitro signal transduction mediated by c-Kit and platelet-derived growth factor receptors. J Pharmacol Exp Ther. 2000;295:139-145.

23. Krystal GW, Honsawek S, Litz J, Buchdunger E. The selective tyrosine kinase inhibitor STI571 inhibits small cell lung cancer growth. Clin Cancer Res. 2000;6:3319-3326.

24. Heinrich MC, Griffith DJ, Druker BJ, Wait CL, Ott KA, Zigler AJ. Inhibition of c-kit receptor tyrosine kinase activity by STI 571, a selective tyrosine kinase inhibitor. Blood. 2000;96:925-932.

25. Rowley JD. A new consistent chromosomal abnormality in chronic myelogenous leukaemia identified by quinacrine fluorescence and Giemsa staining. Nature. 1973;243:290-293

26. Gordon MY, Dowding CR, Riley GP, Goldman JM, Greaves MF. Altered adhesive interactions with marrow stroma of haematopoietic progenitor cells in chronic myeloid leukaemia. Nature. 1987;328:342-344

27. Verfaillie CM, McCarthy JB, McGlave PB. Mechanisms underlying abnormal trafficking of malignant progenitors in chronic myelogenous leukemia. J Clin Invest. 1992;90:1232-1241

28. Chuang TH, Xu X, Kaartinen V, Heisterkamp N, Groffen J, Bokoch GM. Abr and Bcr are multifunctional regulators of the Rho GTP-binding protein family. Proc Natl Acad Sci USA. 1995;92:10282-10286

29. McWhirter JR, Galasso DL, Wang JY. A coiled-coil oligomerization domain of Bcr is essential for the transforming function of Bcr-Abl oncoproteins. Mol Cell Biol. 1993;13:7587-7595

30. Golub TR, Goga A, Barker GF, Afar D, Mclaughlin J, Bohlander SK, Rowley JD, Witte ON, Gilliland DG. Oligomerization of the Abl tyrosine kinase by the Ets protein Tel in human leukemia. Mol Cell Biol. 1996;16:4107-4116

31. Pendergast AM, Quilliam LA, Cripe LD, Bassing CH, Dai Z, Li N, Batzer A, Rabun KM, Der CJ, Schlessinger J, et a. BCR-ABL-induced oncogenesis is mediated by direct interaction with the SH2 domain of the GRB-2 adaptor protein. Cell. 1993;75:175-185

32. Puil L, Liu J, Gish G, Mbamalu G, Bowtell D, Pelicci PG, Arlinghaus R, Pawson T. Bcr-Abl oncoproteins bind directly to activators of the Ras signalling pathway. EMBO J. 1994;13:764-773

33. Afar DE, Goga A, McLaughlin J, Witte ON, Sawyers CL. Differential complementation of Bcr-Abl point mutants with c-Myc. Science. 1994;264:424-426

34. Scita G, Tenca P, Frittoli E, Tocchetti A, Innocenti M, Giardina G, Di Fiore PP. Signaling from Ras to Rac and beyond: not just a matter of GEFs. Embo J. 2000;19:2393-2398.

35. Million RP, Van Etten RA. The Grb2 binding site is required for the induction of chronic myeloid leukemia-like disease in mice by the Bcr/Abl tyrosine kinase. Blood. 2000;96:664-670.

36. Zhang X, Subrahmanyam R, Wong R, Gross AW, Ren R. The NH(2)-Terminal Coiled-Coil Domain and Tyrosine 177 Play Important Roles in Induction of a Myeloproliferative Disease in Mice by Bcr-Abl. Mol Cell Biol. 2001;21:840-853.

37. Sattler M, Mohi MG, Pride YB, Quinnan LR, Malouf NA, Podar K, Gesbert F, Iwasaki H, Li S, Van Etten RA, Gu H, Griffin JD, Neel BG. Critical role for Gab2 in transformation by BCR/ABL. Cancer Cell. 2002;1:479-492

38. Wang JY, Ledley F, Goff S, Lee R, Groner Y, Baltimore D. The mouse c-abl locus: molecular cloning and characterization. Cell. 1984;36:349-356

39. Tybulewicz VL, Crawford CE, Jackson PK, Bronson RT, Mulligan RC. Neonatal lethality and lymphopenia in mice with a homozygous disruption of the c-abl proto-oncogene. Cell. 1991;65:1153-1163

40. Schwartzberg PL, Stall AM, Hardin JD, Bowdish KS, Humaran T, Boast S, Harbison ML, Robertson EJ, Goff SP. Mice homozygous for the ABLm1 mutation show poor viability and depletion of selected B and T cell populations. Cell. 1991;65:1165-1175

41. Li B, Boast S, de los Santos K, Schieren I, Quiroz M, Teitelbaum SL, Tondravi MM, Goff SP. Mice deficient in Abl are osteoporotic and have defects in osteoblast maturation. Nat Genet. 2000;24:304-308.

42. Kharbanda S, Ren R, Pandey P, Shafman TD, Feller SM, Weichselbaum RR, Kufe DW. Activation of the c-Abl tyrosine kinase in the stress response to DNA-damaging agents. Nature. 1995;376:785-788

43. Welch PJ, Wang JY. A C-terminal protein-binding domain in the retinoblastoma protein regulates nuclear c-Abl tyrosine kinase in the cell cycle. Cell. 1993;75:779-790

44. Yuan ZM, Huang YY, Whang Y, Sawyers C, Weichselbaum R, Kharbanda S, Kufe D. Role for c-Abl tyrosine kinase in growth arrest response to dna damage. Nature. 1996;382:272-274

45. Pendergast AM, Gishizky ML, Havlik MH, Witte ON. SH1 domain autophosphorylation of p210 BCR/ABL is required for transformation but not growth factor independence. Mol Cell Biol. 1993;13:1728-1736

46. Barila D, Superti-Furga G. An intramolecular SH3-domain interaction regulates c-Abl activity. Nat Genet. 1998;18:280-282.

47. Schindler T, Bornmann W, Pellicena P, Miller WT, Clarkson B, Kuriyan J. Structural mechanism for STI-571 inhibition of abelson tyrosine kinase. Science. 2000;289:1938-1942.

48. Jackson PK, Paskind M, Baltimore D. Mutation of a phenylalanine conserved in SH3-containing tyrosine kinases activates the transforming ability of c-Abl. Oncogene. 1993;8:1943-1956

49. Pendergast AM, Muller AJ, Havlik MH, Clark R, McCormick F, Witte ON. Evidence for regulation of the human ABL tyrosine kinase by a cellular inhibitor. Proc Natl Acad Sci USA. 1991;88:5927-5931

50. Oda T, Tamura S, Matsuguchi T, Griffin JD, Druker BJ. The SH2 domain of abl is not required for factor-independent growth induced by bcr-abl in a murine myeloid cell line. Leukemia. 1995;9:295-301

51. Ilaria RL, Vanetten RA. The SH2 domain of p210BCR/ABL is not required for the transformation of hematopoietic factor-dependent cells. Blood. 1995;86:3897-3904

52. Anderson SM, Mladenovic J. The BCR-ABL oncogene requires both kinase activity and Src-homology 2 domain to induce cytokine secretion. Blood. 1996;87:238-244

53. Goga A, McLaughlin J, Afar DE, Saffran DC, Witte ON. Alternative signals to RAS for hematopoietic transformation by the BCR-ABL oncogene. Cell. 1995;82:981-988

54. Roumiantsev S, de Aos IE, Varticovski L, Ilaria RL, Van Etten RA. The src homology 2 domain of Bcr/Abl is required for efficient induction of chronic myeloid leukemia-like disease in mice but not for lymphoid leukemogenesis or activation of phosphatidylinositol 3-kinase. Blood. 2001;97:4-13.

55. ten Hoeve J, Arlinghaus RB, Guo JQ, Heisterkamp N, Groffen J. Tyrosine phosphorylation of Crkl in philadelphia(+) leukemia. Blood. 1994;84:1731-1736

56. Oda T, Heaney C, Hagopian JR, Okuda K, Griffin JD, Druker BJ. Crkl is the major tyrosine-phosphorylated protein in neutrophils from patients with chronic myelogenous leukemia. J Biol Chem. 1994;269:22925-22928

57. Nichols GL, Raines MA, Vera JC, Lacomis L, Tempst P, Golde DW. Identification of CRKL as the constitutively phosphorylated 39-kD tyrosine phosphoprotein in chronic myelogenous leukemia cells. Blood. 1994;84:2912-2918

58. Mayer BJ, Hanafusa H. Mutagenic analysis of the v-crk oncogene: requirement for SH2 and SH3 domains and correlation between increased cellular phosphotyrosine and transformation. J Virol. 1990;64:3581-3589

59. Senechal K, Halpern J, Sawyers CL. The Crkl adaptor protein transforms fibroblasts and functions in transformation by the BCR-ABL oncogene. J Biol Chem. 1996;271:23255-23261
60. Heaney C, Kolibaba K, Bhat A, Oda T, Ohno S, Fanning S, Druker BJ. Direct binding of CRKL to BCR-ABL is not required for BCR-ABL transformation. Blood. 1997;89:297-306.
61. McWhirter J, Wang J. Activation of tyrosine kinase and microfilament-binding functions of c-*Abl* by *Bcr* sequences in *Bcr* /*Abl* fusion proteins. Mol Cell Biol. 1991;11:1553-1565
62. McWhirter JR, Wang JY. An actin-binding function contributes to transformation by the Bcr-Abl oncoprotein of Philadelphia chromosome-positive human leukemias. EMBO J. 1993;12:1533-1546
63. Heisterkamp N, Voncken JW, Senadheera D, Gonzalez-Gomez I, Reichert A, Haataja L, Reinikainen A, Pattengale PK, Groffen J. Reduced oncogenicity of p190 Bcr/Abl F-actin-binding domain mutants. Blood. 2000;96:2226-2232.
64. Carlesso N, Frank DA, Griffin JD. Tyrosyl phosphorylation and DNA binding activity of signal transducers and activators of transcription (STAT) proteins in hematopoietic cell lines transformed by BCR/ABL. J Exp Med. 1996;183:811-820
65. Shuai K, Halpern J, Tenhoeve J, Rao XP, Sawyers CL. Constitutive activation of Stat5 by the Bcr-Abl oncogene in chronic myelogenous leukemia. Oncogene. 1996;13:247-254
66. Ilaria RL, Van Etten RA. P210 and P190(BCR/ABL) induce the tyrosine phosphorylation and DNA binding activity of multiple specific STAT family members. J Biol Chem. 1996;271:31704-31710.
67. Okuda K, Golub TR, Gilliland DG, Griffin JD. p210BCR/ABL, p190BCR/ABL, and TEL/ABL activate similar signal transduction pathways in hematopoietic cell lines. Oncogene. 1996;13:1147-1152.
68. Schwaller J, Frantsve J, Aster J, Williams IR, Tomasson MH, Ross TS, Peeters P, Van Rompaey L, Van Etten RA, Ilaria R, Marynen P, Gilliland DG. Transformation of hematopoietic cell lines to growth-factor independence and induction of a fatal myelo- and lymphoproliferative disease in mice by retrovirally transduced TEL/JAK2 fusion genes. Embo J. 1998;17:5321-5333.
69. Mui A, Wakao H, Kinoshita T, Kitamura T, Miyajima A. Suppression of interleukin-3-induced gene expression by a C-terminal truncated STAT5 - role of STAT5 in proliferation. EMBO J. 1996;15:2425-2433
70. Shuai K, Horvath CM, Huang LH, Qureshi SA, Cowburn D, Darnell JE. Interferon activation of the transcription factor Stat91 involves dimerization through SH2-phosphotyrosyl peptide interactions. Cell. 1994;76:821-828.
71. Lin JX, Mietz J, Modi WS, John S, Leonard WJ. Cloning of human Stat5B. Reconstitution of interleukin-2-induced Stat5A and Stat5B DNA binding activity in COS-7 cells. J Biol Chem. 1996;271:10738-10744.
72. Gouilleux F, Pallard C, Dusanter-Fourt I, Wakao H, Haldosen LA, Norstedt G, Levy D, Groner B. Prolactin, growth hormone, erythropoietin and granulocyte-macrophage colony stimulating factor induce MGF-Stat5 DNA binding activity. Embo J. 1995;14:2005-2013.
73. Azam M, Erdjument-Bromage H, Kreider BL, Xia M, Quelle F, Basu R, Saris C, Tempst P, Ihle JN, Schindler C. Interleukin-3 signals through multiple isoforms of Stat5. Embo J. 1995;14:1402-1411.
74. Teglund S, McKay C, Schuetz E, van Deursen JM, Stravopodis D, Wang D, Brown M, Bodner S, Grosveld G, Ihle JN. Stat5a and Stat5b proteins have essential and nonessential, or redundant, roles in cytokine responses. Cell. 1998;93:841-850.
75. Socolovsky M, Fallon AE, Wang S, Brugnara C, Lodish HF. Fetal anemia and apoptosis of red cell progenitors in Stat5a-/-5b-/- mice: a direct role for Stat5 in Bcl-X(L) induction. Cell. 1999;98:181-191.
76. Sexl V, Piekorz R, Moriggl R, Rohrer J, Brown MP, Bunting KD, Rothammer K, Roussel MF, Ihle JN. Stat5a/b contribute to interleukin 7-induced B-cell precursor expansion, but abl- and bcr/abl-induced transformation are independent of stat5. Blood. 2000;96:2277-2283.
77. Sillaber C, Gesbert F, Frank DA, Sattler M, Griffin JD. STAT5 activation contributes to growth and viability in Bcr/Abl- transformed cells. Blood. 2000;95:2118-2125.
78. Onishi M, Nosaka T, Misawa K, Mui AL, Gorman D, McMahon M, Miyajima A, Kitamura T. Identification and characterization of a constitutively active STAT5 mutant that promotes cell proliferation. Mol Cell Biol. 1998;18:3871-3879.
79. Holtschke T, Löhler J, Kanno Y, Fehr T, Giese N, Rosenbauer F, Lou J, Knobeloch K-P, Gabriele L, Waring JF, Bachmann MF, Zinkernagel RM, Morse III. HC, Ozato K, Horak I. Immunodefiency and chronic myelogenous leukemia-like syndrome in mice with a targeted mutation of the ICSBP gene. Cell. 1996;87:307-317

80. Schmidt M, Nagel S, Proba J, Thiede C, Ritter M, Waring JF, Rosenbauer F, Huhn D, Wittig B, Horak I, Neubauer A. Lack of interferon consensus sequence binding protein (ICSBP) transcripts in human myeloid leukemias. Blood. 1998;91:22-29.

81. Hao SX, Ren R. Expression of interferon consensus sequence binding protein (ICSBP) is downregulated in Bcr-Abl-induced murine chronic myelogenous leukemia- like disease, and forced coexpression of ICSBP inhibits Bcr-Abl-induced myeloproliferative disorder. Mol Cell Biol. 2000;20:1149-1161.

82. Toker A. Protein kinases as mediators of phosphoinositide 3-kinase signaling. Mol Pharmacol. 2000;57:652-658.

83. Rameh LE, Cantley LC. The role of phosphoinositide 3-kinase lipid products in cell function. J Biol Chem. 1999;274:8347-8350.

84. Rebecchi MJ, Scarlata S. Pleckstrin homology domains: a common fold with diverse functions. Annu Rev Biophys Biomol Struct. 1998;27:503-528

85. Lemmon MA, Ferguson KM, Schlessinger J. PH domains: diverse sequences with a common fold recruit signaling molecules to the cell surface. Cell. 1996;85:621-624.

86. Gaullier JM, Simonsen A, D'Arrigo A, Bremnes B, Stenmark H, Aasland R. FYVE fingers bind PtdIns(3)P. Nature. 1998;394:432-433.

87. Patki V, Lawe DC, Corvera S, Virbasius JV, Chawla A. A functional PtdIns(3)P-binding motif. Nature. 1998;394:433-434.

88. Rameh LE, Chen CS, Cantley LC. Phosphatidylinositol (3,4,5)P3 interacts with SH2 domains and modulates PI 3-kinase association with tyrosine-phosphorylated proteins. Cell. 1995;83:821-830

89. Serve H, Hsu YC, Besmer P. Tyrosine residue 719 of the c-kit receptor is essential for binding of the p85 subunit of phosphatidylinositol (PI) 3-kinase and for c-kit-associated PI 3-kinase activity in COS-1 cells. J Biol Chem. 1994;269:6026-6030

90. Sun XJ, Rothenberg P, Kahn CR, Backer JM, Araki E, Wilden PA, Cahill DA, Goldstein BJ, White MF. Structure of the insulin receptor substrate IRS-1 defines a unique signal transduction protein. Nature. 1991;352:73-77

91. Sattler M, Salgia R, Okuda K, Uemura N, Durstin MA, Pisick E, Xu G, Li JL, Prasad KV, Griffin JD. The proto-oncogene product p120CBL and the adaptor proteins CRKL and c-CRK link c-ABL, p190BCR/ABL and p210BCR/ABL to the phosphatidylinositol-3' kinase pathway. Oncogene. 1996;12:839-846

92. Gadina M, Sudarshan C, Visconti R, Zhou YJ, Gu H, Neel BG, O'Shea JJ. The docking molecule gab2 is induced by lymphocyte activation and is involved in signaling by interleukin-2 and interleukin-15 but not other common gamma chain-using cytokines. J Biol Chem. 2000;275:26959-26966.

93. Gu H, Maeda H, Moon JJ, Lord JD, Yoakim M, Nelson BH, Neel BG. New role for Shc in activation of the phosphatidylinositol 3-kinase/Akt pathway. Mol Cell Biol. 2000;20:7109-7120.

94. Kapeller R, Cantley LC. Phosphatidylinositol 3-kinase. [Review]. Bioessays. 1994;16:565-576

95. Carpenter CL, Cantley LC. Phosphoinositide 3-kinase and the regulation of growth [Review]. Biochim Biophys Acta Reviews on Cancer. 1996;1288:16

96. Varticovski L, Daley GQ, Jackson P, Baltimore D, Cantley LC. Activation of phosphatidylinositol 3-kinase in cells expressing Abl oncogene variants. Mol Cell Biol. 1991;11:1107-1113

97. Skorski T, Kanakaraj P, Nieborowskaskorska M, Ratajczak MZ, Wen SC, Zon G, Gewirtz AM, Perussia B, Calabretta B. Phosphatidylinositol-3 kinase activity is regulated by bcr/abl and is required for the growth of philadelphia chromosome-positive cells. Blood. 1995;86:726-736

98. Bedi A, Griffin CA, Barber JP, Vala MS, Hawkins AL, Sharkis SJ, Zehnbauer BA, Jones RJ. Growth factor-mediated terminal differentiation of chronic myeloid leukemia. Can Res. 1994;54:5535-5538

99. Bedi A, Zehnbauer BA, Barber JP, Sharkis SJ, Jones RJ. Inhibition of apoptosis by Bcr-Abl in chronic myeloid leukemia. Blood. 1994;83:2038-2044

100. Skorski T, Bellacosa A, Nieborowska-Skorska M, Majewski M, Martinez R, Choi JK, Trotta R, Wlodarski P, Perrotti D, Chan TO, Wasik MA, Tsichlis PN, Calabretta B. Transformation of hematopoietic cells by BCR/ABL requires activation of a PI-3k/Akt-dependent pathway. Embo J. 1997;16:6151-6161.

101. Staal SP. Molecular cloning of the akt oncogene and its human homologues AKT1 and AKT2: amplification of AKT1 in a primary human gastric adenocarcinoma. Proc Natl Acad Sci U S A. 1987;84:5034-5037.

102. Staal SP, Hartley JW. Thymic lymphoma induction by the AKT8 murine retrovirus. J Exp Med. 1988;167:1259-1264.

103. Alessi DR, James SR, Downes CP, Holmes AB, Gaffney PR, Reese CB, Cohen P. Characterization of a 3-phosphoinositide-dependent protein kinase which phosphorylates and activates protein kinase Balpha. Curr Biol. 1997;7:261-269.

104. Stokoe D, Stephens LR, Copeland T, Gaffney PR, Reese CB, Painter GF, Holmes AB, McCormick F, Hawkins PT. Dual role of phosphatidylinositol-3,4,5-trisphosphate in the activation of protein kinase B. Science. 1997;277:567-570.

105. Datta SR, Dudek H, Tao X, Masters S, Fu H, Gotoh Y, Greenberg ME. Akt phosphorylation of BAD couples survival signals to the cell- intrinsic death machinery. Cell. 1997;91:231-241.

106. Brunet A, Bonni A, Zigmond MJ, Lin MZ, Juo P, Hu LS, Anderson MJ, Arden KC, Blenis J, Greenberg ME. Akt promotes cell survival by phosphorylating and inhibiting a Forkhead transcription factor. Cell. 1999;96:857-868.

107. Gesbert F, Sellers WR, Signoretti S, Loda M, Griffin JD. BCR/ABL regulates expression of the cyclin-dependent kinase inhibitor p27Kip1 through the phosphatidylinositol 3-Kinase/AKT pathway. J Biol Chem. 2000;275:39223-39230.

108. Jonuleit T, van der Kuip H, Miething C, Michels H, Hallek M, Duyster J, Aulitzky WE. Bcr-Abl kinase down-regulates cyclin-dependent kinase inhibitor p27 in human and murine cell lines. Blood. 2000;96:1933-1939.

109. Evers EE, Zondag GC, Malliri A, Price LS, ten Klooster JP, van der Kammen RA, Collard JG. Rho family proteins in cell adhesion and cell migration. Eur J Cancer. 2000;36:1269-1274.

110. Schmitz AA, Govek EE, Bottner B, Van Aelst L. Rho GTPases: signaling, migration, and invasion. Exp Cell Res. 2000;261:1-12.

111. Skorski T, Wlodarski P, Daheron L, Salomoni P, Nieborowska-Skorska M, Majewski M, Wasik M, Calabretta B. BCR/ABL-mediated leukemogenesis requires the activity of the small GTP- binding protein Rac. Proc Natl Acad Sci U S A. 1998;95:11858-11862.

112. Krystal G. Lipid phosphatases in the immune system. Semin Immunol. 2000;12:397-403.

113. Rohrschneider LR, Fuller JF, Wolf I, Liu Y, Lucas DM. Structure, function, and biology of SHIP proteins. Genes Dev. 2000;14:505-520.

114. Sattler M, Verma S, Byrne CH, Shrikhande G, Winkler T, Algate PA, Rohrschneider LR, Griffin JD. BCR/ABL directly inhibits expression of SHIP, an SH2-containing polyinositol-5-phosphatase involved in the regulation of hematopoiesis. Mol Cell Biol. 1999;19:7473-7480.

115. Helgason CD, Damen JE, Rosten P, Grewal R, Sorensen P, Chappel SM, Borowski A, Jirik F, Krystal G, Humphries RK. Targeted disruption of SHIP leads to hemopoietic perturbations, lung pathology, and a shortened life span. Genes Dev. 1998;12:1610-1620.

116. Sattler M, Verma S, Shrikhande G, Byrne CH, Pride YB, Winkler T, Greenfield EA, Salgia R, Griffin JD. The BCR/ABL tyrosine kinase induces production of reactive oxygen species in hematopoietic cells. J Biol Chem. 2000;275:24273-24278.

117. Burdon RH. Superoxide and hydrogen peroxide in relation to mammalian cell proliferation. Free Radic Biol Med. 1995;18:775-794.

118. Denu JM, Tanner KG. Specific and reversible inactivation of protein tyrosine phosphatases by hydrogen peroxide: evidence for a sulfenic acid intermediate and implications for redox regulation. Biochemistry. 1998;37:5633-5642

119. Monteiro HP, Stern A. Redox modulation of tyrosine phosphorylation-dependent signal transduction pathways. [Review]. Free. Radic. Biol. Med. 1996;21:323-333

120. Ohba M, Shibanuma M, Kuroki T, Nose K. Production of hydrogen peroxide by transforming growth factor-beta 1 and its involvement in induction of egr-1 in mouse osteoblastic cells. J. Cell. Biol. 1994;126:1079-1088

121. Bae YS, Kang SW, Seo MS, Baines IC, Tekle E, Chock PB, Rhee SG. Epidermal growth factor (EGF)-induced generation of hydrogen peroxide. Role in EGF receptor-mediated tyrosine phosphorylation. J Biol Chem. 1997;272:217-221

122. Sundaresan M, Yu ZX, Ferrans VJ, Irani K, Finkel T. Requirement for generation of H_2O_2 for platelet-derived growth factor signal transduction. Science. 1995;270:296-299

123. Sattler M, Winkler T, Verma S, Byrne CH, Shrikhande G, Salgia R, Griffin JD. Hematopoietic growth factors signal through the formation of reactive oxygen species. Blood. 1999;93:2928-2935

124. Suh Y-A, Arnold RS, Lassegue B, Shi J, Xu X, Sorescu D, Chung AB, Griendling KK, Lambeth JD. Cell transformation by the superoxide-generating oxidase Mox1. Nature. 1999;401:79-82

125. Huang P, Feng L, Oldham EA, Keating MJ, Plunkett W. Superoxide dismutase as a target for the selective killing of cancer cells. Nature. 2000;407:390-395.

126. Rosnet O, Mattei MG, Marchetto S, Birnbaum D. Isolation and chromosomal localization of a novel FMS-like tyrosine kinase gene. Genomics. 1991;9:380-385.

127. Matthews W, Jordan CT, Wiegand GW, Pardoll D, Lemischka IR. A receptor tyrosine kinase specific to hematopoietic stem and progenitor cell-enriched populations. Cell. 1991;65:1143-1152.

128. Rosnet O, Schiff C, Pebusque MJ, Marchetto S, Tonnelle C, Toiron Y, Birg F, Birnbaum D. Human FLT3/FLK2 gene: cDNA cloning and expression in hematopoietic cells. Blood. 1993;82:1110-1119.

129. Small D, Levenstein M, Kim E, Carow C, Amin S, Rockwell P, Witte L, Burrow C, Ratajczak MZ, Gewirtz AM, et al. STK-1, the human homolog of Flk-2/Flt-3, is selectively expressed in CD34+ human bone marrow cells and is involved in the proliferation of early progenitor/stem cells. Proc Natl Acad Sci U S A. 1994;91:459-463.

130. Hannum C, Culpepper J, Campbell D, McClanahan T, Zurawski S, Bazan JF, Kastelein R, Hudak S, Wagner J, Mattson J, et al. Ligand for FLT3/FLK2 receptor tyrosine kinase regulates growth of haematopoietic stem cells and is encoded by variant RNAs. Nature. 1994;368:643-648.

131. Lyman SD, James L, Vanden Bos T, de Vries P, Brasel K, Gliniak B, Hollingsworth LT, Picha KS, McKenna HJ, Splett RR, et al. Molecular cloning of a ligand for the flt3/flk-2 tyrosine kinase receptor: a proliferative factor for primitive hematopoietic cells. Cell. 1993;75:1157-1167.

132. Birg F, Courcoul M, Rosnet O, Bardin F, Pebusque MJ, Marchetto S, Tabilio A, Mannoni P, Birnbaum D. Expression of the FMS/KIT-like gene FLT3 in human acute leukemias of the myeloid and lymphoid lineages. Blood. 1992;80:2584-2593.

133. Carow CE, Kim E, Hawkins AL, Webb HD, Griffin CA, Jabs EW, Civin CI, Small D. Localization of the human stem cell tyrosine kinase-1 gene (FLT3) to 13q12-->q13. Cytogenet Cell Genet. 1995;70:255-257.

134. Armstrong SA, Staunton JE, Silverman LB, Pieters R, den Boer ML, Minden MD, Sallan SE, Lander ES, Golub TR, Korsmeyer SJ. MLL translocations specify a distinct gene expression profile that distinguishes a unique leukemia. Nat Genet. 2002;30:41-47

135. Lisovsky M, Estrov Z, Zhang X, Consoli U, Sanchez-Williams G, Snell V, Munker R, Goodacre A, Savchenko V, Andreeff M. Flt3 ligand stimulates proliferation and inhibits apoptosis of acute myeloid leukemia cells: regulation of Bcl-2 and Bax. Blood. 1996;88:3987-3997.

136. McKenna HJ, Smith FO, Brasel K, Hirschstein D, Bernstein ID, Williams DE, Lyman SD. Effects of flt3 ligand on acute myeloid and lymphocytic leukemic blast cells from children. Exp Hematol. 1996;24:378-385.

137. Piacibello W, Gammaitoni L, Bruno S, Gunetti M, Fagioli F, Cavalloni G, Aglietta M. Negative influence of IL3 on the expansion of human cord blood in vivo long-term repopulating stem cells. J Hematother Stem Cell Res. 2000;9:945-956.

138. Hirayama F, Lyman SD, Clark SC, Ogawa M. The flt3 ligand supports proliferation of lymphohematopoietic progenitors and early B-lymphoid progenitors. Blood. 1995;85:1762-1768.

139. Hudak S, Hunte B, Culpepper J, Menon S, Hannum C, Thompson-Snipes L, Rennick D. FLT3/FLK2 ligand promotes the growth of murine stem cells and the expansion of colony-forming cells and spleen colony-forming units. Blood. 1995;85:2747-2755.

140. Jacobsen SE, Okkenhaug C, Myklebust J, Veiby OP, Lyman SD. The FLT3 ligand potently and directly stimulates the growth and expansion of primitive murine bone marrow progenitor cells in vitro: synergistic interactions with interleukin (IL) 11, IL-12, and other hematopoietic growth factors. J Exp Med. 1995;181:1357-1363.

141. Maraskovsky E, Brasel K, Teepe M, Roux ER, Lyman SD, Shortman K, McKenna HJ. Dramatic increase in the numbers of functionally mature dendritic cells in Flt3 ligand-treated mice: multiple dendritic cell subpopulations identified. J Exp Med. 1996;184:1953-1962.

142. Maraskovsky E, Daro E, Roux E, Teepe M, Maliszewski CR, Hoek J, Caron D, Lebsack ME, McKenna HJ. In vivo generation of human dendritic cell subsets by Flt3 ligand. Blood. 2000;96:878-884.

143. Pulendran B, Banchereau J, Burkholder S, Kraus E, Guinet E, Chalouni C, Caron D, Maliszewski C, Davoust J, Fay J, Palucka K. Flt3-ligand and granulocyte colony-stimulating factor mobilize distinct human dendritic cell subsets in vivo. J Immunol. 2000;165:566-572.

144. Dosil M, Wang S, Lemischka IR. Mitogenic signalling and substrate specificity of the Flk2/Flt3 receptor tyrosine kinase in fibroblasts and interleukin 3-dependent hematopoietic cells. Mol Cell Biol. 1993;13:6572-6585.

145. Marchetto S, Fournier E, Beslu N, Aurran-Schleinitz T, Dubreuil P, Borg JP, Birnbaum D, Rosnet O. SHC and SHIP phosphorylation and interaction in response to activation of the FLT3 receptor. Leukemia. 1999;13:1374-1382.
146. Rottapel R, Turck CW, Casteran N, Liu X, Birnbaum D, Pawson T, Dubreuil P. Substrate specificities and identification of a putative binding site for PI3K in the carboxy tail of the murine Flt3 receptor tyrosine kinase. Oncogene. 1994;9:1755-1765.
147. Zhang S, Fukuda S, Lee Y, Hangoc G, Cooper S, Spolski R, Leonard WJ, Broxmeyer HE. Essential role of signal transducer and activator of transcription (Stat)5a but not Stat5b for Flt3-dependent signaling. J Exp Med. 2000;192:719-728.
148. McKenna HJ, Stocking KL, Miller RE, Brasel K, De Smedt T, Maraskovsky E, Maliszewski CR, Lynch DH, Smith J, Pulendran B, Roux ER, Teepe M, Lyman SD, Peschon JJ. Mice lacking flt3 ligand have deficient hematopoiesis affecting hematopoietic progenitor cells, dendritic cells, and natural killer cells. Blood. 2000;95:3489-3497.
149. Nakao M, Yokota S, Iwai T, Kaneko H, Horiike S, Kashima K, Sonoda Y, Fujimoto T, Misawa S. Internal tandem duplication of the flt3 gene found in acute myeloid leukemia. Leukemia. 1996;10:1911-1918.
150. Kiyoi H, Naoe T, Yokota S, Nakao M, Minami S, Kuriyama K, Takeshita A, Saito K, Hasegawa S, Shimodaira S, Tamura J, Shimazaki C, Matsue K, Kobayashi H, Arima N, Suzuki R, Morishita H, Saito H, Ueda R, Ohno R. Internal tandem duplication of FLT3 associated with leukocytosis in acute promyelocytic leukemia. Leukemia Study Group of the Ministry of Health and Welfare (Kohseisho). Leukemia. 1997;11:1447-1452.
151. Meshinchi S, Woods WG, Stirewalt DL, Sweetser DA, Buckley JD, Tjoa TK, Bernstein ID, Radich JP. Prevalence and prognostic significance of Flt3 internal tandem duplication in pediatric acute myeloid eukemia. Blood. 2001;97:89-94.
152. Rombouts WJ, Blokland I, Lowenberg B, Ploemacher RE. Biological characteristics and prognosis of adult acute myeloid leukemia with internal tandem duplications in the Flt3 gene. Leukemia. 2000;14:675-683.
153. Xu F, Taki T, Yang HW, Hanada R, Hongo T, Ohnishi H, Kobayashi M, Bessho F, Yanagisawa M, Hayashi Y. Tandem duplication of the FLT3 gene is found in acute lymphoblastic leukaemia as well as acute myeloid leukaemia but not in myelodysplastic syndrome or juvenile chronic myelogenous leukaemia in children. Br J Haematol. 1999;105:155-162.
154. Whitman SP, Archer KJ, Feng L, Baldus C, Becknell B, Carlson BD, Carroll AJ, Mrozek K, Vardiman JW, George SL, Kolitz JE, Larson RA, Bloomfield CD, Caligiuri MA. Absence of the wild-type allele predicts poor prognosis in adult de novo acute myeloid leukemia with normal cytogenetics and the internal tandem duplication of FLT3: a cancer and leukemia group B study. Cancer Res. 2001;61:7233-7239
155. Kelly LM, Liu Q, Kutok JL, Williams IR, Boulton CL, Gilliland DG. FLT3 internal tandem duplication mutations associated with human acute myeloid leukemias induce myeloproliferative disease in a murine bone marrow transplant model. Blood. 2002;99:310-318
156. Abu-Duhier FM, Goodeve AC, Wilson GA, Care RS, Peake IR, Reilly JT. Identification of novel FLT-3 Asp835 mutations in adult acute myeloid leukaemia. Br J Haematol. 2001;113:983-988.
157. Yamamoto Y, Kiyoi H, Nakano Y, Suzuki R, Kodera Y, Miyawaki S, Asou N, Kuriyama K, Yagasaki F, Shimazaki C, Akiyama H, Saito K, Nishimura M, Motoji T, Shinagawa K, Takeshita A, Saito H, Ueda R, Ohno R, Naoe T. Activating mutation of D835 within the activation loop of FLT3 in human hematologic malignancies. Blood. 2001;97:2434-2439.
158. Tse KF, Novelli E, Civin CI, Bohmer FD, Small D. Inhibition of FLT3-mediated transformation by use of a tyrosine kinase inhibitor. Leukemia. 2001;15:1001-1010.
159. Levis M, Tse KF, Smith BD, Garrett E, Small D. A FLT3 tyrosine kinase inhibitor is selectively cytotoxic to acute myeloid leukemia blasts harboring FLT3 internal tandem duplication mutations. Blood. 2001;98:885-887.
160. Naoe T, Kiyoe H, Yamamoto Y, Minami Y, Yamamoto K, Ueda R, Saito H. FLT3 tyrosine kinase as a target molecule for selective antileukemia therapy. Cancer Chemother Pharmacol. 2001;48:S27-S30
161. Yu J-C, Apatira M, Li J, Kelly LM, Sternberg DW, Scarborough R, Pandey A, Seroogy J, Gilliland DG, Giese NA. FLT3 antagonism as a strategy for the treatment of acute myeloid leukemia (AML). Blood. 2001;98:721a

162. Allebach J, Levis M, Fai-Tse K, Jones-Brolin S, Ruggeri B, Dionne C, Small D. FLT3-targeted tyrosine kinase inhibitors inhibit proliferation, induce apoptosis, and improve survival in a murine leukemia model utilizing FLT3/ITD-transformed cells. Blood. 2001;89:118a

163. Levis MJ, Allebach J, Tse KF, Zheng R, Baldwin BR, Smith BD, Jones-Brolin S, Ruggeri B, Dionne C, Small D. FLT3-targeted inhibitors kill FLT3-dependent modeled cells, leukemia-derived cell lines, and primary AML blasts in vitro and in vivo. Blood. 2001:721a

164. O'Farrell A, Abrams T, Yuen H, Ngai T, Louie S, Wong L, Heinrich MC, Yee K, Smolich B, Murray L, Mendel D, Cherrington J. SUGEN compounds SU5416 and SU11248 inhibit Flt3 activity: therapeutic application in AML. Blood. 2001;89:118a

165. Yee K, O'Farrell A, Smolich B, Cherrington J, Wait CL, Griffith DJ, McGreevey LS, Heinrich MC. SU5416 and SU5614 inhibit wild-type and activated mutant FLT3 signaling in leukemia cells. Blood. 2001;89:838a

166. Weisberg E, Boulton C, Kelly LM, Manley P, Fabbro D, Meyer T, Gilliland DG, Griffin JD. Inhibition of mutant FLT3 receptors in leukemia cells by the small molecule tyrosine kinase inhibitor PKC412. Cancer Cell. 2002;1:433-443

TARGETING PDGF RECEPTORS IN CANCER – RATIONALES AND PROOF OF CONCEPT CLINICAL TRIALS

Daniel George

Dana-Farber Cancer Institute, Boston, MA, USA

ABSTRACT

The platelet-derived growth factors (PDGF) are a pleotrophic family of peptide growth factors that signal through cell surface, tyrosine kinase receptors (PDGFR) and stimulate various cellular functions including growth, proliferation, and differentiation. To date, PDGF expression has been demonstrated in a number of different solid tumors, from glioblastomas to prostate carcinomas. In these various tumor types, the biologic role of PDGF signaling can vary from autocrine stimulation of cancer cell growth to subtler paracrine interactions involving adjacent stroma and vasculature. The tyrosine kinase inhibitor imatinib mesylate (formerly STI571, Gleevec™, Novartis Pharmaceuticals Corp, East Hanover, NJ) blocks activity of the Bcr-Abl oncoprotein and the cell surface tyrosine kinase receptor c-Kit, and as such was recently approved for several indications in the treatment on chronic myeloid leukemia and gastrointestinal stromal tumors. In both of these examples the target protein was identified by an oncogenic, activating mutation. Imatinib mesylate is also a potent inhibitor of PDGFR kinase and is currently being evaluated for the treatment of chronic myelomonocytic leukemia and glioblastoma multiforme, based upon evidence in these diseases of activating mutations in PDGFR. However, the PDGF pathway may represent a therapeutic target in other solid tumors in which it is not part of the oncogenic transformation. In order to investigate the potential biologic implications of inhibiting PDGFR in these tumor types, clinical trials that investigate both established clinical endpoints of response and benefit, as well as surrogate endpoints that describe the biologic significance of PDGF inhibition in vivo are needed.

INTRODUCTION

Since their discovery, signal transduction growth factor receptors, particularly receptor tyrosine kinases (RTK), have been used for selection of anticancer therapy. Small molecules, antibodies, antisense and other inhibitory agents have been developed, which until recently have demonstrated relatively little evidence of clinical benefit. Of the handful of these agents FDA-approved for cancer indications, the example of imatinib mesylate represents the most successful small molecule that targets a RTK in cancer.

New Trends in Cancer for the 21ˢᵗ Century, edited by
Llombart-Bosch and Felipo, Kluwer Academic/Plenum Publishers, 2003

141

Imatinib mesylate has demonstrated a remarkably high rate of disease response in all stages of CML and continues to result in durable complete responses in early stage (chronic phase) CML[1, 2]. Vital to the success of imatinib mesylate is the selection of a disease population (CML patients) in which a single common mutational event (the translocation of chromosome 9:22) results in an activated tyrosine kinase oncogene (BCR-Abl) that is potently inhibited by the drug. A second example has been demonstrated in metastatic gastrointestinal stromal tumors (GIST), a rare solid tumor with response rates to chemotherapy of < 10%, in which a mutation in the c-Kit RTK results in oncogenic transformation in 95% of cases[3]. Using imatinib mesylate, which also potently inhibits the c-Kit tyrosine kinase receptor, two multicenter studies have demonstrated response rates greater than 50%[4, 5]. These two examples suggest RTKs can represent effective targets in anti-cancer therapy.

Imatinib mesylate is also a potent inhibitor of PDGFR, which may represent the most intriguing potential for expansion into other diseases. Currently, PDGF signaling has been implicated in oncogenic transformation of at least two diseases. In chronic myelomonocytic leukemia (CMML) where the PDGFR is part of a chromosomal translocation involving the TEL gene, and in glioblastoma multiforme (GBM), in which the PDGFB ligand, originally referred to as *c-sis* proto-oncogene, when mutated results in oncogenic transformation through a constitutively active autocrine loop[6]. Based upon these rationales, there are ongoing studies evaluating the clinical efficacy of imatinib mesylate in these cancer patient populations. However, the biology of PDGF signaling is complex and offers some evidence for targeting this pathway in other tumor types. This chapter will outline the rationale for targeting PDGFR in prostate cancer as an example of a common solid tumor type in which PDGF signaling may be functional. Importantly, the concept of targeting growth factor pathways based upon data other than activating mutations or gene amplification is unproven and therefore, any trials testing such a hypothesis must be viewed as a proof of concept study.

PDGF AND PDGF RECEPTORS

In order to understand the rationale for targeting PDGFR in solid tumors, a brief review of the PDGF signaling pathway is needed. The various PDGF and PDGFR isoforms comprise a family of ligands and receptors. PDGF is a 30 kd protein consisting of disulfide-bonded homo- or heterodimers of A and B chains. The A and B chains are 60% homologous and show strict conservation of 8 cysteine residues[7]. These molecules are synthesized as higher molecular weight precursors that are subjected to proteolytic processing. All three combinations of subunits occur: AA, AB, and BB. The recently discovered PDGF C isoform occurs as a homodimer (PDGF CC); it is not known whether it can also form heterodimers with other PDGF chains[8].

The PDGF receptors occur as α and β homodimers and α/β heterodimers and belong to the RTK family of receptors. The extracellular portions of these proteins are characterized by the presence of 5 immunoglobulin-like domains, created by regularly spaced disulfide bonds. The receptor chains share 30% similarity in their amino acid sequences.The intracellular portions of each receptor contains a conserved tyrosine kinase domain into which is inserted an interrupting sequence of approximaly 100 amino acids. Similar "kinase inserts" are present in the homologous CSF-1 receptor and c-Kit receptors, and putative binding sites for the SH2 domains of substrates for these receptors [9, 10]. The α receptor can bind to all dimeric PDGF isoforms (AA, BB, AB and CC), whereas the β receptor chain preferentially binds the B isoform (Fig 1).

Platelet-derived Growth Factor (PDGF): Ligands and Receptors

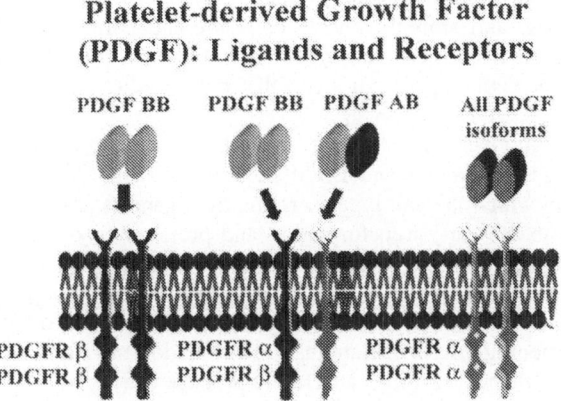

Figure 1. PDGF: Ligands and receptors. Several PDGF isoforms bind to two related receptors. The specificity in assembly of different dimeric receptor complexes of PDGF isoforms is shown.

Upon binding of the dimeric ligand to the extracellular portions of the two PDGF receptor chains, a receptor homodimer or heterodimer is formed, which induces autophosphorylation of cytosolic receptor tyrosine residues. Multiple SH2 domain-containing signal transduction molecules are recruited and bind to the phosphorylated receptors, thereby initiating various signaling pathways which ultimately lead to cell growth, changes in cell morphology, and prevention of apoptosis[11-13]. The originally identified target cells for PDGF are fibroblasts and smooth muscle cells, but many other normal cell types express PDGF receptors, including renal mesangial cells, testicular Leydig cells, neurons, Schwann cells and retinal pigment epithelial cells of the CNS[14].

PDGF plays an important role in normal physiology. For example, during embryonic development, PDGF signaling is critical in the formation of connective tissues in various organs[15]. In adult tissues, a primary function of PDGF is to stimulate wound healing, via chemotaxis and mitogenesis of fibroblasts, and secretion of extracellular matrix components. Importantly, PDGF β receptors are expressed on capillary endothelial cells and PDGF has been shown to have pro-angiogenic effects, recruiting and stabilizing pericytes onto immature blood vessels [16]. Macrophages, T-lymphocytes, myeloid lineage hematopoietic cells and mammary epithelium also express PDGFR β. Conversely, platelets, astrocytes, and liver sinusoidal epithelium express only PDGFR α. Finally, PDGF has been shown to have an important role in the control of the interstitial fluid pressure, most likely by stimulating interactions between connective tissue cells and the extracellular matrix[15]. In several preclinical studies PDGFR inhibition results in a decrease in interstitial pressures and possibly a normalization of blood flow into tumor beds[17, 18].

PDGF IN CANCER

Whereas normal PDGF function is critical for normal embryonic development and adult homeostasis, as in wound healing, overactivity of the PDGF/PDGFR axis has been implicated in several disorders characterized by excessive cell growth. These include fibrotic conditions, plaque formation during atherosclerosis, and certain malignancies [15]. Glial cells, fibroblasts, and smooth muscle cells are the normal physiologic targets of PDGF. Tumors derived from these cell types have therefore been analyzed for autocrine stimulation, defined as signaling within a cell that both produces the ligand and expresses its receptor.

In the case of glioblastomas, a large fraction of analyzed tumors demonstrated coexpression of PDGF α receptor and PDGF A or B chains[19, 20]. Dysregulated autocrine PDGF stimulation, in which the cell type secreting the ligand is also the target cell (Fig 2), is felt to contribute to the early transformation and progression of these tumors. For this reason imatinib mesylate is being evaluated in clinical trials for treatment of adult and pediatric glioblastoma. Coexpression of PDGF and PDGF receptors, suggestive of autocrine growth stimulation, has also been observed in various other types of human tumors including meningiomas, melanomas, neuroendocrine tumors, ovarian cancer, pancreatic cancer, gastric cancer, lung cancer, and prostate cancer[15].

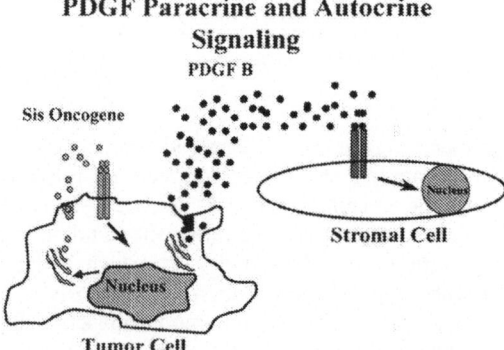

Figure 2. Autocrine and paracrine PDGF effects on tumor development. Coexpression of PDGF and PDGF receptors in various types of human tumors is consistent with autocrine growth stimulation. Many common solid tumors display PDGF—producing tumor cells and PDGF β receptor—expressing stromal fibroblasts leading to a paracrine PDGF effect.

Mutational Activation of PDGF Receptors in Tumors

The mechanisms of dysregulated PDGF and PDGF receptor expression and function have not been fully elucidated. As mentioned earlier, mutation of the proto-oncogene c-sis can lead to overexpression of the PDGF B ligand. In addition, overexpression of PDGF α receptor in glioblastoma is associated with gene amplification of the PDGF receptor[19, 21]. Another example of gene amplification leading to dysregulation of a signal transduction pathway and a therapeutic target in cancer is the HER-2/neu (Erb B2) protein in breast cancer. In the case of HER-2 positive breast cancer, trastuzumab (Herceptin) demonstrated modest clinical activity alone but greater benefit when combined with cytotoxic chemotherapy, and led to recent FDA approval for treatment of advanced breast cancer in combination with chemotherapy [Slamon, 2001 #23].

Chromosomal translocation represents yet another mechanism by which functional target proteins are dysregulated in tumors. The Bcr-Abl fusion protein in CML, arising from a 9:22 translocation that creates the Bcr-Abl oncogene represents the clearest example of this mechanism. Another promising example of a transforming chromosomal translocation occurs in CMML, in which a fusion oncogene is generated by the merger of the promoter and 5' end of the TEL gene with the 3' end of the PDGF β receptor gene including its functionally active kinase domain[22, 23]. This TEL-PDGFRβ fusion protein results in a ligand-independent, constitutively active form of the PDGF β receptor and oncogenic transformation.

A fourth potential mechanism of signal transduction dysregulation in cancer involves transforming viruses that can infect tissues and result in carcinoma in situ and tumorigenesis. Potentially, transforming viruses may identify other potential therapeutic targets for cancer treatment but as yet remain unproven. One example indirectly involving PDGF signaling is the E5 oncoprotein of bovine papilloma virus type 1. In this model, the E5 protein causes oligomerization of the PDGF β receptor, thereby inducing its constitutive activation in the absence of ligand[24]. Whether homologous human viral proteins exhibiting similar dysregulation of PDGF signaling in human cancers is a functional target for therapy remains unknown.

Paracrine PDGF Effects and Tumor Angiogenesis

Paracrine stimulation is essentially a local hormonal effect occurring within a tissue in which a ligand from one cell activates receptor signaling in a different cell type within the same tissue (Fig 2). Release of ligands that feed back to the original cell can create an intercellular interaction known as a paracrine loop. Paracrine loops are responsible for many of the physiologic functions of PDGF signaling that occur normally in tissues. In addition, these same paracrine interactions occur in many tissues that make up a solid tumor—stromal cells, blood vessels, and tumor parenchymal cells per se— and function in a complex and interdependent way. Many common solid tumors, including colorectal adenocarcinoma, lung carcinomas, and breast carcinomas, contain both PDGF-producing cells and PDGF β receptor-expressing stromal fibroblasts[15].

The multi-step process of angiogenesis is a prominent example of paracrine interactions in tumors. Angiogenesis is critical for tumor growth and may be mediated either directly or indirectly. Direct angiogenic activity of the PDGF BB and PDGF β receptor isoforms involves recruitment and differentiation of pericytes, the cells that stabilize immature blood vessels and contribute to their functional integrity[25, 26]. Indirect stimulation may be mediated via induction of other growth factors such as vascular endothelial growth factor (VEGF). Furthermore, pericytes, through PDGF signaling, may also enhance tumor growth by regulating tumor interstitial fluid pressure and transcapillary transport[17].

PROSTATE CANCER AND PDGF RECEPTOR EXPRESSION

Ligand and Receptor Expression

Prostate cancer is the most common form of non-cutaneous solid tumor and second most common cause of death from cancer in American men. The growth of normal prostate epithelium and primary prostate cancer is influenced by a number of growth factors, many of which function by binding to receptor tyrosine kinases. Immunohistochemical analysis of PDGF A and B chain, and PDGF α and β receptors in epithelial and stromal prostate tumor cells indicates that PDGF A and α receptor are expressed in these cells at varying levels. However, most studies agree that a subset of prostate tumors and stroma contain a high level of PDGF and PDGFR expression. In contrast, the normal cells surrounding the tumor lesions do not express PDGF A and PDGFR α receptor[27, 28]. Interestingly, these two proteins are also expressed in a precursor lesion in prostate cancer known as prostatic intraepithelial neoplasia (PIN). This observation suggests that de novo expression occurs early in the transformation process and may be causally related to it.

Bone marrow is the predominant metastatic site for prostate cancer and bone marrow metastases account for the majority of prostate cancer morbidity and mortality. Chott and colleagues assessed the role of growth factors and their cognate receptors in metastatic androgen-independent prostate cancer, by reverse-transcriptase polymerase chain reaction (RT-PCR) in a series of bone marrow samples freshly isolated marrow from patients with prostate cancer[29].

Using degenerate primers to amplify the conserved tyrosine kinase domain, several receptor and nonreceptor tyrosine kinase were identified in metastatic prostate cancer. The PDGF α receptor and the Jak 1 kinase were present in the majority of samples. This assay was not quantitative and does not establish that PDGF receptor is the most abundant kinase, only that it is the most frequently detected by this method. Immunohistochemistry of the bone marrow biopsies containing metastatic prostate cancer confirmed the presence of these kinases, and no staining was observed in the stroma, suggesting that expression was confined to the tumor cells[29].

Recent studies using gene expression microarray analysis also suggest the presence of PDGF receptor expression in prostate tumors. In one report of 21 prostate tumors, PDGFR b was part of a five-gene model that accurately predicted for disease progression (Fig 3)[30]. In addition, PDGFR β was one of a handful of genes, whose expression correlated with gleason score in two separate expression data bases (P. Febbo, personal communication). While no functional role has clearly been established for PDGFR β in prostate cancer progression, this data would support this hypothesis.

Clinical Trial of PDGFR Inhibitors in Prostate Cancer

These preclinical findings led to the first clinical trial of a putative PDGF receptor antagonist in metastatic androgen-independent prostate cancer. The PDGF receptor inhibitor, SU101 was evaluated in a multi-institutional, Phase II trial in patients with hormone-refractory prostate cancer[31]. The patient population included individuals in advanced stage disease, many of whom had already undergone a number of treatments including chemotherapy.

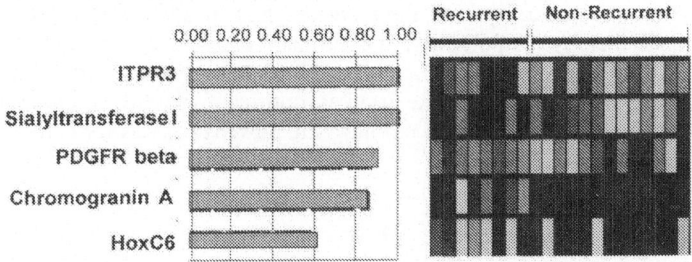

Figure 3. Genes Used to Build an Outcome Prediction Model. The genes most commonly used in the 5-gene model are shown above. The expression of each gene (rows) in each recurrent or non-recurrent sample (columns) is represented by the number of standard deviations above (grey) or below (black) the mean for that gene across all 21 samples (From Cancer Cell 2002, 1:203-209).

The 39 evaluable patients continued on primary androgen ablation with luteinizing hormone-releasing hormone analogues or orchiectomy while SU101 was administered as a weekly IV infusion following a four day loading dose. This treatment regimen achieved only modest overall clinical benefits. One explanation for the low response rate in the study is that the short half-life of SU101 produces only transient blockade of PDGF-mediated signaling, and that prolonged receptor inhibition may be necessary for clinical benefit. Another possible limitation is that clinical response was evaluated solely by reduction in prostate-specific antigen (PSA) levels, with a positive response being defined as a 50% decline in PSA from pretreatment levels sustained over a four week period[32].

Immunohistochemistry for PDGF α and β receptors was performed on fresh samples and archived biopsies. This analysis showed a high level of PDGF receptor expression on tumor epithelial cells that did not differ between the primary and metastatic sites, even for samples obtained from the same patients (Fig 4). These findings suggest that PDGF receptors are consistently expressed during disease progression and that they may serve as an appropriate therapeutic target for all stages of disease.

Phase II trial of imatinib mesylate in hormone-refractory prostate cancer

With the goal of treating hormone-refractory prostate cancer patients with imatinib mesylate, a multi-institutional study encompassing 8 centers in the US and Canada enrolled 40 such patients. The trial was closed to accrual in May 2001. Patients received 400 mg of imatinib mesylate daily. The primary endpoint of the study was the PSA response, with secondary endpoints of safety, time to disease progression, and plasma VEGF levels also measured. The results of this study are being finalized and will be published in the near future. Preliminarily, the results demonstrate that several patients experienced relative declines in their serum PSA levels compared to pretreatment baseline levels, but no patient showed a durable decline of greater than 50%.

While this study was designed as a preliminary evaluation of the efficacy of imatinib mesylate in patients with prostate cancer, it has several limitations. First, as in the previous

SU101 study, the patient population had very advanced prostate cancer. Many patients had undergone previous local therapy, and their disease had in all cases progressed despite previous hormonal therapy. Importantly, the primary endpoint, PSA levels, might not reflect the biological activity of imatinib mesylate in prostate cancer. Further, it is also not known whether the single 400 mg dose used is optimal for solid tumors like prostate cancer. Finally, as an initial study it will not have the power to assess for cytostatic effects, including time to disease progression.

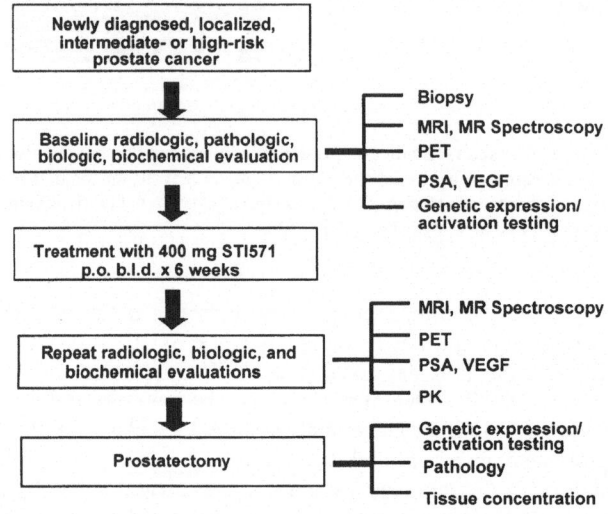

Figure 4. Study design for a phase II trial for patients newly diagnosed with prostate cancer.

Pilot study in newly diagnosed patients

In order to address some of the limitations of this Phase II trial, another pilot study has been initiated. This is a study of imatinib mesylate in newly diagnosed prostate cancer patients, with localized, untreated disease prior undergoing radical prostatectomy. These patients must have intermediate or high risk for disease relapse based on their PSA, Gleason score and clinical stage[33].

Before starting treatment, a baseline radiographic evaluation with positron emission tomography (PET) and magnetic resonance imaging (MRI) will be performed. Biopsies will also be performed to obtain fresh tissue for molecular and gene expression assays. Patients will be treated for 6 weeks or more depending on their ability to tolerate the drug. Radiographic and biologic assays will be repeated after 6 weeks, at which time patients will undergo prostatectomy. They will receive imatinib mesylate up to the day of surgery in order to ascertain the tissue concentration of drug. Gene expression profiling will also be evaluated at that time. Since PDGF plays an important role in both angiogenesis and wound healing, imatinib mesylate will be discontinued in the postoperative period.

The primary endpoint of this study is safety and tolerability. An important secondary objective is the pharmacodynamic assessment of the effects of imatinib mesylate in prostate cancer, using novel applications of technology in this setting. Pathologic evaluation by histology, gleason grade, microvessel density, apoptosis and proliferation serve as the basis for determination of response. Changes in pharmacodynamic assessments will then be correlated with pathologic response. For example, functional imagine techniques with MRI will assess changes in disease volume by 3D volumetrics, MRI spectroscopy and water diffusion will be used to measure apoptosis in vivo, and dynamic flow MRI will help to define a surrogate measure of angiogenesis. $F^{18}DG$ PET will be used to assess changes in tumor metabolism. All of these studies will be correlated with pathologic findings. Finally, molecular analysis of PDGFR phosphorylation status and downstream surrogates of signaling (Akt and MAPK) will be evaluated and correlated with possible drug effects.

Another ambitious aspect of this project is to examine gene expression alterations that occur in these patients, given the significance of PDGFR β expression in prior studies by this modality. It will be technically challenging to get enough tissue for gene array analysis by needle biopsies, but, clearly, obtaining this information may be very useful to ascertain which patients are likely to benefit from imatinib mesylate.

CONCLUSION

PDGF receptors represent an attractive therapeutic target in prostate cancer as they are frequently expressed in these cancers. Their functional role in prostate cancer is still under intense investigation, but it is clear that they are specifically inhibited by the tyrosine kinase inhibitor imatinib mesylate. This inhibitor appears to have a favorable therapeutic index, since in normal tissues PDGF receptor is expressed at very specific developmental stages (embryogenesis) and in response to stress (wound healing).

Imatinib mesylate has been approved for the treatment of CML and is now in clinical trials for patients with prostate cancer. Results from these trials should provide insight on the suitability of PDGF receptor as a therapeutic target. It is hoped that the development of gene expression profiling will help to identify those patients most likely to respond to therapy in the future. Once it is established that pharmacodynamic assessments can gauge the effects of imatinib mesylate and help with patient selection, other settings, including patients with more advanced disease, will be considered.

References

1. Druker BJ, Talpaz M, Resta DJ, et al. Efficacy and safety of a specific inhibitor of the BCR-ABL tyrosine kinase in chronic myeloid leukemia. N Engl J Med 2001; 344:1031-7.
2. Druker BJ, Sawyers CL, Kantarjian H, et al. Activity of a specific inhibitor of the BCR-ABL tyrosine kinase in the blast crisis of chronic myeloid leukemia and acute lymphoblastic leukemia with the Philadelphia chromosome. N Engl J Med 2001; 344:1038-42.
3. Joensuu H, Roberts PJ, Sarlomo-Rikala M, et al. Effect of the tyrosine kinase inhibitor STI571 in a patient with a metastatic gastrointestinal stromal tumor. N Engl J Med 2001; 344:1052-6.
4. Demetri GD, von Mehren M, Blanke CD, et al. Efficacy and safety of imatinib mesylate in advanced gastrointestinal stromal tumors. N Engl J Med 2002; 347:472-80.

5. van Oosterom AT, Judson I, Verweij J, et al. Safety and efficacy of imatinib (STI571) in metastatic gastrointestinal stromal tumours: a phase I study. Lancet 2001; 358:1421-3.
6. Johnsson A, Heldin CH, Wasteson A, et al. The c-sis gene encodes a precursor of the B chain of platelet-derived growth factor. Embo J 1984; 3:921-8.
7. Betsholtz C, Johnsson A, Heldin CH, et al. cDNA sequence and chromosomal localization of human platelet-derived growth factor A-chain and its expression in tumour cell lines. Nature 1986; 320:695-9.
8. Li X, Ponten A, Aase K, et al. PDGF-C is a new protease-activated ligand for the PDGF alpha-receptor. Nat Cell Biol 2000; 2:302-9.
9. Koch CA, Anderson D, Moran MF, Ellis C, Pawson T. SH2 and SH3 domains: elements that control interactions of cytoplasmic signaling proteins. Science 1991; 252:668-74.
10. Yarden Y, Escobedo JA, Kuang WJ, et al. Structure of the receptor for platelet-derived growth factor helps define a family of closely related growth factor receptors. Nature 1986; 323:226-32.
11. Wennstrom S, Hawkins P, Cooke F, et al. Activation of phosphoinositide 3-kinase is required for PDGF-stimulated membrane ruffling. Curr Biol 1994; 4:385-93.
12. Wennstrom S, Siegbahn A, Yokote K, et al. Membrane ruffling and chemotaxis transduced by the PDGF beta-receptor require the binding site for phosphatidylinositol 3' kinase. Oncogene 1994; 9:651-60.
13. Bos JL. Ras-like GTPases. Biochim Biophys Acta 1997; 1333:M19-31.
14. Deuel TF. Polypeptide growth factors: roles in normal and abnormal cell growth. Annu Rev Cell Biol 1987; 3:443-92.
15. Ostman A, Heldin CH. Involvement of platelet-derived growth factor in disease: development of specific antagonists. Adv Cancer Res 2001; 80:1-38.
16. Sundberg C, Ljungstrom M, Lindmark G, Gerdin B, Rubin K. Microvascular pericytes express platelet-derived growth factor-beta receptors in human healing wounds and colorectal adenocarcinoma. Am J Pathol 1993; 143:1377-88.
17. Pietras K, Ostman A, Sjoquist M, et al. Inhibition of platelet-derived growth factor receptors reduces interstitial hypertension and increases transcapillary transport in tumors. Cancer Res 2001; 61:2929-34.
18. Heuchel R, Berg A, Tallquist M, et al. Platelet-derived growth factor beta receptor regulates interstitial fluid homeostasis through phosphatidylinositol-3' kinase signaling. Proc Natl Acad Sci U S A 1999; 96:11410-5.
19. Fleming TP, Saxena A, Clark WC, et al. Amplification and/or overexpression of platelet-derived growth factor receptors and epidermal growth factor receptor in human glial tumors. Cancer Res 1992; 52:4550-3.
20. Guha A, Dashner K, Black PM, Wagner JA, Stiles CD. Expression of PDGF and PDGF receptors in human astrocytoma operation specimens supports the existence of an autocrine loop. Int J Cancer 1995; 60:168-73.
21. Hermanson M, Funa K, Hartman M, et al. Platelet-derived growth factor and its receptors in human glioma tissue: expression of messenger RNA and protein suggests the presence of autocrine and paracrine loops. Cancer Res 1992; 52:3213-9.
22. Carroll M, Tomasson MH, Barker GF, Golub TR, Gilliland DG. The TEL/platelet-derived growth factor beta receptor (PDGF beta R) fusion in chronic myelomonocytic leukemia is a transforming protein that self-associates and activates PDGF beta R kinase-dependent signaling pathways. Proc Natl Acad Sci U S A 1996; 93:14845-50.
23. Jousset C, Carron C, Boureux A, et al. A domain of TEL conserved in a subset of ETS proteins defines a specific oligomerization interface essential to the mitogenic properties of the TEL-PDGFR beta oncoprotein. Embo J 1997; 16:69-82.
24. DiMaio D, Lai CC, Klein O. Virocrine transformation: the intersection between viral transforming proteins and cellular signal transduction pathways. Annu Rev Microbiol 1998; 52:397-421.
25. Crosby JR, Seifert RA, Soriano P, Bowen-Pope DF. Chimaeric analysis reveals role of Pdgf receptors in all muscle lineages. Nat Genet 1998; 18:385-8.
26. Lindahl P, Johansson BR, Leveen P, Betsholtz C. Pericyte loss and microaneurysm formation in PDGF-B-deficient mice. Science 1997; 277:242-5.
27. Fudge K, Bostwick DG, Stearns ME. Platelet-derived growth factor A and B chains and the alpha and beta receptors in prostatic intraepithelial neoplasia. Prostate 1996; 29:282-6.
28. Fudge K, Wang CY, Stearns ME. Immunohistochemistry analysis of platelet-derived growth factor A and B chains and platelet-derived growth factor alpha and beta receptor expression in benign prostatic hyperplasias and Gleason-graded human prostate adenocarcinomas. Mod Pathol 1994; 7:549-54.

29. Chott A, Sun Z, Morganstern D, et al. Tyrosine kinases expressed in vivo by human prostate cancer bone marrow metastases and loss of the type 1 insulin-like growth factor receptor. Am J Pathol 1999; 155:1271-9.
30. Singh D, Febbo PG, Ross K, et al. Gene expression correlates of clinical prostate cancer behavior. Cancer Cell 2002; 1:203-9.
31. Ko YJ, Small EJ, Kabbinavar F, et al. A multi-institutional phase ii study of SU101, a platelet-derived growth factor receptor inhibitor, for patients with hormone-refractory prostate cancer. Clin Cancer Res 2001; 7:800-5.
32. Bubley GJ, Carducci M, Dahut W, et al. Eligibility and response guidelines for phase II clinical trials in androgen-independent prostate cancer: recommendations from the Prostate-Specific Antigen Working Group. J Clin Oncol 1999; 17:3461-7.
33. D'Amico AV, Whittington R, Malkowicz SB, et al. Biochemical outcome after radical prostatectomy, external beam radiation therapy, or interstitial radiation therapy for clinically localized prostate cancer. Jama 1998; 280:969-74.

IMMUNE-PROMOTED TUMOR CELL INVASION AND METASTASIS

New considerations in cancer therapy

Emilio Barberá Guillem and James W. Sampsel

Available information shows that the immune system does not spontaneously reject malignant tumors. In addition, medical maneuvers to stimulate an immune response against established tumors do not show repetitive good results. Apparently, malignant tumor cells escape immune recognition and attack through multiple molecular mechanisms. Laboratory experiments show that properly stimulated specific CD8+ T cells, some CD4+ T cells, NK cells, and macrophages are capable of killing tumor cells. But, even in experimentally controlled conditions, a regular, complete, reliable and applicable tumor immune rejection has not been achieved yet. The birth of monoclonal antibodies, easy to produce in the laboratory and with very restricted target recognition, initiated a wave of expectation in the anti-cancer immune therapy believers. The "magic bullet" concept became popular, many new tumor antigens were discovered and new anti-tumor antigen antibodies developed. Thirty years after monoclonal antibodies introduction, few if any of those antibodies have shown a reliable anticancer curative effect. A question is raised looking at this defeating scenario: Is the immune system prepared to reject tumors? The plain answer to this question is another question: Why not? The immune system recognizes damaged cells and eliminates them in a continuous process of tissue repair. If tumor cells are identified as damaged cells the immune system should eliminate them. Nevertheless, in normally differentiated tissues, after elimination of damaged cells, a process of cell substitution and remodeling takes place based on recruitment of reserve cells and stem cells. Normal tissue repair involves, among other features, immune system cells and blood cells. Bone marrow derived scavenger cells remove cell debris. A controlled inflammatory cellular infiltration guaranties local replacement of connective matrix, cell motility/translocation, and neoangiogenesis. Apparently, tumor tissue replacement doesn't need stem cells while tumor cells can divide infinitely. Therefore, the elimination of tumor cells is a mater of imbalance: if the elimination process is faster the tumor disappear, but if the replacement process is faster the tumor grows. In addition, the particular performance of tumor cells disturbs the repair process and, in consequence, tumor connective matrix replacement, cell relocation, and neoangiogenesis are in chaos.

[1] Emilio Barbera Guilllem, 1555 Picardae Court, Powell, OH 43065, USA
[2] James W. Sampsel, 860 W4th, st., Marysville, OH 43040, USA

New Trends in Cancer for the 21st Century, edited by
Llombart-Bosch and Felipo, Kluwer Academic/Plenum Publishers, 2003

In the early 70s researchers observed that the existence in the host of a competent antitumor immune response was not always correlated with the slowest tumor growth. In vitro test showed that T cells were able to identify and specifically kill tumor cells[1, 2], although they reported that serum of the cancer patients contain "blocking factors" capable of inhibiting those anti-tumor cell actions[3]. Blocking factors were identified as immune complexes composed of antigenic tumor derived glycoproteins and their specific antibodies[4-6]. Unfortunately, the main research group sustaining this theory, suddenly lost interest in the subject, and in the late 80s blocking factors disappeared from the scientific literature without trails.

However, parallel reports were highlighting possible tumor stimulatory effects of the anti-tumor immune response[7-9]: (A) Experiments of tumorigenesis induced by injection of Moloney murine sarcoma virus (M-MuSV) showed that, compared to naïve mice, previously immunized mice with inactivated virus were more susceptible to develop the specific sarcoma. That specific susceptibility was abrogated by irradiation of mice prior to M-MuSV challenge[10]. These last results sustained the concept that anti-tumor antigen immune response can promote tumor. (B) Experiments of methylcholanthrene induced tumors showed similar results when immunized mice developed more and faster tumors[11]. (C) Extensive experiments with isotransplants (approximately 20,000) of different tumors (27 diverse types) including leukemia, sarcomas, carcinomas, all of strictly spontaneous origin, revealed that prior "immunization" of recipients with homologous lethally irradiated cells increased their tumor receptivity[12], reinforcing the concept that the immune response against tumor antigens can promote tumor establishment[13]. In all of those studies the mechanism behind that tumor promoting effect was not proved or even suggested.

In the 90s, new experiments on immune responses, taking place during the growth of solid tumors transplanted in syngeneic hosts, showed that host immune responses are fully compatible with progressive tumor development[14]. Although both B cell and T cell responses were detected in tumor, those results strongly suggested that anti-tumor antibodies might provide a sort of protection to tumor cells[15].

ANTI-TUMOR B CELL RESPONSE FACILITATES TUMOR PROGRESSION

Experiments of tumor implants in B cell knockout (KO) mice (μMT/μMT mutated mice) were illustrative of the existence of tumor protective mechanisms associated with B cell anti-tumor immune response. In our hands, about 80% of B cell KO mice do not develop tumors after challenge with isogeneic tumor cell doses capable of developing tumors in 100% of normal mice (Fig. 1A). Consistent results were obtained in other laboratories using B cell reconstituted SCID mice: Tumors grew more slowly in and were rejected more frequently by the mice lacking B cells[16]. No explanation was given for that association of facts.

Other experiments reinforce the association between responder B cells and faster tumor progression: Normal C3H mice intrasplenically injected with 10^5 Met129 mammary tumor cells all develop liver metastases in 10 days. If these mice are partially depleted of B cells by intravenous injection of anti-IgM antibody, the metastasis outcome is drastically reduced (Fig. 1B). Transfusion of two million 99% pure B lymphocytes (B200+, CD19+ cells positively selected by immune-magnetic methods), obtained from normal isogeneic mice, 24h after tumor challenge, do not modify those results. However, transfusion of the same amount, purity and timing of B lymphocytes obtained from mice carrying the same tumor for more than 14 days dramatically increases the metastatic outcome (Fig. 1C)[17]. Mice injected with B lymphocytes obtained from mice bearing different kind of tumor show intermediate results. These experiments show that B lymphocytes becomme capable of tumor promotion, with certain level of specificity, after being in a host developing a tumor. Apparently, the host develops B cell response against different tumor antigens, some of them specific and others common to many tumors types (example Thomsen Frederichreich antigens). Transplanted B cells from identical tumors identify more antigens and more clones could be activated compared to B cells from different tumor type. That suggests a link between specific B cell involvement and degree of tumor promotion.

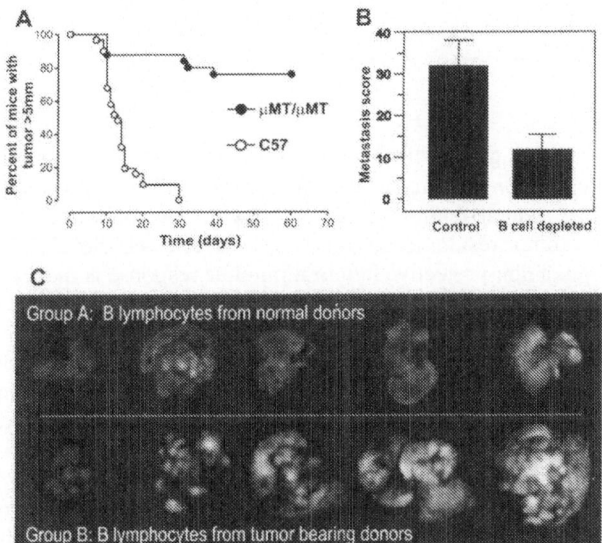

Figure 1. (A) One million Lewis lung carcinoma (3LL) cells injected subcutaneously develop tumors in 30 days in 100% of the immune competent mice (empty circles). Same dose of cells do not develop tumor in 80% of B cell knockout mice (mMT/mMT) (solid circles). (B) Intrasplenically injected tumor cells develop less metastases in immune competent mice receiving B cell depleting doses of anti-IgM antibodies (50% reduced circulating B cells). (C) Increased liver metastasis in mice receiving B cell transfusions from tumor bearing isogeneic mice. Controls receive same numbers of B cells from normal isogeneic donors.

Contradicting results have been reported from experiments of lung metastasis models impairing B cells. In rats, in which B lymphocytes express CD45RA, tail vein injection of tumor cells mixed with anti-CD45RA IgG increases the amount of lung metastases compared to rats injected with tumor cells alone. In those published experiments, separate administration of identical doses of that antibody did not replicate the data. Although that model had important flaws, the data were interpreted as a proof of early involvement (a window of 24h) of B cells in antitumor surveillance[18], theory that has been recently opposed by others[19]. Our experiments of tail vein injection of B16F10 melanoma cell in isogeneic C57BL-μMT/μMT mice do not support those data: These mice always develop less lung metastasis compared to normal C57BL mice (Table 1).

Table 1. B16F10 metastatic melanoma cells (105) intrasplenically injected in B lymphocyte KO mice (mMT/mMT) produce in 21 days low rates of metastasis, compared to normal immune competent mice (wt).

		Mice with metastasis / Mice injected		Metastases per mm' of lung surface area	
		C57BL wt	C57BL μMT/μMT	C57BL wt	C57BL μMT/μMT
Tumor cell dose Tail vein inj.	10⁴ Cells	6/6	0/6	8	0
	10⁴ Cells	6/6	3/6	14	5

Experiments from other groups also using μMT/μMT mice are consistent with our data, and disclose the progression of a reciprocal interaction between CD4+ cells and B cells after tumor challenge, which facilitates tumor growth: The presence of B cells in the priming phase of the tumor results in disabled CD4+ T cell help for CTL mediated tumor immunity, and instead, a non-protective humoral immune response is induced[20].

There are many unexplained observations showing that CD4+ lymphocyte depleted mice have increased resistance to metastasis[21]. Elimination of certain subsets of T lymphocytes (specifically V alpha 3+ regulatory T cells) also reduces chances of metastasis[21]. An explanation of that phenomenon was obtained from experiments on mouse tumor implants, which showed that CD4+ lymphocyte depletion indirectly enhances tumor rejection by impairing the concomitant B cell response[22].

However. other experiments challenge this last hypothesis as the only possible mechanism linking B cell response to faster tumor growth and increased metastasis. Data obtained from experiments of T47-D human breast carcinoma cells implanted in SCID beige and in nu/nu beige mice. SCID beige mice have a deficient NK activity and neither T nor B immune response. Athymic nu/nu beige mice, deficient in NK activity, do not have T cell immune response but have B cells capable of producing IgM and certain amounts and qualities of IgG. As predicted according to the above-described data, nu/nu mice develop tumors much faster than SCID mice (Fig. 2A)[23]. None of these mice have an effective CTL or NK population; therefore, the differences in tumor growth cannot be attributed to a T cell impairment induced by B cells neither in SCID nor in nu/nu models. These experiments actually pointed towards a positive action of tumor growth support in the presence of a B cell response.

ANTI-TUMOR ASSOCIATED ANTIGEN IgGs ARE INVOLVED IN THE TUMOR IMMUNE-PROMOTION PHENOMENON

Early data mentioned above pointed to immune-complexes formed by tumor antigens and specific IgG as responsible for establishing a sort of tumor cell tolerance[1-6]. Nevertheless, considering the proposed direct promotion of tumor growth and metastasis by

B cell immune response, we decided to study the role of IgG in this phenomenon using models of tumor cells spontaneously expressing well known tumor associated antigens (TAA) and existing specific monoclonal anti-TAA immunoglobulins (Ig). So, different tumor cells spontaneously expressing and secreting sialyl-Tn tumor associated antigens (sTn)[24] were used in all experiments. B72.3 monoclonal IgG1 that recognizes clustered sTn epitopes[25] was used as counterpart. SCID and nu/nu beige mice were used to avoid interferences with CTL or NK cells.

Tumor cells were implanted subcutaneously and 2, 4 and 6 days after tumor challenge, same doses of pure specific monoclonal IgG or irrelevant IgG dissolved in saline were injected intraperitoneally. In SCID mice injected with T47-D cells secreting sTn+ material, three 100 µg doses of B72.3 IgG significantly accelerated tumor growth in 100% of treated mice (Fig 2B) compared to the group treated with irrelevant IgG[23] Similar results were obtained from experiments with nu/nu mice. In nu/nu mice injected with T47-D cells, the same three 100 µg doses of B72.3 IgG also significantly increased tumor growth speed compared to the group treated with irrelevant IgG (Fig 2C). Here, in both experiments, the isolated tumor promoting effect of the specific anti-TAA IgG points to a direct involvement of this specific IgG in an undefined mechanism that provides tumor help, independently of the CTL or NK function.

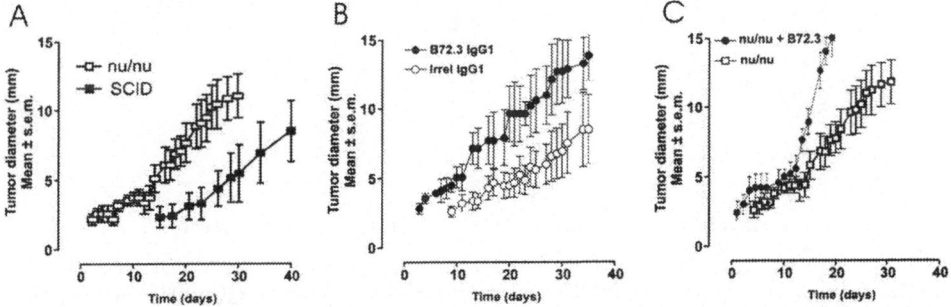

Figure 2. (A) T47-D human breast carcinoma cells subcutaneously injected in athymic nu/nu beige (capable of developing anti-tumor antibodies) develop faster tumors (empty squares) compared to SCID beige mice (which do not generate anti-tumor antibodies) which develop slow growing tumors (solid squares). (B)T47-D human breast carcinoma cells subcutaneously injected in SCID beige mice develop slow growing tumors (empty circles). Same implants develop faster tumors when SCID receive injected exogenous anti-tumor antibodies (B72.3 IgG1, solid circles). (B) T47-D cell subcutaneously injected in athymic nu/nu beige mice develop faster growing tumors (empty squares). Tumor growth is accelerated when the nu/nu mice receive supplements of injected exogenous anti-tumor antibodies (B72.3 IgG1, solid circles).

Some tumor cells expressing Fc receptors, are capable of IgG ligation, responding to the presence of immune complexes containing IgG by secreting cytokines and increasing proliferation rates[26]. This could explain the tumor growth promoting effect of specific IgG. However, in our experience only some tumors express FcγRI, and compared to the general appearance and magnitude of tumor promotion imposed by IgG injection this cannot stand as the sole mechanism behind the immune-promoted tumor growth phenomenon.

Experiments with FcR negative tumor cells confirm this suspicion: T47-D breast carcinoma cell or SW620 colon carcinoma cells, both human and positive for sTn were mixed with 10% mouse hybridoma cells secreting B72.3 IgG1 (ATCC HB-8108). As a control, the same carcinoma cells were mixed with 10% hybridoma cells of identical plasmocytoma base but secreting 9D9 IgG1 (ATCC CRL-1703), a monoclonal antibody specific for bovine low density lipoprotein (LDL), without cross reactivity for mouse tissues or those tumor cells. One million cells per mice of these mixtures were injected subcutaneously in groups of SCID beige mice. In this model without endogenous IgG, hybridoma cells played the role of TAA specific IgG source, like tumor infiltrating plasma cells frequently observed in fast growing tumors and metastases[27]. In these conditions tumor cells mixed with the specific hybridoma developed extremely fast growing and metastatic tumors. On the other hand, tumor cells mixed with the irrelevant hybridoma did not grow or were much slower and did not metastasize (Fig 3).

Not discarding the possible CTL-inhibitory actions of B lymphocytes or antibodies in an immune competent host, it seems evident that at least certain IgG specific for TAA, released by lymphocytes or plasma cells, promote tumor progression independently of CTL, NK, and other candidates of cellular tumor rejection.

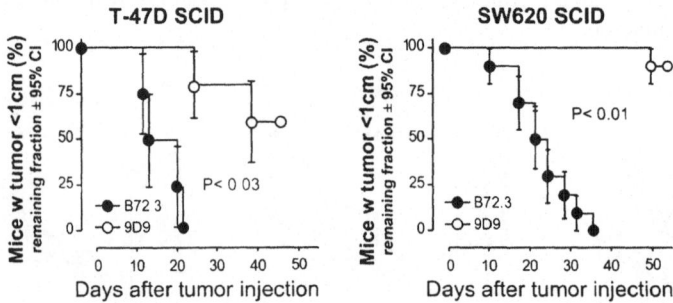

Figure 3. Highly angiogenic T47-D human mammary adenocarcinoma (A) and low angiogenic SW620 human colon carcinoma (B) growing in SCID mice in the presence of irrelevant IgG (9D9). Tumors grew faster in the presence of specific anti-tumor IgG (B72.3).

TUMORS GROWING IN HUMANS FREQUENTLY SHOW B CELL INVOLVEMENT

Many studies report the presence of certain titers of antibodies reacting with tumor-associated membrane bound or secreted antigens in the sera of cancer patient. These include viral antigens, altered glycoproteins and different gene products generated by alternative splicing, alternative promoter usage, or allelic polymorphism[28-30]. Most of these antibodies only detect molecules present in tumor cells but not normal or embryonic tissues[29-31]. Others also react with molecules present in hyperplasic tissues, like polyps, or in inflammatory lesions such as diverticulitis, and Crohn's disease[32]; those also can be found in some normal individuals[33-35]. Antitumor antibodies are present in patients of practically all kind of tumors, including melanoma, neural tumors[29], squamous cell carcinomas[30], adenocarcinomas of lung[31], breast[36], and colorectal[37]. The amount of these antibodies has been associated with tumor load and evolution time of the tumor, being also detectable after tumor removal, and preceding the clinical detection of recurrent tumors[29]. Although countless reports insist on the existence of anti-tumor antibodies in different cancer patients and different stages of the tumor[38], there are not enough repetitive and consistent data to affirm that the humoral antitumor immune response has or has not a value in rejecting tumor or suppressing tumor progression.

Histological studies of clinical cases undoubtedly show B cell involvement in tumor pathology. Lymph nodes anatomically related to the tumor frequently show follicular hyperplasia[39]. Detailed histochemical studies demonstrated that the tumor-associated antigens such as TAG-72 and CEA are presented in the germinal centers of tumor-involved lymph nodes[40, 41]. Although tumor-associated antigens may be seen in lymph node sinuses, MO, and in metastatic cells, it is notorious that these tumor-associated antigens are massively presented on the follicular dendritic cell network of the germinal centers (Fig. 4), which show concomitant B cell hyperplasia and signs of B cell proliferation.

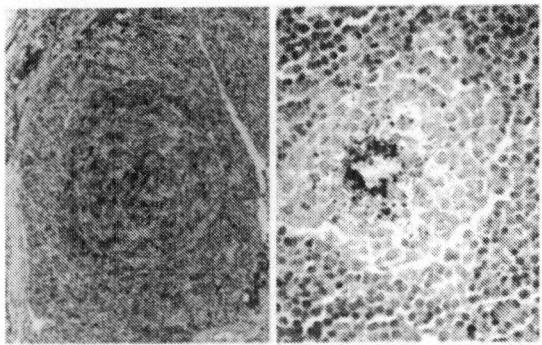

Figure 4. A) Tumor associated antigen TAG72 (brawn, immune-peroxidase staining) presented on follicular dendritic cells in germinal centers of tumor draining lymph nodes (human colon cancer). B. Autorradiographic picture of similar lymph node from a patient treated with I125-anti-TAG72 MAb, showing radioactive accumulation in the germinal centers (black spots).

Tracing deposits of tumor antigen with specific radiolabeled monoclonal antibodies in cancer patients provided reinforcing clinical data about the anti-tumor reactive character of regional lymph showing marked follicular hyperplasia[42], and linked high numbers of lymph nodes presenting tumor-associated antigen with high risk of tumor recurrence[43]. However, germinal centers presenting certain tumor associate antigen have been reported in other non-cancer pathology with ambiguous interpretations[44, 45]. Although most clinical and pathology studies strongly suggest a relationship between tumor behavior and regional lymph node B cell response[46-48], like serum circulating anti-tumor antibodies, the tumor rejecting significance of those follicular hyperplasic images remains unexplored and controversial, and mechanistic/molecular studies of these phenomena are seldom or non existent.

Nevertheless, we found that administration of radioactive monoclonal antibodies against tumor-associated antigens, such as TAG-72, presented on follicular dendritic cells. followed by surgical reduction of radiolabeled lymph nodes, is related to a lower rate of tumor recurrence (Fig. 5)[49]. That association is difficult to explain as an exclusive consequence of metastasis clearance while actually, most (about 80%) of the radiolabeled tumor antigen detectable spots are antigen presenting structures, which do not contain tumor cells, and many metastases do not have detectable amounts of label and are overlooked[50]. Thus, knowing that germinal center structures are needed to support the generation of memory B cells and to permit existing memory B cells to express an isotype switched memory Ig response following sustained soluble antigenic challenge[51,52], it is understandable that those germinal centers were involved in sustaining a specific Ig production against soluble specific tumor associated antigens. Based on these facts, we suggest that the combination of surgical removal plus the long lasting, short distance, irradiation of specific germinal centers by antigen-mediated concentration of I_{125}-labeled antibody (Fig. 4B) can induce a transitory decline of the specific anti-tumor B cell/Ig response in favor of a more effective T cell rejection of residual tumor cells[49].

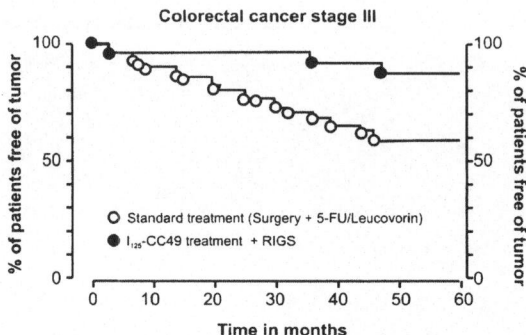

Figure 5. Clinical results of 24 colon cancer patients, all stage III, treated with I_{125}-anti-TAG72 MAb (CC49), and selective lymphadenectomy by radio-immune-guided surgery (RIGS).

There follows our efforts to further test this hypothesis. We developed a C57BL mice model of tumor recurrence based on intradermal implantation of a solid invasive carcinoma (10^6 Lewis lung carcinoma cells, 3LL), followed by surgical tumorectomy when the tumor reaches 5 mm in diameter, and analysis of the survival consequences. Ninety five percent of normal immunocompetent C57BL mice treated with this protocol developed primary tumor at the implantation site, and 100% developed local or distant recurrent lethal tumors after surgical removal of the primary, all in a time period of 30 days (Fig. 6A). The same protocol was applied to C57BL Lymphotoxin alpha -/- mice (LTalpha -/-) (Fig. 6B). LTalpha signaling is critically required for germinal center formation and for the IgM and IgG responses to both T dependent and T independent type 2 Ags.[52]. LT alpha -/- mice, rendered deficient in LT alpha by gene targeting, have no detectable lymph nodes or Peyer's patches, profound defects in development of follicular dendritic cell networks, germinal center formation, and T/B cell segregation in lymphatic organs. Follicular dendritic cell clusters and germinal centers are absent from the peripheral lymphoid tissues of LTalpha-/- mice, which produce high levels of antigen-specific IgM, but very low levels of IgG after immunization[53]. Although thymus development is normal, and peripheral blood contain CD4+ and CD8+ T cells in a normal ratio[54], LTalpha -/- mice develop CD8+ T cells with inadequate expression of the IL-12 receptor, impaired cytotoxic and cytokine-mediated effector functions linked to defective CC7R signaling[55, 56], resulting in enhanced susceptibility to viral infections[55]. In addition, while membrane-bound LTalpha is critical for NK cell early in ontogeny[57], these LTalpha -/- mice exhibit impaired NK cell development and recruitment and reduced ability of tumor cell destruction[58]. Our model of tumor recurrence on LTalpha-/-showed that, in spite of the global immune deficiency of these mice, more than 25% never develop primary tumor, and from those that develop tumor, more than 50% never recur (Fig. 6B). Both primary and recurrent tumors grow slower in LTalpha -/- mice compared to normal mice (Fig 6B). Tumor recurrence, both local and distant (metastasis), requires tumor cell invasion, thus the reduced tumor recurrence in these mice is indicative of an impaired tumor cell invasion. That increased resistance against tumor growth and invasion showed in LTalpha -/- cannot be attributed to the enhancement of the CTL and NK functions, which are depressed in those mice compared to normal mice, thus the lack of LTalpha and the reduction of specific IgG remain as major candidates responsible for that increased anti-tumor resistance: (A) Secretion or surface presentation of LTalpha by activated CD4+ T helper type 1 cells (Th1), and activated B cells have been considered essential in the development of chronic inflammation infiltrates by influencing the local expression of chemokines and adhesion molecules such as E-selectin adhesion molecule (ELAM), vascular cell adhesion molecule (VCAM), intercellular adhesion molecule (ICAM), mucosal addressin cellular adhesion molecule (MAdCAM), and peripheral node addressin (PNAd)[59]. Therefore, the tumor invasion inhibitory effect shown by LTα-/- hosts could be a consequence of a reduced inflammatory response surrounding tumor cells[60, 61].(B) The absence of germinal centers in these mice allows class switching but no further affinity maturation of IgG, which requires prolonged availability of antigen exposed by follicular dendritic cells[62]; therefore, as mentioned above, the absence of sufficient high affinity anti-tumor IgG could be behind the impaired tumor invasive behavior observed in LTalpha -/- host.

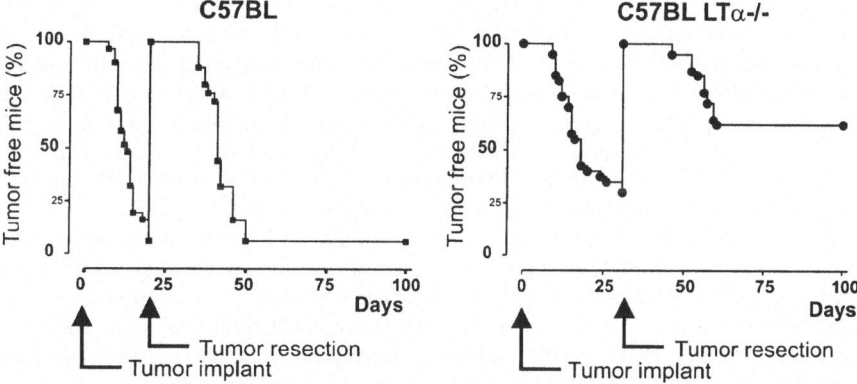

Figure 6. Tumor recurrence (local and metastasis) in normal immune competent hosts versus B cell deficient host (LTα-/-). A) All mice with strong humoral anti-tumor immune response developed the implanted tumor, and a recurrent tumor after surgical removal of the first tumor. B) 30% of the mice without functional germinal centers rejected the implanted tumor, and from the group that developed the tumor, more than 30% never developed recurrent tumor.

ANTIBODIES PROMOTE TUMOR CELL SPREAD THROUGH GRANULOCYTES AND MACROPHAGES

Theoretically, anti-tumor antibodies, specifically IgG, can favor malignant tumor progression through typical mechanisms of the inflammatory process. A continuous succession of connective matrix degradation and neo-angiogenesis maintain tumor invasion and metastasis, and both auto-sustained by malignantly transformed tumor cells. However, these functions, connective matrix degradation and neo-angiogenesis are also physiological processes involved in tissue repair and remodeling, reliant on of inflammatory cell involvement, mainly monocyte/macrophages (MOs) and neutrophil polymorphonuclear cells (PMNs). MOs express the receptors for IgG: FcgammaRI (CD64), FcgammaRII (CD32), and FcgammaRIII (CD16). In the case of tumors secreting or shedding antigenic molecules, MOs assume the clearance of IgG immune complexes (ICs) through those Fcgamma receptors. In parallel, ICs induce inflammation by activating MO expression of inflammatory cytokines and matrix metalloproteases (MMPs), enzymes capable of degrading every component of the extracellular matrix[64, 65]. The existence and persistence of tumor associated antigens and specific IgG activate a cascade of feedback reactions, which ensures the amplification of the IgG production and ICs formation until there is complete clearance of the antigen. Phagocytosis or cytokine activated MOs can induce a strong IFN-gamma dominant Th1 cell response and, in reciprocity, IFN-gamma upregulates on MO the surface expression of FcgammaRI[64]. This could exert certain antitumor activity. However, when ICs are ligated to Fcgamma receptors of activated MOs, their phenotype changes (type 2 activated MO), and there is induced an IL-4 dominant T cell response increasing antibody production[66]. In reciprocity, Th2 cells provide IL-10, which blocks the MO expression of antigen-presenting major histocompatibility complex (MHC) II and the costimulatory B7 molecules. This impairs effective anti-tumor T cell activation, and it induces the expression of more Fcgamma receptors specially CD16. The expression of CD16 should enable MOs to carry out antibody-dependent cell-mediated cytotoxicity (ADCC) against tumor cells[67]. However, in the presence of IgG-ICs, binding to and transmitting survival signals to the MOs, allow these cells to complete the type-2 differentiation process and survive for long periods of time, extending the inflammation course. This last effect is counterbalanced in the absence of TAA and IgG-ICs while this MO differentiation step is largely undercut by the capacity of IL-10 to induce MO apoptosis[68]. Only signals delivered by ICs through the FcgammaRIIb (CD16B), expressed on some stages of the macrophage differentiation[69], can down-regulate FcgammaR-mediated phagocytosis and immune complex-induced inflammation[70].

Together with MO, PMN accumulation is a hallmark of immune complex-mediated inflammatory reaction. PMN trafficking involves transendothelial migration into tissue interstitium. Complement activation induced by IgG-ICs deposition is an important event leading to PMN recruitment. Complement activation product C5a plays an important role in chemoattracting PMNs, and regulates adhesion molecules, chemokines, and cytokines expression. The process of PMNs recruitment and translocation is initiated and modulated by the production of early response MO cytokines and chemokines. MO secreted chemokines such as MO inflammatory protein (MIP)-2 and cytokine-inducible neutrophil chemoattractant (CINC) recruit PMNs[70, 71]. Neutrophil recruitment results from the capture of circulating PMNs by activated endothelial cells. Immobilized ICs can support by themselves rapid attachment of PMNs to endothelial cells, under physiologic flow conditions, through the PMN expressed Fcgamma receptor CD16[72]. In addition, MO released cytokines such as TNF-alpha and IL-1 upregulate the expression of intracellular adhesion molecule-1 (ICAM-1) and E-selectin, setting the optimal conditions for PMN migration through endothelium[71, 73]. Moreover, cytokine priming deeply modulate PMNs responsiveness to ICs. For example, insoluble ICs activated both primed or unprimed PMNs through CD16 to release enzymes of the granule (degranulation), while soluble complexes do not activate degranulation of unprimed PMNs[72, 74].

Both MO and PMNs are common infiltrators of the tumor tissue, and tumor shed antigens are embedding the tumor connective matrix (Fig 7). The repetitive observation of important amounts of IgG in the tumor matrix either in experimental tumors or human tumors (Fig 7) led us to investigate the importance of tumor associated antigens-IgG ICs role in tumor biology. A modified test of matrigel tumor cell invasion provided illustrative information about the importance of this processes[75]. Briefly, in this test a 100-200 μm thick layer of matrigel separates two cell culture chambers (Fig 8). The matrigel layer includes a preset proportion of either mouse naïve T lymphocytes, or MO, or PMNs, or combinations. The upper cell culture chamber contains human invasive tumor cells secreting sTn tumor associated antigen (sTn-TAA). The lower cell culture chamber contains free of complement media with either mouse anti-sTn IgG, or mouse irrelevant IgG (Fig 8). When the test is in progress, IgG of the lower chamber and sTn-TAA from the upper chamber (secreted by the tumor cells) diffuse through the matrigel film. Irrelevant IgG does not couple sTn-TAA and no complexes are formed. However, anti-sTn IgG and sTn-TAA form a gradient of precipitated complexes in the matrigel film, which activate the matrigel-resident cells. Human tumor cells of the upper chamber have enough migration power to slowly (24-48 h) penetrate the matrigel film and form a few colonies in the lower chamber. Precise mouse or human specific antibodies and PCR probes permit separately analysis of the cytokine response of either mouse (inflammatory cells) or human cells (tumor cells). Appropriate experimental combinations provided controls and tests of the importance of tumor associated antigen-IgG ICs (TAA-IgG-ICs) participation in tumor cell invasion. In the presence of TAA-IgG-ICs, combined MO and PMNs populations multiply up to 30 times IL-1 and up to 10 times IL-6 secretion by MO (Fig 9A and 9B). A 40 times increased tumor cell migration followed that powerful inflammatory response (Fig 10). When either the specific IgG or the TAA was absent, tumor cell migration was in the normal range. Moreover, invasive tumor cells not secreting the specific antigen showed basal migration rates in the presence of IgG, MO, and PMNs. However, when in the upper chamber soluble antigen matching the IgG idiotype was added, tumor cells not secreting that antigen multiply 20-30 times the migration rate (Fig 10B). These results confirmed the ICs role in promoting tumor cell invasion in the presence of the MO/PMN tandem. Basically, any IgG-IC included in the tumor cell vicinity is capable of triggering inflammatory responses on MO and PMNs leading to increased tumor cell invasiveness, but tumor cell secreted antigens have more chances based on proximity[75, 76]. The Fcgamma receptors involvement in these phenomena was disclosed in similar experiments when the IgG-Fab fraction was substituted for IgG. IgG-Fab fraction did not induce cytokine secretion or tumor cell migration, and Fcgamma receptor blockade impaired both cytokine secretion and tumor cell migration enhancements[75, 76].

These experiments point up diffusible TAA-anti-TAA ICs as the trigger and sustainer of a peri-tumor cell inflammatory infiltration and process leading to an exacerbated local matrix degradation, tumor cell motility, and tumor cell invasion[75, 76].

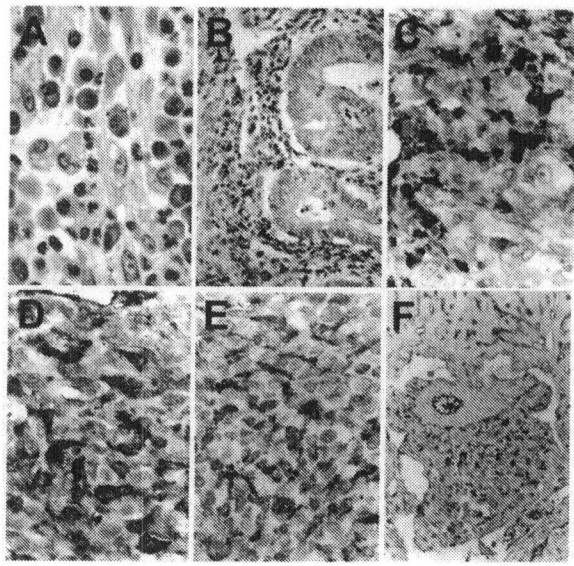

Figure 7. A) Inflammatory cell infiltrate in a human breast carcinoma. B) Macrophage and PMN infiltrating the connective matrix of a human colon carcinoma (brawn, anti-CD11b immune staining). C) IgG1 positive cells (brawn, peroxidase immune staining) infiltrating the tumor matrix in a human breast carcinoma. D) Extensive infiltrate of macrophages containing IgG in experimental mammary adenocarcinoma. E) Infiltrate of macrophages containing IgG in metastases of experimental mammary adenocarcinoma. F) Infiltrate of macrophages containing IgG and endothelial cells of the peripheral sinusoids coated with IgG in liver metastasis of experimental mammary adenocarcinoma.

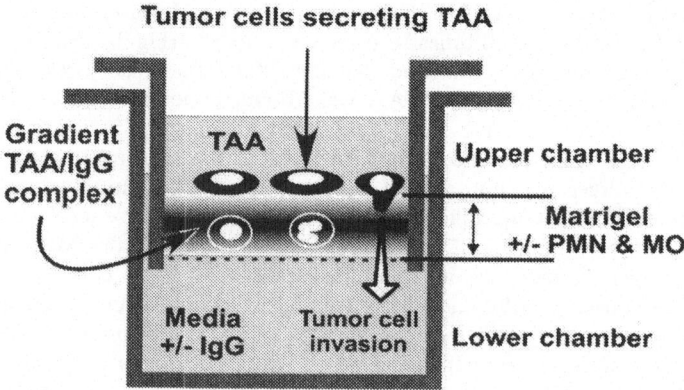

Figure 8. In vitro experimental model of tumor cell and inflammatory cell interaction in the connective matrix.

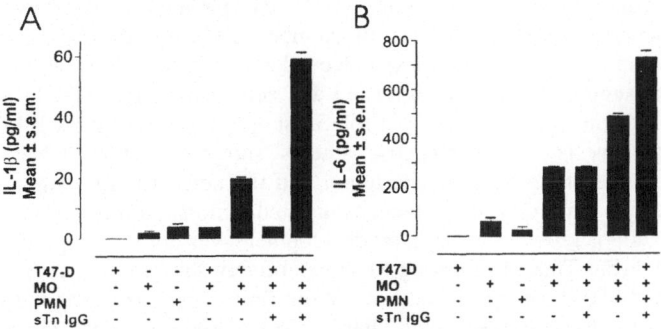

Figure 9. Modulation of the inflammatory response by interactions of tumor cells and inflammatory cell. Additional effect of complexes including tumor associated antigen and the specific IgG. In vitro model.

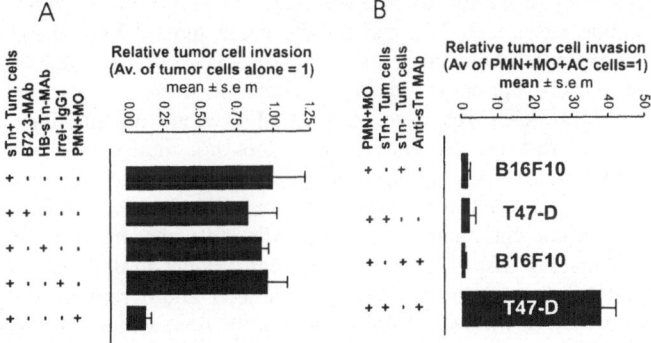

Figure 10. Tumor cell invasion promotion by inflammatory cells and immune complexes composed of tumor associated antigen and the specific anti-tumor associated antigen IgG.

ANTIBODIES PROMOTE TUMOR NEOANGIOGENESIS THROUGH GRANULOCYTES AND MACROPHAGES

In normal tissue repair it has been demonstrated that the recruitment of MO constitutes the main source of VEGF and the fundamental step for the establishment of an effective angiogenesis[77]. Experiments inhibiting VEGF demonstrate that neoangiogenesis is a bottleneck in the malignant process; while by impairing angiogenesis the tumor growth could be totally suppressed[78-81]. Knowing that tumor cells produce VEGF, we broadly assume that the tumor cells are sufficient to promote enough vessel formation for the fast growing neoplastic tissue[81-85]. However, there is a certain discrepancy in accepting the exclusivity of the tumor cell supplying sufficient vascular stimulating factors for necessary tumor neoangiogenesis, while other normal cells included in the tumor tissue also secrete VEGF[86-89]. Hypoxia, ICs, chemokines, and NO, common in the tumor environment, are capable of inducing MO recruitment and MO-VEGF expression[90-95]. Actually, high VEGF expression has been frequently observed in tumor infiltrating MO (TIMs)[92-94], and increased tumor angiogenesis has been reported after monocyte recruitment into the tumor[92].

TIMs are abundant in all kind of tumors[67, 93]. Morphometric and flow cytometry analysis in experimental tumors showed that the number of MO infiltrating the tumor mass is proportional to tumor volume (Fig 11A) independently of the tumor age or volume[97]. These observations suggested that MO, attracted and activated by IgG-ICs, in addition of supporting tumor cell invasion might play a role in supporting tumor growth by inducing inflammatory angiogenesis[95]. Morphometric studies showed us that TIMs are more concentrated in the interphase between the tumor and the normal tissue, among capillary sprouts (Fig 11C). In experimental subcutaneous injected tumors, our results showed that in early stages of the tumor growth the capillary development was always proportional to MO concentration (Fig 11B). These infiltrating MOs repetitively showed endocytosed material containing TAA and anti-TAA IgG in human tumors (Fig 11D) supporting the possibility that in the *in vivo* tumor environment both phagocytosis of cell debris and the presence of immune complexes (formed with TAA and anti-TAA IgG) may promote the secretion of very important amounts of VEGF. The same *in vitro* test mentioned above, showed that tumor cells in contact or proximity to MO stimulate the secretion of MO-VEGF, but not vice versa, and importantly, each MO can secrete much more VEGF than certain tumor cells (Fig 12). The example of the common tumor associated sTn antigen was illustrative. ICs made of repeated sTn epitopes and anti-sTn-IgG (in these experiments B72.3 IgG1 MAb) can activate MO VEGF response. Anti-sTn-IgG alone did not increase the MO-VEGF release showing that the presence of IgG does not induce that MO secretion of VEGF. ICs formed with sTn-TAA and specific IgG act as moderate stimulators of the MO VEGF response. However, the concurrence of tumor cells shedding antigenic debris, the specific anti-tumor antigen IgG, and infiltrating PMN cells can dramatically increase the MO release of VEGF (Fig 12). Therefore, the locally concentrated immune complexes composed of shed tumor antigens and the specific IgG could represent a fundamental primer and/or maintainer of the MO/PMN tandem activation, which can produce enough VEGF to support angiogenesis needed for tumor growth[97]. These results substantiate the importance of TIM as a source of VEGF in the tumor tissue.

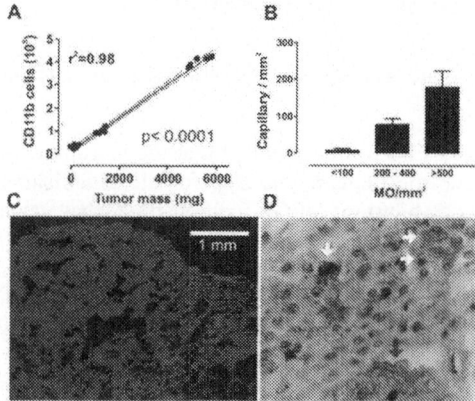

Figure 11. A) Correlation of number of infiltrating macrophages and tumor mass in mouse experimental tumors. B) Correlation of number of infiltrating macrophages and number of new capillaries in the tumor (neoangiogenesis). C) Accumulation of the macrophage infiltration (red areas) in the "growing tumor - normal tissue" interface. D) Infiltrating macrophages of a human colon carcinoma containing tumor associated antigen TAG72 (white arrows). Many tumor cells contain TAG72 (black arrow).

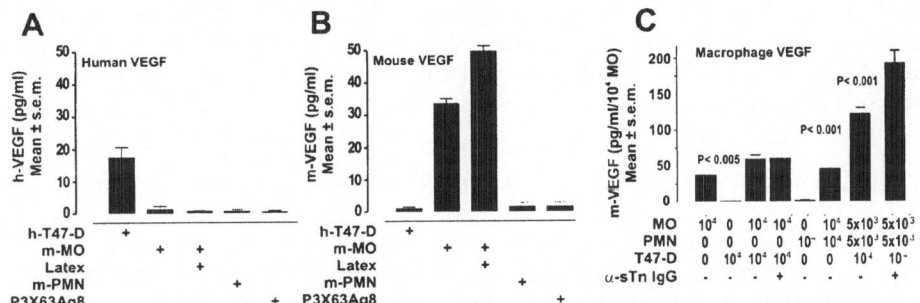

Figure 12. Macrophage VEGF modulation by tumor cells, other inflammatory cells and immune complexes composed of tumor associated antigen and the specific IgG. A) VEGF secretion of tumor cells. B) VEGF secretion of inflammatory cells. C) Modulation of the monocyte secreted VEGF under different experimental conditions.

RT-PCR analysis of the MO mRNA before and after such stimulus showed an unchanged pattern of VEGF gene expression: VEGF-A and B were expressed but not C or D. This suggest that MO may control the establishment of new blood supply in the growing tumor, but not new lymphatic capillaries, which basically are VEGF-C controlled[98, 99].

The results from *in vivo* experiments were consistent with these interpretations. The number of capillaries per unit of tumor volume and the daily growth rate of tumors were related to the serum concentration of anti-sTn IgG. Tumors growing in SCID mice, which do not develop specific IgG response, had very low vascular network and very slow growth. However, tumor growing in SCID mice injected with exogenous ANTI-STN-IGGIgG, specific for the tumor-associated antigen sTn, showed much higher capillary density and faster tumor growth. Such tumor enhancing effect was not observed in SCID mice injected with the same doses of irrelevant IgG isotype which proves that increase of angiogenesis is related to the specific recognition of tumor associated antigens by the specific IgG. Moreover, nu/nu mice capable of developing a B cell response, mainly IgM based, produced a certain serum concentration of endogenous anti-sTn IgG, and these mice developed tumors with a significantly higher density of capillaries as compared to tumors developed in SCID mice. With identical numbers and classes of tumor cells implanted in nu/nu beige mice or in SCID beige mice, tumors grew faster in nu/nu mice. When nu/nu mice had an exogenous source of anti-sTn-IgG supplied by injection, the results showed a higher concentration of serum anti-sTn IgG and dramatically increased tumor vascularization. That effect was also specific, because the same carcinoma growing in nu/nu mice injected with irrelevant IgG, had the same capillary density as the controls. Neither of these mouse types, SCID or nu/nu beige, have NK cells or effective T cells. Therefore, the difference in tumor growth could not be attributed to a different tumor rejection capacity. The only possible effectors for a tumor rejection in these mouse types were the MO and the PMN cells. The microscopy examination, however, showed no suspicion of efficient tumor rejection associated with the MO/PMN infiltration. On the contrary, the MO/PMN infiltrate was always associated with neo-angiogenesis.

Therefore *In vitro* data suggest that immune complexes involving shed tumor antigens and specific IgG constitute a powerful enhancer of VEGF production by MO infiltrate.

Considering that those immune-complexes can also induce the release of chemo-attractant factors by stromal cells, it is understandable that the immune-complexes could further sustain the tumor infiltration by more stromal cells, establishing a feedback process of infiltration-inflammation-angiogenesis.

THE TUMOR PROMOTING SIDE EFFECT OF THE ANTI-TUMOR IMMUNE RESPONSE

For a long time the puzzling tumor-promoting role of the anti-tumor humoral immune response, or specifically the surprising anti-tumor resistance of B cell deficient animals, have been "some think not to talk about". New experimental data in this field show that there is no magic or misinterpretation on that apparent tumor help provided by the humoral immune response; like in any exacerbated autoimmune process, the inflammatory response induced by antigens and antibodies in the tumor context brings, as a side effect, two powerful vectors for tumor progression: connective matrix degradation and neoangiogenesis. Probably due to a lack of appeal of this kind of bad news, these data have been neglected in favor of more gleaming positive experiments where tumor cells are actually defeated by the thought and expected anti-tumor effectors. However, the data were there, have been slowly escalating, and to ignore them is reckless.

Today existing data underline a set of important conclusions:

A) Any diffusible tumor associated antigen, shed, secreted or separate from the tumor cell by any kind of mechanism will not be full effective for complement or antibody-dependent cell-mediated cytotoxicity.

B) IgG targeting this type of TAA may form ICs capable to stimulate MO and PMNs infiltration/activation in the vicinity of the tumor cell growing colonies.

C) These accumulated and activated inflammatory cells can induce certain level of tumor cell destruction, but also very important connective matrix degradation, neoangiogenesis, and tumor cell motility induction, which favor tumor cell invasion and metastasis.

A delicate balance destruction/promotion is therefore inherent in the humoral anti-tumor immunity. As a result, immune therapy approaches based on the enhancement of IgG production, or exogenous humanized IgG administration, against tumor antigens should be cautiously studied considering: (A) The nature and behavior of the targeted TAA, (B) possible genetic modifications of the IgG Fc segment[99], and (C) complementary anti-inflammatory therapeutic strategies including B cell control.

References

1. Hellstrom I, Hellstrom KE, Pierce GE, Yang JP. Cellular and humoral immunity to different types of human neoplasms. Nature. 220(174): 1352-4. 1968.
2. Hellstrom I, Hellstrom KE, Sjogren HO, Warner GA. Demonstration of cell-mediated immunity to human neoplasms of various histological types. Int J Cancer. 7(1): 1-16. 1971.
3. Sjogren HO, Hellstrom I, Bansal SC, Hellstrom KE. Suggestive evidence that the "blocking antibodies" of tumor-bearing individuals may be antigen-antibody complexes. Proc Natl Acad Sci U S A. 68(6):1372-5. 1971.
4. Sjogren HO, Hellstrom I, Bansal SC, Warner GA, Hellstrom KE. Elution of "blocking factors" from human tumors, capable of abrogating tumor-cell destruction by specifically immune lymphocytes. Int J Cancer. 9(2): 274-83. 1972.

5. Tamerius J, Nepom J, Hellstrom I, Hellstrom KE. Tumor-associated blocking factors: isolation from sera of tumor-bearing mice. J Immunol. 116(3): 724-30. 1976.

6. Nepom JT, Hellstrom I, Hellstrom KE. Antigen-specific purification of blocking factors from sera of mice with chemically induced tumors. Proc Natl Acad Sci U S A. 74(10): 4605-9. 1977.

7. Prehn RT, Lappe MA. An immunostimulation theory of tumor development. Transplant Rev. 7:26-54. 1971.

8. Prehn RT. The immune reaction as a stimulator of tumor growth. Science. 176(31): 170-1. 1972.

9. Prehn RT. Immunomodulation of tumor growth. Am J Pathol. 77(1): 119-122. 1974.

10. Murasko DM, Prehn RT. Stimulatory effect of immunization on tumor induction by Moloney murine sarcoma virus. J Natl Cancer Inst. 61(5):1323-7. 1978.

11. Lawler EM, Prehn RT. Influence of immune status of host on immunogenicity of tumors induced with two doses of methylcholanthrene. Cancer Immunol Immunother. 13(3):194-7. 1982.

12. Hewitt HB, Blake ER, Walder AS. A critique of the evidence for active host defense against cancer, based on personal studies of 27 murine tumors of spontaneous origin. Br J Cancer. 33(3): 241-59. 1976.

13. Prehn RT. Stimulatory effects of immune reactions upon the growths of untransplanted tumors. Cancer Res. 54(4): 908-14. 1994.

14. Manson LA. Anti-tumor immune responses of the tumor-bearing host: the case for antibody-mediated immunologic enhancement. Clin Immunol Immunopathol. 72(1): 1-8. 1994.

15. Manson LA. The role of anti-tumor antibody in progressive tumor growth. Transplant Proc. 16(2): 524-7. 1984.

16. Monach PA, Schreiber H, Rowley DA. CD4+ and B lymphocytes in transplantation immunity. II. Augmented rejection of tumor allografts by mice lacking B cells. Transplantation. 55(6): 1356-61. 1993.

17. Barbera-Guillem E, Nelson MB, Barr B, Nyhus JK, May KF Jr, Feng L, Sampsel JW. B lymphocyte pathology in human colorectal cancer. Experimental and clinical therapeutic effects of partial B cell depletion. Cancer Immunol Immunother 48(10): 541-9. 2000.

18. Quan N, Zhang Z, Demetrikopoulos MK, Kitson RP, Chambers WH, Goldfarb RH, Weiss JM. Evidence for involvement of B lymphocytes in the surveillance of lung metastasis in the rat. Cancer Res. 59(5): 1080-9. 1999.

19. Shingu K, Helfritz A, Kuhlmann S, Zielinska-Skowronek M, Jacobs R, Schmidt RE, Pabst R, von Horsten S. Kinetics of the early recruitment of leukocyte subsets at the sites of tumor cells in the lungs: natural killer (NK) cells rapidly attract monocytes but not lymphocytes in the surveillance of micrometastasis. Int J Cancer. 99(1): 74-81. 2002.

20. Qin Z, Richter G, Schuler T, Ibe S, Cao X, Blankenstein T. B cells inhibit induction of T cell-dependent tumor immunity. Nat Med. 4(5): 627-30. 1998.

21. Mandelboim O, Vadai E, Fridkin M, Katz-Hillel A, Feldman M, Berke G, Eisenbach L.Regression of established murine carcinoma metastases following vaccination with tumour-associated antigen peptides. Nat Med. 1(11): 1179-83. 1995.

22. Wang R, Taniguchi M.Limited T cell antigen receptor repertoire in tumor-infiltrating lymphocyte and inhibition of experimental lung metastasis of murine melanoma by anti-TCR antibody. J Immunol. 154(4): 1797-803. 1995.

23. Emilio Barbera-Guillem, Julie K. Nyhus, Chris C. Wolford, Chad R. Friece, and James W. Sampsel,Vascular endothelial growth factor secretion by tumor infiltrating macrophages essentially supports tumor angiogenesis, and IgG immune-complexes potentiate the process. Cancer Res. In publication. 2002

24. Koeppen HK, Singh S, Stauss HJ, Park BH, Rowley DA, Schreiber H. CD4-positive and B lymphocytes in transplantation immunity. I. Promotion of tumor allograft rejection through elimination of CD4-positive lymphocytes. Transplantation. 55(6): 1349-55. 1993.

25. O'Boyle KP, Goya V, Zuckier LS, Chun S, Bhargava K. Expression of human tumor mucin-associated carbohydrate epitopes, including sialylated Tn, and localization of murine monoclonal antibodies CC49 and B72.3 in a syngeneic rat colon carcinoma model. J Immunother Emphasis Tumor Immunol. 16(4): 251-61. 1994.

26. Nelson MB, Nyhus JK, Oravecz-Wilson KI, Barbera-Guillem E. Tumor cells express FcgammaRI which contributes to tumor cell growth and a metastatic phenotype. Neoplasia. 3(2): 115-24 2001.

27. Horst HA, Horny HP Tumor-infiltrating lymphoreticular cells. Histologic and immunohistologic investigations performed on metastasizing squamous cell carcinomas of the head and neck. Cancer. 1991 Dec 1;68(11):2397-402.

28. Tjiong MY, Zumbach K, Schegget JT, van der Vange N, Out TA, Pawlita M, Struyk L. Antibodies against human papillomavirus type 16 and 18 E6 and E7 proteins in cervicovaginal washings and serum of patients with cervical neoplasia. Viral Immunol. 14(4): 415-24. 2001.
29. Behrends U, Jandl T, Golbeck A, Lechner B, Muller-Weihrich S, Schmid I, Till H, Berthold F, Voltz R, Mautner JM. Novel products of the HUD, HUC, NNP-1 and alpha-internexin genes identified by autologous antibody screening of a pediatric neuroblastoma library. Int J Cancer. 100(6): 669-77. 2002.
30. Sofen H, O'Toole C. Anti-squamous tumor antibodies in patients with squamous cell carcinoma. Cancer Res. 38(1): 199-203. 1978.
31. Brichory F, Beer D, Le Naour F, Giordano T, Hanash S. Proteomics-based identification of protein gene product 9.5 as a tumor antigen that induces a humoral immune response in lung cancer. Cancer Res. 61(21): 7908-12. 2001.
32. Berczi I, McMorris LS, Thoriakson TK, Thoriakson RH, Kellen JA, Sehon AH. Detection of tumor antibodies in patients with gastrointestinal carcinomas by a solid-phase radioimmunoassay. J Natl Cancer Inst. 63(3): 553-66. 1979.
33. Knuth A, Lloyd KO, Lipkin M, Oettgen HF, Old LJ. Natural antibodies in human sera directed against blood-group-related determinants expressed on colon cancer cells. Int J Cancer. 32(2): 199-204. 1983.
34. Butschak G, Karsten U. Isolation and characterization of thomsen-friedenreich-specific antibodies from human serum. Tumour Biol. 23(3): 113-22. 2002.
35. von Mensdorff-Pouilly S, Gourevitch MM, Kenemans P, Verstraeten AA, van Kamp GJ, Kok A, van Uffelen K, Snijdewint FG, Paul MA, Meijer S, Hilgers J. An enzyme-linked immunosorbent assay for the measurement of circulating antibodies to polymorphic epithelial mucin (MUC1). Tumour Biol. 19(3): 186-95. 1998.
36. von Mensdorff-Pouilly S, Verstraeten AA, Kenemans P, Snijdewint FG, Kok A, Van Kamp GJ, Paul MA, Van Diest PJ, Meijer S, Hilgers J. Survival in early breast cancer patients is favorably influenced by a natural humoral immune response to polymorphic epithelial mucin. J Clin Oncol. 18(3): 574-83.2000.
37. Scanlan MJ, Welt S, Gordon CM, Chen YT, Gure AO, Stockert E, Jungbluth AA, Ritter G, Jager D, Jager E, Knuth A, Old LJ. Cancer-related serological recognition of human colon cancer: identification of potential diagnostic and immunotherapeutic targets. Cancer Res. 62(14): 4041-7. 2002.
38. Lee YT, Sheikh KM, Quismorio FP Jr, Friou GJ. Circulating anti-tumor and autoantibodies in breast carcinoma: relationship to stage and prognosis. Breast Cancer Res Treat. 6(1):57-65 1985.
39. Meyer EM, Grundmann E. Lymph node reactions to cancer. Klin Wochenschr 60(21) :1329-38. 1982.
40. Mariani-Costantini R, Muraro R, Ficari F, Valli C, Bei R, Tonelli F, Caramia F, Frati L. Immunohistochemical evidence of immune responses to tumor-associated antigens in lymph nodes of colon carcinoma patients. Cancer . 67(11): 2880-6. 1991.
41. Michalak T, Krawczynski K, Harlozinska A, Potomski J, Albert Z. Localization of carcinoembryonic antigen in mesenteric lymph nodes of patients with gastrointestinal cancer. Neoplasma. 30(1): 67-72. 1983.
42. Triozzi PL, Kim JA, Aldrich W, Young DC, Sampsel JW, Martin EW Jr. Localization of tumor-reactive lymph node lymphocytes in vivo using radiolabeled monoclonal antibody. Cancer. 73(3):580-9. 1994.
43. Arnold MW, Young DC, Hitchcock CL, Schneebaum S, Martin EW Jr. Radioimmunoguided surgery in primary colorectal carcinoma: an intraoperative prognostic tool and adjuvant to traditional staging. Am J Surg. 170(4): 315-8. 1995.
44. Potomski J, Harlozinska A, Starzky H, Richter R, Wozniewski A. Correlation between immunohistochemical localization of carcinoembryonic antigen (CEA) and histological estimation of carcinomas, normal mucosae and lymph nodes of the digestive tract in humans. Arch Immunol Ther Exp (Warsz). 27(1-2): 177-86 1979.
45. Loy TS, Haege DD. B72.3 immunoreactivity in benign abdominal lymph nodes associated with gastrointestinal disease. Dis Colon Rectum. 38(9): 983-7. 1995.
46. Cernea C, Montenegro F, Castro I, Cordeiro A, Gayotto L, Ferraz A, de Carlucci D Jr. Prognostic significance of lymph node reactivity in the control of pathologic negative node squamous cell carcinomas of the oral cavity. Am J Surg. 174(5): 548-51. 1997.
47. Herr HW, Bean MA, Whitmore WF. Jr. Prognostic significance of regional lymph node histology in cancer of the bladder. J Urol . 115(3): 264-7. 1976.
48. Riegrova D, Jansa P. Prognostic significance of reactive changes in regional lymph nodes in gastric and mammary carcinomas. Neoplasma. 29(4): 481-6. 1982.

49. Barbera-Guillem E, Arnold MW, Nelson MB, Martin EW Jr. First results for resetting the antitumor immune response by immune corrective surgery in colon cancer. Am J Surg. 176(4): 339-43. 1998.

50. Hitchcock CL, Arnold MW, Young DC, Schneebaum S, Martin EW Jr. TAG-72 expression in lymph nodes and RIGS. Dis Colon Rectum. 39(4): 473-5. 1996.

51. Fu YX, Huang G, Wang Y, Chaplin DD. Lymphotoxin-alpha-dependent spleen microenvironment supports the generation of memory B cells and is required for their subsequent antigen-induced activation. J Immunol. 164(5): 2508-14. 2000.

52. Wang J, Foster A, Chin R, Yu P, Sun Y, Wang Y, Pfeffer K, Fu YX. The complementation of lymphotoxin deficiency with LIGHT, a newly discovered TNF family member, for the restoration of secondary lymphoid structure and function. Eur J Immunol . 32(7): 1969-79. 2002.

53. Ryffel B, Di Padova F, Schreier MH, Le Hir M, Eugster HP, Quesniaux VF. Lack of type 2 T cell-independent B cell responses and defect in isotype switching in TNF-lymphotoxin alpha-deficient mice. J Immunol 1997 Mar 1;158(5):2126-33)

54. Fu YX, Huang G, Wang Y, Chaplin DD.B lymphocytes induce the formation of follicular dendritic cell clusters in a lymphotoxin alpha-dependent fashion. J Exp Med. 187(7): 1009-18. 1998.

55. De Togni P, Goellner J, Ruddle NH, Streeter PR, Fick A, Mariathasan S, Smith SC, Carlson R, Shornick LP, Strauss-Schoenberger J, et al. Abnormal development of peripheral lymphoid organs in mice deficient in lymphotoxin. Science. 264(5159): 703-7. 1994.

56. Kumaraguru U, Davis IA, Deshpande S, Tevethia SS, Rouse BT. Lymphotoxin alpha-/- mice develop functionally impaired CD8+ T cell responses and fail to contain virus infection of the central nervous system. J Immunol. 166(2):1066-74. 2001.

57. Eo SK, Kumaraguru U, Rouse BT. Plasmid DNA encoding CCR7 ligands compensate for dysfunctional CD8+ T cell responses by effects on dendritic cells. J Immunol. 167(7): 3592-9. 2001.

58. Elewaut D, Brossay L, Santee SM, Naidenko OV, Burdin N, De Winter H, Matsuda J, Ware CF, Cheroutre H, Kronenberg M. Membrane lymphotoxin is required for the development of different subpopulations of NK T cells. J Immunol 2000 Jul 15;165(2):671-9.

59. Ito D, Back TC, Shakhov AN, Wiltrout RH, Nedospasov SA. Mice with a targeted mutation in lymphotoxin-alpha exhibit enhanced tumor growth and metastasis: impaired NK cell development and recruitment. J Immunol. 163(5): 2809-15. 1999.

60. Ruddle NH. Lymphoid neo-organogenesis: lymphotoxin's role in inflammation and development. Immunol Res. 19(2-3): 119-25. 1999.

61. Bevilacqua MP, Nelson RM Endothelial-leukocyte adhesion molecules in inflammation and metastasis. Thromb Haemost. 70(1): 152-4. 1993.

62. Chen WS, Wei SJ, Liu JM, Hsiao M, Kou-Lin J, Yang WK. Tumor invasiveness and liver metastasis of colon cancer cells correlated with cyclooxygenase-2 (COX-2) expression and inhibited by a COX-2-selective inhibitor, etodolac. Int J Cancer. 2001 Mar 15;91(6):894-9.

63. Wang Y, Huang G, Wang J, Molina H, Chaplin DD, Fu YX. Antigen persistence is required for somatic mutation and affinity maturation of immunoglobulin. Eur J Immunol. 30(8): 2226-34. 2000.

64. Anderson F, Game BA, Atchley D, Xu M, Lopes-Virella MF, Huang Y. IFN-gamma pretreatment augments immune complex-induced matrix metalloproteinase-1 expression in U937 histiocytes. Clin Immunol. 102(2): 200-7. 2002.

65. Warner RL, Lewis CS, Beltran L, Younkin EM, Varani J, Johnson KJ. The role of metalloelastase in immune complex-induced acute lung injury. Am J Pathol. 158(6): 2139-44. 2001.

66. Anderson CF, Mosser DM.A novel phenotype for an activated macrophage: the type 2 activated macrophage. J Leukoc Biol. 72(1): 101-6. 2002.

67. van Ravenswaay Claasen, H.H., Kluin, P.M., and Fleuren, G.J. Tumor infiltrating cells in human cancer. On the possible role of CD16+ macrophages in antitumor cytotoxicity. Lab. Invest. 67(2): 166-174, 1992.

68. Wang ZQ, Bapat AS, Rayanade RJ, Dagtas AS, Hoffmann MK.Interleukin-10 induces macrophage apoptosis and expression of CD16 (FcgammaRIII) whose engagement blocks the cell death programme and facilitates differentiation. Immunology. 102(3): 331-7. 2001.

69. Cameron AJ, McDonald KJ, Harnett MM, Allen JM. Differentiation of the human monocyte cell line, U937, with dibutyryl cyclicAMP induces the expression of the inhibitory Fc receptor, FcgammaRIIb. Immunol Lett. 83(3): 171-9. 2002.

70. Tridandapani S, Siefker K, Teillaud JL, Carter JE, Wewers MD, Anderson CL. Regulated expression and inhibitory function of Fcgamma RIIb in human monocytic cells. J Biol Chem. 277(7): 5082-9. 2002.

71. Guo RF, Ward PA. Mediators and regulation of neutrophil accumulation in inflammatory responses in lung: insights from the IgG immune complex model (1,2). Free Radic Biol Med. 33(3): 303-10. 2002.

72. Anderson CF, Mosser DM. Cutting edge: biasing immune responses by directing antigen to macrophage Fc gamma receptors. J Immunol. 168(8): 3697-701. 2002.

73. Coxon A, Cullere X, Knight S, Sethi S, Wakelin MW, Stavrakis G, Luscinskas FW, Mayadas TN.Fc gamma RIII mediates neutrophil recruitment to immune complexes. A mechanism for neutrophil accumulation in immune-mediated inflammation. Immunity. 14 (6): 693-704. 2001.

74. Fossati G, Bucknall RC, Edwards SW. Insoluble and soluble immune complexes activate neutrophils by distinct activation mechanisms: changes in functional responses induced by priming with cytokines. Ann Rheum Dis. 61(1): 13-9. 2002.

75. Nyhus JK, Wolford CC, Friece CR, Nelson MB, Sampsel JW, Barbera-Guillem E. IgG-recognizing shed tumor-associated antigens can promote tumor invasion and metastasis. Cancer Immunol Immunother. 50(7): 361-72. 2001.

76. Barbera-Guillem E, May KF Jr, Nyhus JK, Nelson MB. Promotion of tumor invasion by cooperation of granulocytes and macrophages activated by anti-tumor antibodies. Neoplasia. 1(5): 453-60. 1999.

77. Swift, M.E., Kleinman, H.K., and DiPietro, L.A. Impaired wound repair and delayed angiogenesis in aged mice. Lab. Invest. 79(12): 1479-1487, 1999.

78. Presta, L.G., Chen, H., O'Connor, S.J., Chisholm, V., Meng, Y.G., Krummen, L., Winkler, M., and Ferrara, N. Humanization of an anti-vascular endothelial growth factor monoclonal antibody for the therapy of solid tumors and other disorders. Cancer Res., *57(20):* 4593-4599, 1997.

79. Saleh, M., Stacker, S.A., and Wilks, A.F. Inhibition of growth of C6 glioma cells *in vivo* by expression of antisense vascular endothelial growth factor sequence. Cancer Res., *56(2):* 393-401, 1996.

80. Borgstrom, P., Hillan, K.J., Sriramarao, P., and Ferrara, N. Complete inhibition of angiogenesis and growth of microtumors by anti-vascular endothelial growth factor neutralizing antibody: novel concepts of angiostatic therapy from intravital videomicroscopy. Cancer Res., *56(17):* 4032-4039, 1996.

81. Rak, J., Mitsuhashi, Y., Bayko, L., Filmus, J., Shirasawa, S., Sasazuki, T., and Kerbel, R.S. Mutant ras oncogenes up regulate VEGF/VPF expression: implications for induction and inhibition of tumor angiogenesis. Cancer Res., *55(20):* 4575-4580, 1995.

82. Yoshiji, H., Gomez, D.E., Shibuya, M., and Thorgeirsson, U.P. Expression of vascular endothelial growth factor. its receptor, and other angiogenic factors in human breast cancer. Cancer Res., *56(9):* 2013-2016, 1996.

83. Detmar, M., Velasco, P., Richard, L., Claffey, K.P., Streit, M., Riccardi, L., Skobe, M., Brown, L.F. Expression of vascular endothelial growth factor induces an invasive phenotype in human squamous cell carcinomas. Am. J. Pathol., *156(1):* 159-167, 2000.

84. Kondo, Y., Arii, S., Mori, A., Furutani, M., Chiba, T. and Imamura, M. Enhancement of angiogenesis, tumor growth, and metastasis by transfection of vascular endothelial growth factor into LoVo human colon cancer cell line. Clin. Cancer Res., *6(2):* 622-630, 2000.

85. Aonuma, M., Saeki, Y., Akimoto, T., Nakayama, Y., Hattori, C., Yoshitake, Y., Nishikawa, K., Shibuya, M., and Tanaka, N.G. Vascular endothelial growth factor overproduced by tumour cells acts predominantly as a potent angiogenic factor contributing to malignant progression. Int. J. Exp. Pathol., *80(5):* 271-281, 1999.

86. Verheul, H.M., Hoekman, K., Luykx-de Bakker, S., Eekman, C.A., Folman, C.C., Broxterman, H.J., and Pinedo, H.M. Platelet: transporter of vascular endothelial growth factor. Clin. Cancer Res., *3(12 Pt 1):* 2187-2190, 1997.

87. Wartiovaara, U., Salven, P., Mikkola, H., Lassila, R., Kaukonen, J., Joukov, V., Orpana, A., Ristimaki, A., Heikinheimo, M., Joensuu, H., Alitalo, K., and Palotie, A. Peripheral blood platelets express VEGF-C and VEGF, which are released during platelet activation. Thromb. Haemost., *80(1):* 171-175, 1998.

88. Salven, P., Orpana, A., and Joensuu, H. Leukocytes and platelets of patients with cancer contain high levels of vascular endothelial growth factor. Clin. Cancer Res., 5(3): 487-491, 1999.

89. Huang YQ, Li JJ, Hu L, Lee M, Karpatkin S. Thrombin induces increased expression and secretion of VEGF from human FS4 fibroblasts, DU145 prostate cells and CHRF megakaryocytes. Thromb Haemost. 86(4): 1094-8. 2001.

90. Xiong, M., Elson, G., Legarda, D., and Leibovich, S.J. Production of vascular endothelial growth factor by murine macrophages: regulation by hypoxia, lactate, and the inducible nitric oxide synthase pathway.Am. J. Pathol., *153(2):* 587-598, 1998.

91. Lu, B., Rutledge, B. J., and Gu, L. Abnormalities in monocyte recruitment and cytokine expression in monocyte chemoattractant protein 1-deficient mice. J. Exp. Med., 187: 601-608, 1998.
92. Takayuki Ueno, Masakazu Toi,1 Hisashi Saji, Mariko Muta, Hiroko Bando, Katsumasa Kuroi, Morio Koike, Hidekuni Inadera, and Kouji Matsushima. Significance of Macrophage Chemoattractant Protein-1 in Macrophage Recruitment, Angiogenesis, and Survival in Human Breast Cancer. Clin. Cancer Res., 6: 3282-3289, 2000.
93. Shanley, T.P., Schmal, H., Warner, R.L., Schmid, E., Friedl, H.P., and Ward, P.A. Requirement for C-X-C chemokines (macrophage inflammatory protein-2 and cytokine-induced neutrophil chemoattractant) in IgG immune complex-induced lung injury. J. Immunol., 158(7): 3439-3448, 1997.
94. Kranz, A., Mattfeldt, T., and Waltenberger, J. Molecular mediators of tumor angiogenesis: enhanced expression and activation of vascular endothelial growth factor receptor KDR in primary breast cancer. Int. J. Cancer, 84(3): 293-298, 1999.
95. Goede, V., Brogelli, L., Ziche, M., and Augustin, H.G. Induction of inflammatory angiogenesis by monocyte chemoattractant protein-1. Int. J. Cancer, 82(5): 765-770, 1999.
96. Brunda, M.J., Sulich, V., Wright, R.B., and Palleroni, A.V. Tumoricidal activity and cytokine secretion by tumor-infiltrating macrophages. Int. J. Cancer, 48(5): 704-708, 1991.
97. Barbera-Guillem, E., Nyhus, J.K., Wolford, C.C., Friece C.R., and Sampsel J.W. Vascular endothelial growth factor secretion by tumor infiltrating macrophages essentially supports tumor angiogenesis, and IgG immune-complexes potentiate the process. Cancer Res. (In press). 2002.
98. Jeltsch, M., Kaipainen, A., Joukov, V., Meng, X., Lakso, M., Rauvala, H., Swartz, M., Fukumura, D., Jain, R.K., and Alitalo, K. Hyperplasia of lymphatic vessels in VEGF-C transgenic mice. Science, 276(5317): 1423-1425, 1997.
99. Skobe, M., Hawighorst, T., Jackson, D.G., Prevo, R., Janes, L., Velasco, P., Riccardi, L., Alitalo, K., Claffey, K., and Detmar, M. Induction of tumor lymphangiogenesis by VEGF-C promotes breast cancer metastasis. Nat. Med., 7(2): 192-198, 2001.

IMPROVEMENTS OF SURVIVAL IN NINE PHASE II CLINICAL STUDIES WITH DIFFERENT TYPES OF CANCER UPON ANTI-TUMOR VACCINATION WITH AN AUTOLOGOUS TUMOR CELL VACCINE MODIFIED BY VIRUS INFECTION TO INTRODUCE DANGER SIGNALS

Volker Schirrmaker

German Cancer Research Center, Division of Cellular Immunology,

Im Neuenheimer Feld 280, D-69120 Heidelberg, Germany

INTRODUCTION

The host immune response to foreign challenge requires the coordinated action of both the innate and aquired arms of the immune system. The innate immune response not only provides the first line of defence against microorganisms but also the biological context - the "danger signal" – that instructs the adaptive immune system to mount a response[1]. The adaptive reponse is mediated by T and B lymphocytes that have undergone germline gene-rearrangements of their antigen specific receptors. This second line of defence is characterized by exquisite specificity and long-lasting memory.

Recognition of pathogens is mediated by a set of germline encoded receptors that are referred to as pattern recognition receptors (PRR). Toll-like receptors (TLR)[2] function as PRR and are essential for translating the recognition of microbial components to activation of the immune system. Activation of TLR leads to the release of several inflammatory mediators, including chemokines, from resident tissue macrophages and dendritic cells (DCs), and modulates the expression of chemokine receptors on dendritic cells. These TLR mediated events are essential for both the recruitment of immature DCs to sites of pathogen entry and their ultimate journey back to lymph nodes to activate naïve T cells. In addition, chemokines released by resident tissue cells after TLR-activation guide these activated T cells into the site of pathogen entry and/or replication. In this way, chemokines link innate immune cell activation in the tissue to the recruitment of antigen-specific T cells generated in secondary lymphoid organs[3].

In this review I like to discuss recent issues about links between innate and adaptive immunity and how this knowledge is translated in our research to improve host immune responses against tumors. We exploit the use of virus infection to introduce danger signals

New Trends in Cancer for the 21st Century, edited by
Llombart-Bosch and Felipo, Kluwer Academic/Plenum Publishers, 2003

into tumor cells to activate innate immune responses and to improve adaptive anti-tumor immune responses in connection with long term immunological memory.

Introduction of danger signals into tumor cells by virus infection

About 20 years ago we started this work in the ESb lymphoma animal tumor model. Postoperative vaccination with virus-modified – but not with unmodified - ESb cells was able to cause protection from metastases in about 50 % of syngeneic mice[4]. In those studies we had selected for this purpose an avian RNA paramyxovirus, namely Newcastle Disease Virus (NDV). Since this was a good choice we continued to use NDV also for clinical application. Different virulent strains of NDV cause Newcastle Disease in a wide variety of birds, most notably in chickens. NDV can also infect humans, but in this mammalian host this virus causes only mild symptoms of conjunctivitis or laryngitis. The observations that NDV can replicate up to 10,000 times better in human cancer cells than in most normal human cells has prompted much interest in this virus as a potential anti-cancer agent. NDV has been labelled as a complementary and alternative medicine (CAM) and much detailed information can be found at a respective home-page of the National Cancer Institute, USA (http://www.nci.nih.gov/cancerinfo/pdq/cam/NDV).

Newcastle Disease Virus (NDV)

Fig. 1 shows a schematic representation of the structure of the virus and its genome. The genetic material of NDV is negative stranded RNA rather than DNA. Initial binding of NDV to a host cell takes place through the interaction of hemagglutinin-neuraminidase (HN) molecules in the virus coat with sialic acid- containing molecules, such as gangliosides, on the surface of most cells. Most strains of NDV can make infectious progeny viruses only in some types of non-human cells (e.g. chicken embryo cells) thereby allowing these strains to be maintained. NDV is an enveloped virus. Progeny virus particles are released from infected cells by budding at the plasma membrane. In this process, single copies of the NDV genome become wrapped in an outer coat, the envelope, that is made from the host cells' plasma membrane. Two specific virus proteins, HN and F, the fusion protein, are the main NDV proteins found in the outer coat of isolated virus particles and also at the plasma membrane of infected cells.

Fig. 2 illustrates how it is possible to distinguish via flow cytometry (FACS) analysis between a cell in which virus infection and replication took place and a cell in which the virus did not replicate. True infection and virus replication occurs in tumor cells upon infection with live virus (Fig. 2 A). 24 hrs after virus infection and staining with anti-HN or anti-F antibodies, tumor cells show a pattern of high viral antigen density (HAD) while upon treatment with NDVwhich had been inactivated by UV light (NDV-UV) (Fig. 2 B) the FACS histogram reveals only cells with low viral antigen density (LAD) (i.e. cells with cell surface adsorbed virus)[5].

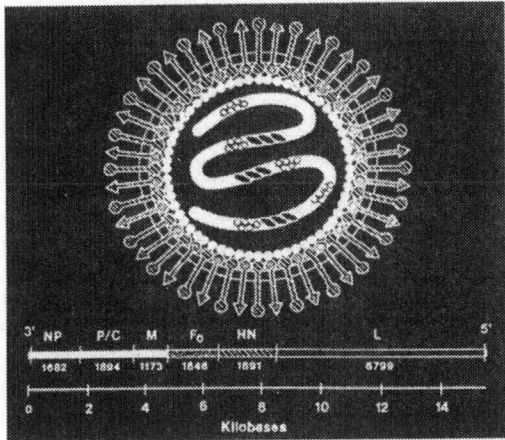

Fig. 1. Diagram of the structure of NDV. The lipid bilayer of the virus envelope contains the two membrane integrated viral attachment glycoproteins hemagglutinin-neuraminidase (HN) and fusion protein (F). F is synthesized as inactive precursor (Fo) and gains fusion function by a post-translational cleavage process that is mediated by cellular trypsin-like enzymes which remove about 100 amino acids from the N-terminals of Fo. The genetic map consists of a negative strand RNA encoding 6 genes.

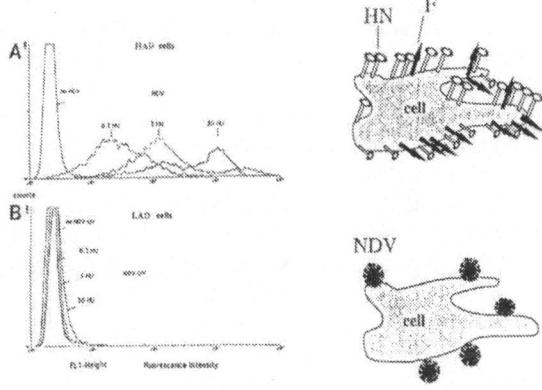

Fig. 2. Replication of NDV Ulster in human tumor cells: Independence of viral replication from host cell proliferation and sensitivity of viral replication to UV-irradiation. Cells of a human melanoma line were pre-irradiated with 200 Gy before they were infected with increasing amounts of NDV. The amounts are expressed as hemagglutinating units (HU) per 10^7 cells. In parallel, the cells were coincubated with corresponding amounts of NDV which had been pre-treated for 5 min. by UV-light exposure (NDV-UV). Two days later, the cells were stained for viral HN-cell surface expression and analysed by FACScan cytometry. Note that in the absence of cell proliferation the whole population of cells can be infected by NDV. As a consequence of intra-cytoplasmic viral replication there was a dose dependent increase of viral antigen density at the cell surface of the tumor cells. Thus we can distinguish cells in which NDV replication occurred as cells with high viral antigen density (HAD) (A) from cells to which NDV could only bind with low antigen density (LAD) (B). When normal PBMC are infected with live NDV Ulster as the tumor cells in A, only LAD cells can be seen. The difference in cell surface expression of the two viral proteins HN and F by LAD and HAD cells is schematically illustrated on the right side.

Why we selected NDV

We selected NDV not only because of its tumor selective replication properties but also because we wanted to avoid the use of viruses which had the chance to adapt to mammalian hosts during evolution. In this process most mammalian viruses have developed immune escape mechanisms. A number of pox-viruses and herpes viruses encode secreted chemokine receptor homologues which, by neutralizing locally produced chemokines, may impair the influx of dendritic cell precursors into infected tissues[6]. Immune escape may also be achieved by downregulation of MHC-class I molecules and upregulation of anti-apoptotic factors in infected cells as known for adenoviruses[7]. Cytomegalovirus (CMV), Measles virus (MV) and HIV are human pathogens known to induce immuno-suppression in humans[8]. Recently it was shown that infection of dendritic cells by murine CMV induces functional paralysis and prevents delivery of the signals required for T cell activation[9].

Why we selected a non-lytic NDV strain and autologous tumor cells

Lytic strains of NDV are able to make infectious progeny virus in human cells whereas non-lytic strains are not. The former strains can produce active F molecules while the latter strains only produce uncleaved inactive Fo molecules. The budding of progeny viruses that contain activated F molecules in their outer coats causes the plasma-membrane of NDV infected cells to fuse with the plasma membrane of neighbouring cells, leading to the production of large, inviable fused cells known as syncytia. The preferential killing of cancer cells via lytic virus is known as *"oncolysis"*. Thus, lytic strains of NDV are also *oncolytic strains*. In contrast, non-lytic strains of NDV kill infected cells more slowly, with death apparently being the result of disruption of normal host cell metabolism and induction of apoptosis.

We selected the non-lytic strain Ulster for reasons of safety during application in cancer patients and also because we intended to develop a virus infected whole cell cancer vaccine consisting of intact viable irradiated cancer cells. NDV Ulster has a monocyclic abortive replication cycle in tumor cells[12]. This replication involves the formation of double-strand RNA (dsRNA) which functions as a danger signal and activates TLR[10]. Thus we tried to link the expression of tumor associated antigens (TAA) with danger signals.

Protective anti-tumor immunity in the ESb mouse lymphoma model could be induced only under special immunization protocols and was highly specific for the autologous tumor line[13]. We decided to use autologous tumor cells also because these represent the closest possible match to a patients' tumor. Autologous tumor cells might express not only common TAA but also individually unique TAA derived from mutations or other genetic alterations. The use of whole tumor cells eliminates the need to first identity the respective TAA. It has been the experience of many tumor immunologists that whole cell vaccines can stimulate the immune system more efficiently than oncolysates[11]. NDV Ulster is first adsorbed to the tumor cells in vitro (1 h binding), then the virus-modified tumor vaccine is injected thus allowing for virus replication in vivo at the site of vaccine application. Vaccines consisting of tumor cells infected with a non-lytic strain of NDV should remain in the body long enough to generate effective immune responses which are mostly based on T cell mediated immunity[14]. Viral replication in the tumor cells takes about 6-40 hours[5], a time sufficient to generate delayed type hypersensitivity (DTH) skin responses which are dependent on antigen-specific memory T cells.

During this time period of 6-40 hours, the infected tumor cells will produce progeny NDV virus particles. Although these are non-infectious due to uncleaved Fo molecules[5] they are able to stimulate in PBMC innate immune responses such as the release of IFN-α and activation of monocytes (see below). In this way we may achieve a link between innate and adaptive immune responses.

CONSEQUENCES OF HUMAN TUMOR CELL INFECTION BY NDV ULSTER

Gamma-irradiated human breast carcinoma, colon-carcinoma or glioblastoma cells from defined cell lines were modified either by true infection with live NDV Ulster or, for control, by mere cell-surface adsorption of replication deficient NDV-UV. Modification with live but not inactive NDV induced in all human tumor cells the production of interferon-β (IFN-β), interferon-α (IFN-α) and of the chemokines RANTES and IFN-γ-inducible protein-10 (IP-10). In addition, infection by live NDV induced upregulation of HLA-ABC molecules on all tumor lines tested and HLA-DR-molecules on breast-carcinoma lines. Two cell adhesion molecules, ICAM-I (CD54) and LFA-3 (CD58), were also upregulated on human tumor cells after infection with live NDV. 48-72 hours after infection of the irradiated tumor cells with live NDV, many tumor cells were dead or in early or late stages of apoptosis[15].

Apoptosis is often characterized as a non-inflammatory cell death. In the setting of virus or bacterial infection, apoptosis might, however, promote inflammatory responses and lead to antigen cross-priming. In the case of NDV infected human tumor cells we demonstrated the induction of pro-inflammatory cytokines, interferons and chemokines. These induced molecules definitely change the signalling microenvironment of cognitive APC-T cell interactions at the site of tumor vaccine application. They may also provide maturation signals *in vivo* for DCs so that immature DCs, which engulfed the apoptotic bodies from ATV-NDV vaccine, may become immunogenic rather than tolerogenic. dsRNA has been showed to lead to maturation, activation and protection of DCs[16].

A broad spectrum of human tumor cells can be modified by infection with NDV efficiently. The list of successfully infected cells includes 13 different human tumor cell types, 33 established cell lines, at least 40 primary cultures and more than 400 non-cultured freshly separated tumor cells as they are used for production of the autologous human live cell vaccine ATV-NDV[5].

Fig. 3 illustrates these different effects of human tumor cell infection by NDV Ulster[15]. The biological consequence of such virus infection of tumor cells is perceived as "dangerous" by the immune system because of the following danger signalling molecules: 1) viral HN molecules (see below), 2) dsRNA[10] 3) IFN α, β (see below), 4) chemokines (see Introduction).

RESISTANCE OF NORMAL CELLS TO INFECTION BY NDV

In contrast to tumor cells in which NDV regularly replicates, this virus does not replicate in normal cells. To compare virus infection of human T-lymphoma cells with that of corresponding normal cells, T cells from the peripheral blood of healthy donors were isolated, infected with increasing amounts of NDV, incubated for 1-2 days and then analysed by FACS. On the normal lymphocytes, we only detected LAD type cells while in lymphoma cells we saw HAD cells. Further tests revealed that NDV Ulster does not replicate even in embryonic normal liver cells from the original host, the chicken. After 3 subpassages in such cell cultures there was no cytopathic effect nor was there cell surface hemadsorption activity[5].

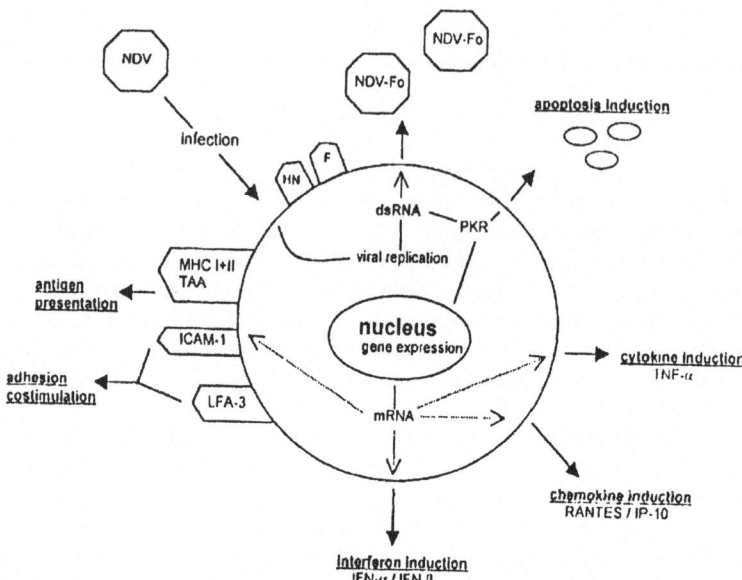

Fig. 3. Diagram of the biological effects of NDV infection of human tumor cells: the biological context perceived as "dangerous". The infection leads to the introduction of viral surface antigens (HN and F), to secretion of cytokines, chemokines and type 1 interferons, to modulation of surface molecules (HLA) and cell adhesion molecules and to induction of apoptosis. dSRNA = double strand RNA; PKR = protein kinase dsRNA-binding; HN = hemagglutinin-neuraminidase, F = viral fusion protein, NDV-Fo = non-infectious virus particles produced by the tumor cells.

Why normal cells resist NDV infection while tumor cells do not remains to be investigated. At present we see a difference in the IFN-α response. While normal human peripheral blood mononuclear cells (PBMC) make high titers of IFN-α after stimulation with non-infectious NDV-UV this is not the case with tumor cells. IFN-α is an anti-viral factor which can quickly induce a state of virus resistance in other cells. The resistance of normal cells to virus infection induced by interferons includes three main pathways: i) the Mx pathway, which involves Mx proteins and leads to inhibition of transcription, ii) the 2-5 A system, which involves 2-5A synthetases and leads to RNA cleavage and iii) the dsRNA-dependent protein kinase (PKR) pathway which finally leads to inhibition of protein synthesis and transcriptional control[17].

While normal PBMC produce IFN-α immediately after cell surface contact with inactivated NDV, tumor cells produce IFN-α only after true virus infection. It is possible that the difference between normal cells and tumor cells with regard to sensitivity to NDV infection has to do with the differences in kinetics and magnitude of the respective IFN-α

responses (Table 1) and also perhaps, with differences in responsiveness to IFN-α, starting from type I interferon receptor signalling via downstream events involving interferon regulatory factor transcription factors[18] and any of the above virus resistance mechanism pathways.

ACTIVATION BY NDV OF NATURAL INTERFERON-PRODUCING CELLS (NIPC)

Table 1. PBMC contain a small fraction of so-called natural interferon-producing cells (NIPC) capable of producing high amounts of IFN-α upon contact with virus or virus infected cells[19]. NDV Ulster as well as NDV-UV turned out to be excellent inducers in PBMC of IFN-α production (Table 1). The cells responsive in PBMC to NDV were shown to represent a novel dendritic cell- like subset of CD64[+]/CD16[+] blood monocytes[20]. Viral replication was not required and antibodies against HN but not F molecules of NDV were able to block these responses[21]. To determine the molecular viral components of NDV which induce this important innate immune response we transfected Baby Hamster Kidney (BHK) cells with plasmids containing either HN or F genes linked to a Semliki Forest Virus replicase for high efficiency gene expression. Upon contact with BHK-cells expressing HN but not F at their cell surface (Fig. 4 A), human PBMC produced IFN-α (Fig. 4 A). Thus, NDV and its cell surface HN molecules, upon interaction with NIPC, activate these dendritic-like cells, which were suggested to connect innate with adaptive immune responses. Upon activation, NIPC produce 1000 x more IFN-α than other blood cells, migrate to inflamed lymph nodes, activate macrophage scavengers and NK cells and promote the survival of activated T cells[19].

Table 1. Differences in the IFN-α responsiveness to NDV of human normal cells and tumor cells

	IFNα (pg/ml) [1]	
	normal cells	tumor cells
representative example:	adherent PBMC [2]	MCF-7 [3]
+ UV-inactivated NDV Ulster	86 431	< 10
+ live NDV Ulster	77 210	55
effects	independent on viral replication	dependent on viral replication
IFN-α titers	high	low

[1] Cells (PBMC or MCF-7) were co-incubated for 3 days with 60 hemagglutinating units (HU) per 10[7] cells of either live or UV-inactivated NDV and then supernatants were tested by ELISA for IFN-α content. [2] The major cell type producing IFN α in PBMC is the natural interferon producing cell NIPC. [3] a human breast carcinoma cell line

Studies with mutated HN molecules revealed that it is a lectin-like cell binding domain within the molecule and not so much its neuraminidase activity which is important for its IFN-α inducing capacity[22]. Thus, this innate immune response, like others[23], is due to a lectin- carbohydrate recognition event[22].

Further experiments with HN-transfectants showed that this molecule, when expressed at cell surfaces can also function as an additional adhesion molecule so that not only NIPC but also other cells, including T-lymphocytes, bind better. Figure 4 B shows that many more CD4 T lymphocytes bind to HN-transfectants than to wild type fibroblast or neo-gene transfected control cells. The increased adhesion could be blocked by anti- HN and not by anti-F monoclonal antibody[24].

We furthermore demonstrated that viral HN-molecules when expressed on peptide-MHC class I presenting stimulator cells will augment the induction of peptide specific CD8 cytolytic T lymphocytes (CTL). A greater than 6-fold increase in peptide specific CTL-responses was observed in cultures restimulated with peptide pulsed fibroblasts which co-expressed viral HN due to either infection or transfection[25].

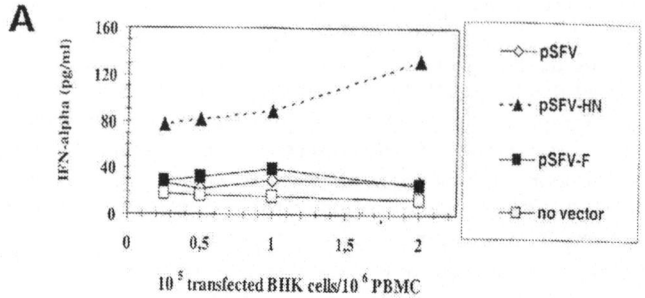

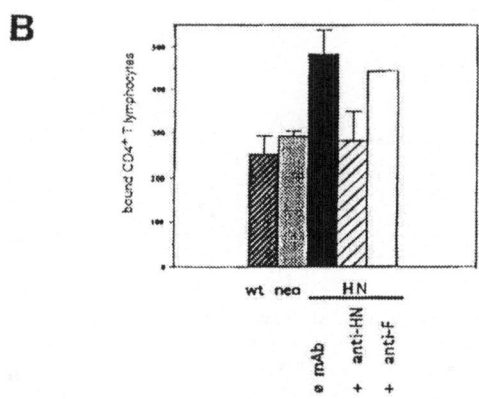

Fig. 4. HN-molecules on transfected cell lines are biologically active. They induce in PBMC interferon-α (A) and they facilitate the adhesion of CD4 T-lymphocytes (B). (A) Induction of interferon-α in PBMC by Baby Hamster Kidney (BHK) cells transfected with a Semliki-Forest Virus (SFV) replicase vector containing either HN or F. 1x10⁶ PBMC were co-cultured for 24 hours with the indicated numbers of BHK cells which had been precultured for 40 hours to allow for gene expression. The supernatants of the co-cultures were collected and interferon-α production determined by ELISA. (B) Increased binding capacity of HN-transfected mouse fibroblasts and blocking of cell adhesion by anti-HN monoclonal antibody. Ltk⁻ wild type (wt) or neogene control transfectants (neo) or HN transfectants (HN) were grown to confluency . The HN-transfectants were incubated with the indicated antibodies or without them and then washed. Then all the cells were coincubated with murine CD4 T cells for 1 hour. After removing unbound cells, the adherent cells were counted.

IFN-α as a danger signal

The release of high cytolytic T lymphocytes amounts of IFN-α by NIPC and plasmacytoid dendritic cells indicates that these cells of the innate immune system have sensed "danger". It has only recently become clear that IFN–α has an important adjuvant function in the immune response. It activates dendritic cells[26, 27], induces TRAIL in NK cells[28] and the IL-12 receptor □ chain in T cells[29]. Together with IL-12, IFN-α polarizes the T cell towards a cell-mediated Th1 response characterized by DTH and CTL activity. In addition, IFN-α induces the upregulation of molecules which are important for antigen recognition (e.g. HLA), cell-cell interaction (e.g. cell adhesion molecules, CAM) and cytotoxicity (e.g. TRAIL)[15] (see also Fig. 3).

ACTIVATION BY NDV OF ANTITUMOR CYTOXICITY IN MONOCYTE/MACROPHAGES

Tumor necrosis-factor related apoptosis inducing ligand (TRAIL) is a type II integral membrane protein belonging to the tumor-necrosis factor (TNF) family. TRAIL induces apoptotic cell death in a wide range of tumor cells and virus infected cells but generally not in normal cells. When human PBMC were either non-treated or treated with NDV Ulster, cultured for 24 hours and then stained with a biotin-conjugated anti-TRAIL antibody, FACS-analysis revealed that TRAIL was upregulated on NDV treated PBMC. Additional gating on either CD14 monocytes or CD3 T-lymphocytes revealed that TRAIL was upregulated on both cell types[21]. TRAIL induction by NDV could be blocked by anti-HN but not by anti-F monoclonal antibodies.

The avirulent, lentogenic strains Ulster and La Sota of NDV were shown to be capable of inducing in mouse macrophages antitumor cytotoxicity, both in vitro and in vivo[30]. The activated macrophages showed a broader cytotoxic activity against tumor cells than cytotoxic T lymphocytes. In vitro experiments revealed that NDV activated in mouse macrophages NF-κb and stimulated nitric oxide (NO) production[31]. Much of the observed anticancer activity of murine NDV activated macrophages could be attributed to the production and release of TNF–α. In addition, NDV-activated macrophages showed anti-cancer activity in vivo when they were injected into mice carrying murine metastatic mammary carcinoma or Lewis-lung carcinoma tumors[30].

ACTIVATION BY *NDV ONCOLYSATES* OF APC FUNCTION OF DENDRITIC CELLS

Dendritic cells (DCs) are the most important professional antigen-presenting cells (APC) and were recently shown to play an important role in tumor antigen processing and initiation of specific T-lymphocyte responses. We evaluated the effects of infecting human tumor cells with NDV on the antigen-presentation capacity of DCs and on their ability to stimulate autologous breast cancer reactive memory T cells. DC from breast-cancer patients were pulsed with lysates from the MCF-7 breast-cancer line (Tu-L) or from NDV infected MCF-7 cells (TuN-L, *viral oncolysates*) and compared for stimulatory capacity in an ELISPOT response of autologous memory T cells from the bone-marrow of the same patients[32]. DC pulsed with *viral oncolysates* showed increased expression of costimulatory molecules and induced significantly higher ELISPOT responses in comparison to Tu-L pulsed DC. Supernatants from co-cultures of memory T cells and TuN-L pulsed DC contained increased titers of IFN–α and IL-15 (Fig. 5). IL-15 supports memory CD8 T cell proliferation and maintenance through interaction with IL-15 receptor α chains on these cells[33].

To analyze potential danger signals derived from NDV infection, we employed modern proteomics technology such as MALDI mass-spectrometry of differentially expressed proteins and Western blot analysis. NDV infection resulted in a number of differences in protein expression including a heat-shock protein (HSP-27) which became phosphorylated[32]. These new results suggest that a DC preparation pulsed with *viral oncolysate* includes danger signals (e.g. IFN-α, ds RNA, chemokines, HSP molecules) and is superiour for memory T cell stimulation to a DC preparation pulsed with lysates from non-infected tumor cells.

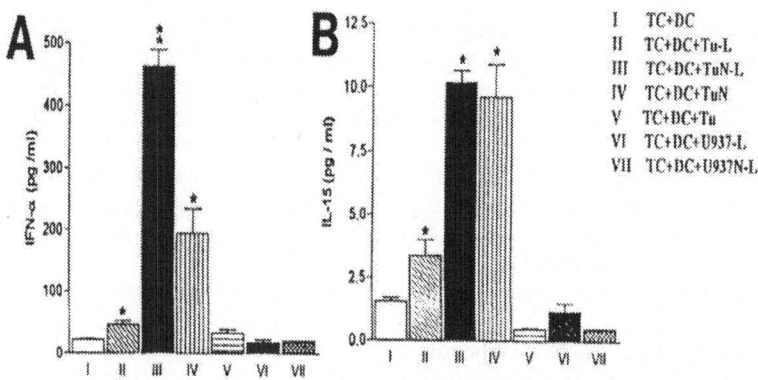

Fig. 5. Dendritic cells pulsed with viral oncolysates potently stimulate autologous T cells from cancer patients. Concentrations of IFN-α (A) and IL-15 (B) measured by ELISA after 40 h in the supernatants of co-cultures between 5×10^6 bone marrow T cells from breast cancer patients and 1×10^6 autologous DC as APC. DC were either unpulsed (group I) or pulsed with lysate from the MCF-7 breast carcinoma line (Tu-L; group II) or with lysate from 24 h NDV infected MCF-7 cells (TuN-L; group III). The response of the following two groups are derived from T cells that were co-cultured with DC and live irradiated MCF-7 cells (Tu; group V) or NDV infected MCF-7 cells (TuN; group IV). The responses of the next two groups represent specificity controls. In these we produced Tu-L (group VI) or TuN-L (group VII) from the promonocytic cell line U-937. Statistical comparisons were made with group I. * $p<0.05$; ** $p<0.005$. Means ± SD was calculated from 4 (IFN-α) and 3 (IL-15) patients and experiments, each experiment consisted of triplicates.

ANTI-RUMOR VACCINATION WITH DENDRITIC CELLS PULSED WITH VIRAL ONCOLYSATES

Having seen that cancer patients memory T cells can be reactivated quite efficiently with autologous dendritic cells upon pulsing them with *viral oncolysates* from NDV infected tumor cells we decided to evaluate the potential of this approach for antitumor vaccination. My clinical colleague, Dr. Ahlert (http://www.biotech-praxislab.de/), who has many years of experience with antitumor vaccination with NDV infected autologous tumor cells (ATV-NDV) is presently evaluating the potential of this approach.

Evidence for memory T cells in the bone marrow of cancer patients

Secondary immune responses by memory T cells are faster and stronger than primary responses. Their requirements for activation are less strict (lower dependency on co-stimulation) and they release a broader spectrum of cytokines and are multifunctional after re-activation. Thus, memory T cells are superior to naïve T cells for protective immunity. There is a programmed development of effector and memory CD8 T cells and different subsets of memory T cells, namely "central" and "effector" memory cells, have recently been distinguished. Of special interest are also stem cell-like properties of memory T cells: Upon response to homeostatic signals they have a self-renewal capacity[34].

In previous animal tumor experiments we had discovered that the bone marrow is a special compartment with regard to the establishment of tumor dormancy and immunological memory[14, 35]. Following inoculation of live or irradiated lacZ gene transfected tumor cells into mice, beta-galactosidase stained tumor cells could be detected in frozen sections or cytospin preparations from different organs. In immunocompetent animals we saw a correlation between the persistence of dormant tumor cells at low levels in the bone marrow correlating with long-term protective immune memory[14]. We could break-down the status of tumor dormancy in situ by CD8 T cell depletion[36]. In immunocompetent tumor dormant mice, 21 % of the bone marrow derived tumor cells were positive for the proliferation marker Ki67. The fraction of Ki67 positive tumor cells in diseased bone marrow of immune compromised mice was 40 % and in absence of immune CD8 T cells the frequency of BM residing tumor cells increased by two orders of magnitude. These findings suggested that tumor dormancy in this model was due to active immune control of tumor cells by CD8 T cells in the bone marrow, keeping them at a low level without elimination[35, 36].

These observations then lead us to investigate the situation in cancer patients. In an analysis of 84 primary operated breast cancer patients and 11 healthy donors, we found that the bone marrow of most patients contained memory T cells with specificity for tumor associated antigens. Patients bone marrow and peripheral blood contained CD8 T cells which specifically bound TAA derived HLA/peptide tetramers. In short term culture with autologous dendritic cells prepulsed with tumor lysates, patients' memory T cells from bone marrow (but not from peripheral blood) could be specifically reactivated to interferon-γ producing and cytotoxic effector cells[37].

In order to be able to evaluate in vivo the effectiveness of ex vivo re-activated memory T cells from bone-marrow we established a new human tumor xenotransplant system in NOD/SCID mice. More than 97 % of implanted pieces from freshly operated breast cancer patients engrafted in these mice maintained their original histomorphology as well as expression patterns of tumor markers and cytokines[38]. A single transfer of restimulated bone marrow T cells into NOD/SCID mice caused regression of autologous tumor xenotransplants. This was associated with infiltration by human T cells and tumor cell apoptosis and necrosis[37].

MEMORY T CELL STIMULATION IN VITRO WITH ATV-NDV

While naïve T cells can only be primed by antigens which are cross-presented by professional host APC such as dendritic cells, memory T cells can also be activated directly by a tumor vaccine presenting TAA together with costimulatory signals. In pre-clinical animal tumor models we had investigated tumor cell properties that are required to trigger a secondary syngeneic MHC class I restricted tumor specific CD8 CTL response in vitro. Irradiated trypan-blue excluding live tumor cells were superiour in stimulatory capacity to equivalent or even higher amounts of dead cells or crude membrane preparations (oncolysates). Disruption of tumor cells by freeze/thawing led to a complete loss of CTL stimulatory capacity[39]. Also in tumor bearing animals, *viral oncolysates* did not stimulate a secondary tumor specific CTL response in the peritoneal cavity whereas whole-cell vaccines did[39]. γ-irradiated viable tumor cells as whole-cell vaccines could stimulate in situ syngeneic antitumor CTL and delayed type-hypersensitivity (DTH)-reactivity whereas tumor cell lysates elicited only DTH-reactivity[40].

In order to examine in human autologous mixed lymphocyte-tumor cell cultures (AMLTC) the effect of NDV infection of tumor stimulator cells on different T cell subsets, we tested the upregulation of CD69 and CD25 (IL-2 receptor α-chain) on T cells as markers for early and late T cell activation[24]. PBMC from a patient suffering from larynx-carcinoma were co-cultured with irradiated autologous tumor cells which had been NDV-infected or not. As shown in Fig. 6, NDV infected tumor stimulator cells caused upregulation of the CD69 on 25 % of CD8 T cells and of both CD69 and CD25 on 10 % of CD4 T cells. Stimulation by non-modified autologous tumor cells lead to no change in the expression of the examined T cell activation markers.

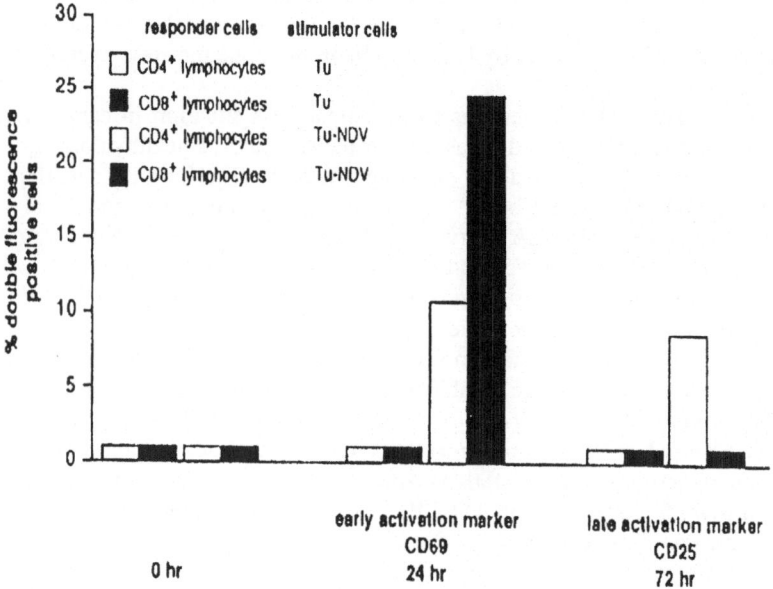

Fig. 6. Induction of T cell activation markers CD69 and CD25 on patient-derived CD3 T cells from PBMC after stimulation with NDV infected autologous larynx carcinoma cells. PBMC from a patient suffering from larynx carcinoma were cocultured with irradiated autologous tumor cells – NDV infected or not – up to 3 days. Expression of activation markers was measured by double immunofluorescence staining and FACS flow cytometry.

We furthermore demonstrated in an autologous human anti melanoma CD4 T helper clone that NDV infection of autologous melanoma cells induces a B7-1/B7-2-independent T cell costimulatory activity and thereby prevents in the clone the induction of anergy by the tumor cell[41]. Proliferation assays showed that the T cell clone, upon contact with autologous melanoma cells was rendered non-reactive and remained unresponsive even to subsequent stimulation by interleukin-2. NDV infection of the melanoma cell line not only completely restored the proliferative response, comparable to the stimulation by cross-linking with anti-CD3/anti-CD28 monoclonal antibodies, but also inhibited the induction of anergy. Electrophoretic mobility shift assays of cell lysates from the clone revealed the induction of the CD28 responsive complex by coincubation with NDV infected melanoma cells[42].

CLINICAL STUDIES WITH ATV-NDV

We now summarize how we translated our vaccine concept into the clinic and what we achieved. The specific component of each vaccine for human application are patient derived (autologous) live tumor cells (ATV). These are infected by NDV and inactivated by 200 Gy γ-irradiation to produce the vaccine ATV-NDV. Tumor cells are isolated from freshly operated tumor specimens by mechanical dissection and enzymatic dissociation and can be stored, after controlled freezing, in liquid nitrogen. While the first clinical studies[42, 43] employed total dissociated cells (including non-tumor cells such as stroma cells and tumor infiltrating lymphocytes (TIL)), we later[44, 45] introduced a further tumor cell purification procedure and removed TIL by immuno-magnetic beads. In some other studies[46-48] cell-culture adapted autologous tumor cells were used instead. All studies were approved beforehand by local ethical commissions. When the clinical decision was made that a patient should receive ATV-NDV vaccine, an ampule containing 10^7 frozen dissociated cells was thawed. Then, if necessary, the above cell purification procedure was applied, followed by virus infection and γ-irradiation. Both preparation steps require about 6 hours of laboratory work and now follow standard operating procedures (SOPs). Establishment of primary cultures from ovarian carcinoma[46], pancreatic and stomach carcinoma[47] and from glioblastoma[48] was possible in the majority of tumor samples.
The intradermal vaccinations were well tolerated and could be repeated many times without causing serious problems. A few patients developed mild fever and/or mild headache for 1-2 days. There was no evidence for autoimmune phenomena such as vasculitis, rheumatoid arthritis or lymphatic disorders. ATV-NDV vaccinations induced local immune responses in the skin associated with itching, swelling (cellular induration) and erythema within 24-48 hrs without dermal necrosis. Up to the third vaccination, patients showed increased skin reactivity to the vaccine. A DTH challenge test with non-modified autologous tumor cells, performed before the first and after the last vaccination, revealed increased DTH reactivity after the last vaccination in comparison to before vaccination[42-44, 48]. Systemic immune reactions could also be seen. These included swelling of certain lymph nodes, often in proximity to the operated tumor[45], increased anti-tumor T cell responsiveness of blood samples after vaccination and mobilization of TIL into tumor tissue[48].
The major clinical Phase II studies with ATV-NDV which were performed in cooperation with clinical colleagues in Germany since 1990 are summarized in Table 2. Details can be obtained from the respective original publications (42-48). The list includes

9 Phase II studies performed with 8 different important human cancers (with carcinomas from colon, rectum, pancreas, stomach, breast and ovary and with melanoma and glioblastoma) in which a total number of 382 patients were involved. The first studies were conducted in locally advanced colorectal cancer and in metastatic colorectal cancer in which the vaccinated groups in comparison to historical controls showed improved overall survival (OS) or disease-free survival (DFS), respectively. Studies in locally advanced colorectal cancer (Duke's C)[44] and in primary operated early breast cancer[45] revealed that the quality of the tumor vaccine is very important to achieve a clinical benefit. The tumor cell number and the viability of the cells turned out to be independent statistically significant parameters of quality and efficacy of this type of tumor vaccine, thus corroborating our preclinical results from animal tumor models[4, 39, 40].

Table 2. Clinical studies with NDV infected autologous tumor cell vaccine (ATV-NDV) in which a therapeutic benefit is suggested.

Type of Cancer	Type of study	Comparison group	No. of patients (n)	concurrent therapy	benefit[3]	reference
1) Colorectal, metastatic	Phase II trial	pair-matched case control	23	no	improved DFS	34
2) Colorectal, locally advanced	Phase II trial	pair-matched case control	57	no	improved OS	40
3) Breast, early	Phase II trial	internal control, retrospective analysis	63	yes [1]	improved OS	36
4) Ovary, metastatic	Phase II trial	historical control	82	yes [1]	improved [4] DFS	37
5) Renal, metastatic	Phase II trial	historical control	40	yes [2]	improved OS (11 patients with CR or PR)	35
6) Pancreas, stage G3	Phase II trial	historical control	9	yes [1]	improved OS[4]	38
7) Stomach	Phase II trial	historical control	7	yes [1]	improved OS [4]	38
8) Melanoma, recurrent, metastatic	Phase II trial	internal control, retrospective analysis	41	yes [1]	improved OS	38
9) Glioblastoma multiforme	Phase II trial	pair-matched case control	50	no	improved DFS and OS [4] (2 patients with CR)	39
		total n =	382			

[1]Chemotherapy, radiation therapy, hormonal therapy, given as in the control, in addition to vaccination. [2]Cytokine therapy given in addition to vaccination in therapy group. [3]DFS = disease free survival; OS = overall survival; CR = complete response; PR = partial response. [4]ATV-NDV in these studies consisted of cell-culture adapted autologous tumor cells while in all other studies the tumor cells were isolated from fresh operated specimens without cell culture.

Fig. 7 shows an example from what we achieved clinically with an optimal vaccine formulation in primary operated breast cancer patients. ATV-NDV vaccine was given in two different formulations with high and low cell numbers and viability respectively to two cohorts of more than 30 patients with similar risk factors. The study was started 1991 together with Dr. T. Ahlert and the three year survival data were published[45]. Figure 1 now shows the Kaplan Meier curves after a prolonged median observation period of 5.2 years for long-term survival (A) and recurrence-free survival (B). The analysis was performed by Focus (Düsseldorf) under financial support of the Dietmar Hopp-Stiftung (Walldorf). There was a highly significant long-term survival benefit and also a significant benefit in recurrence-free survival in group A which received an optimal formulation of a vaccine containing at least 1.5×10^6 viable tumor cells and at least 33 % overall cell viability. There were only 5 patients dead in group A as compared to 16 in group B which could only receive a suboptimal vaccine formulation. The survival in group B corresponds to expectation of patients with similar risk factors under standard therapy without vaccination. Probability of survival at 4 years was 63 % for group B and 94 % for group A. This 31 % difference suggests that antitumor vaccination with ATV-NDV in the adjuvant situation can improve long-term survival probability in breast cancer.

Meanwhile it was possible with financial support from the Dietmar Hopp Stiftung (Walldorf, Germany) to perform in primary operated breast-cancer patients a small prospective randomised controlled study with 30 patients. Results are not yet available.

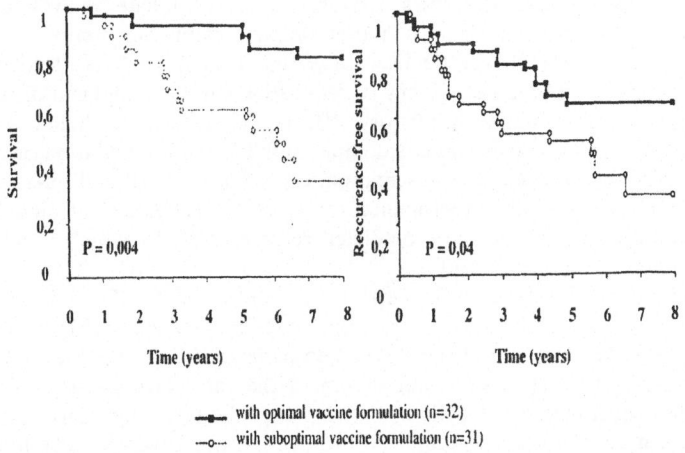

A- Overall postoperative survival of breast cancer patients   B- Recurrence-free survival of breast cancer patients

P = 0,004

P = 0,04

Time (years)   Time (years)

—■— with optimal vaccine formulation (n=32)
—○— with suboptimal vaccine formulation (n=31)

Fig. 7. Improvement of survival in breast cancer. Primary operated breast cancer patients received postoperative vaccinations with ATV-NDV in two different formulations given to two cohorts of more than 30 patients with similar risk factors. The Figure shows the Kaplan Meier estimates after a prolonged median observation period of 5.2 years for long-term survival (A) and recurrence-free survival (B). There was a highly significant long-term survival benefit and also a significant benefit in recurrence free survival in the group which received an optimal formulation (at least 1.5×10^6 viable infected tumor cells and at least 33 % overall cell viability). There were only 5 patients dead in this group as compared to 16 in the other group. The survival in the group with suboptimal vaccine formulation corresponds to expectation of patients with similar risk factors under standard therapy without vaccination.

GENERAL CONSIDERATIONS AND CONCLUSIONS

We here present a new concept of immunotherapy of cancer which aims at the activation of cancer reactive memory T cells which we demonstrated to pre-exist in the bone marrow of cancer patients. A boost with an appropriate tumor vaccine is expected to cause a transition from central to effector memory T cells and to cytotoxic effector CD8 T cells that infiltrate tumor tissue of metastases. The antitumor cytotoxic effect should reduce the tumor burden below a threshold that can be further controlled by a pool of long-term memory T cells.

In an animal tumor model we observed a connection between tumor dormancy and long-term protective immune memory. These and other observations suggested that dormant tumor cells are a source of persisting TAA and that this helps to maintain TAA specific long-term memory.

The maintenance of long-term polyclonal antitumor memory is considered of utmost importance for improvement of long-term survival of cancer patients. Defective maintenance of memory below the threshold for immunological protection would allow the uncontrolled regrowth of remaining tumor cells. Tumor dormancy has also been described in breast cancer. Some patients do not develop recurrence in spite of disseminated tumor cells at the time of diagnosis. Other patients develop secondary tumors very late, maybe ten years after successful therapy, suggesting break-down of some control mechanism. Such individual differences in prognosis may be due to differences in immune control via memory T cells.

In our strategy of active immunotherapy we designed the tumor vaccine ATV-NDV in which we link multiple danger signals with multiple tumor antigens from individual patient-derived tumor cells. This allows activating multiple innate as well as adaptive immune responses. An important facet of the autologous whole cell tumor vaccine is the choice of the virus, namely Newcastle Disease Virus. This is well tolerated in patients, shows tumor selectivity and high efficiency of replication (in the cytoplasm of tumor cells) and induces pleiotropic immunostimulatory effects. These are mediated through the induction of interferons, cytokines and chemokines and through upregulation of cell surface molecules of importance for antigen presentation, cell adhesion, cell-cell interaction and T cell co-stimulation. We provide experimental evidence for activation of memory T cells from cancer patients and for an NDV mediated release of IL-15 which is an important survival factor for CD8 memory T cells.

In all of the 9 phase II clinical trials performed with this ATV-NDV vaccine (Table 2) we observed significant prolongations of either overall survival (OS) or disease free survival (DSF) or both. In some of the vaccinated patients it was possible to demonstrate complete or parial tumor remission and in others the long-term persistence of cancer reactive immunological memory T cells even years after the last vaccination. Although we are aware of the need of further randomised prospective trials we consider nine phase II clinical studies with significant improvements of survival and involving several hundreds of patients as a rather convincing demonstration of i) clinical benefit and ii) effectivity of this type of tumor vaccine.

The preparation of this type of vaccine requires a somewhat sophisticated technology but it is certainly less demanding than any of the gene therapy cancer vaccines. On one hand the concept is individually tailored to each patient on the other hand it does not seem to be restricted to particular types of cancer and to have rather broad applicability. Clinical benefits are suggested for 8 different human cancers including colorectal and breast carcinomas and highly aggressive types such as pancreatic carcinoma and glioblastoma.

Acknowledgement

This work would not have been possible without the dedicated help and contributions of many basic scientists and clinicians. Their names can be obtained from the list of the quoted references.

References

1. Gallucci S., Matzinger, P: Danger signals: SOS to the immune system. Curr. Opin. Immunol. 13: 114-119 (2001).
2. Akira S., Takeda K., Kaisho T: Toll-like receptors: critical proteins linking innate and acquired immunity. Nat. Immunol. 2: 675-680, (2001).
3. Luster A.D. The role of chemokines in linking innate and adaptive immunity. Curr. Opin. Immunol. 14: 129-135 (2002).
4. Heicappell R., Schirrmacher V. von Hoegen P. et al. Prevention of metastatic spread by postoperative immunotherapy virally modified autologous tumor cells. I. Parameters for optimal therapeutic effects. Int. J. Cancer 37: 569-577 (1986).
5. Schirrmacher V., Haas, C., Bonifer, R., Ahlert, T., Gerhards R. and Ertel C. Human tumor cell modification by virus infection: an efficient and safe way to produce cancer vaccine with pleiotropic immune stimulatory properties when using Newcastle Disease Virus. Gene Ther. 6: 63-73, (1999).
6. Tortorella, D., Gewurz, B.E., Furman, M.H. Schust, D.J. and Ploegh, H.L. Viral subversion of the immune system. Annu. Rev. Immunol. 18: 861-926, (2000).
7. Wold, W.S., Doronin, K., Toth, K., Kuppuswang, M., Lichtenstein DL and Tollefson, E.A. Immune responses to adenoviruses: viral evasion mechanisms and their implications for the clinic. Curr. Opin. Immunol. 11: 380-386 (1999).
8. Naniche D. and Oldstone MBA. Generalized immunosuppression: how viruses undermine the immune response. Cell Mol. Life Sci. 57: 1399-1407 (1999).
9. Andrews DM, Andoniou E., Granucci, F., Ricciardi-Castagnoli P. and Degli-Esposti A. Infection of dendritic cells by murine cytomegalovirus induces functional paralysis. Nat. Immunol. 2: 1077-1084 (2001).
10. Alexopoulou L, Holt A.C., Medzhitov R. and Flavell R.A. Recognition of double-stranded RNA and activation of NF-kappa B by Toll-like receptor. Nature 413: 732-738 (2001).
11. Kobayashi H., Sendo F., Shirai, T., Kaji H., Kodama T. and Saito H. Modification in growth of transplantable rat tumors exposed to Friend virus. J. Natl. Cancer Inst. 42: 413-419 (1969).
12. Ahlert, T., Schirrmacher V. Isolation of a human melanoma adapted Newcastle Disease Virus mutant with highly selective replication patterns. Cancer Res. 50: 5962-5968 (1990).
13. Bosslet, K., Schirrmacher, V. and Shantz, G. Tumor metastases and cell-mediated immunity in a model system in DBA/2 mice. VI. Similar specificity patterns of protective anti-tumor immunity in vivo and of cytolytic T cells in vitro. Int. J. Canc. 24: 303-313 (1979).
14. Khazaie, K., Prifti, S., Beckhove, P., Griesbach, A., Russell, S. Collins, M. and Schirrmacher, V. Persistence of dormant tumor cells in the bone marrow of tumor-cell-vaccinated mice correlates with long term immunological protection. Proc. Natl.Acad. Sci. 91, 7430-7434 (1994).
15. Washburn B. and Schirrmacher V. Human tumor cell infection by Newcastle Disease Virus leads to upregulation of HLA and cell adhesion molecules and to induction of interferons, chemokines and finally apoptosis. Int. J. Oncol. 21: 85-93 (2002).
16. Cella M., Salio, M., Sakkakibara, Y., Langen, H, Julkunen, I and Lanzavecchia A. Maturation, activation and protection of dendritic cells induced by double-stranded RNA. J. Exp. Med. 189: 821-829 (1999).

17. Stark, G.R., Kerr, I.M., Williams, BRG, Silverman, R.H. and Schreiber R.D. How cells respond to interferons. Ann. Rev. Biochem. 67: 227-264 (1998).
18. Sato, M., Taniguchi T., Tanaka N. The interferon system and interferon regulatory factor transcription factors – studies from gene knockout mice. Cytokine & Growth Factor Rev. 12: 133-142 (2001).
19. Kadowaki, N., Antonenko, S., Lau, J.Y. and Liu Y.J. Natural interferon alpha/beta-producing cells link innate and adaptive immunity. J. Exp. Med. 192: 219-226 (2000).
20. Grage-Griebenow, E., Zawatzky, R., Kahlert, H., Brade, L., Flad, H.D., and Ernst M. Identification of a novel dendritic cell-like subset of CD64+/CD16$^+$ blood monocytes. Eur. J. Immunol. 31, 48-56 (2001).
21. Zeng J., Fournier, P., Schirrmacher V. Induction of interferon-α and tumor necrosis factor-related apoptosis-inducing ligand in human blood mononuclear cells by hemagglutinin-neuraminindase but not F protein of Newcastle Disease Virus. Virol. 287: 19-30 (2002).
22. Zeng, J., Fournier, P., Schirrmacher V. Stimulation of human natural interferon-α response via paramyxovirus hemagglutinin lectin-cell interaction. J. Mol. Med. 80: 443-451 (2002).
23. Fujita T. Evolution of the lectin-complement pathway and its role in innate immunity. Nature Rev. 2: 346-353 (2002).
24. Haas, C., Ertel C., Gerhards, R., Schirrmacher V. Introduction of adhesive and costimulatory immune functions into tumor cells by infection with Newcastle Disease Virus. Int. J. Oncol. 13: 1105-1115 (1998).
25. Ertel, C., Millar N.S., Emmerson, P.T., Schirrmacher V. and von Hoegen P. Viral hemagglutinin augments peptide-specific cytotoxic T cell responses. Eur. J. Immunol. 23: 2592-2596 (1993).
26. Pulendran, B., Banchereau J., Maraskovsky E., Maliszewski C. Modulating the immune response with dendritic cells and their growth factors. Trends Immunol. 22: 41-47 (2001).
27. Le Bon, A., Schiavoni, G., D'Agostino, G., Gresser, I., Belardelli, F., Tough, D.F. Type I interferons potently enhance humoral immunity and can promote isotype switching by stimulating dendritic cells in vivo. Immunity 14, 461-470 (2001).
28. Sato, K., Hida, S., Takayanagi, H., Yokochi T., Kayagaki N., Takeda, K., Yagita, H., Okumura K., Tanaka N. Taniguchi T., Ogasawara K. Antiviral response by natural killer cells through TRAIL gene induction by IFN-alpha/beta. Eur. J. Immunol. 31: 3138-3146 (2001).
29. Rogge, L., Barberis-Maino, L., Biffi, M., Passini, N., Presky, D.H., Gubler, U., Sinigaglia E. Selective expression of an interleukin-12 receptor component by human T helper 1 cells. J. Exp. Med. 185: 825-831 (1997).
30. Schirrmacher, V., Bai, L., Umansky, V. Yu L, Xing Y., Qian Z. Newcastle Disease Virus activates macrophages for anti-tumor activity. Int. J. Oncol. 16: 363-373 (2000).
31. Umansky, V., Shatrov, VA, Lehmann, V. and Schirrmacher V. Induction of nitric oxide synthesis in macrophages by Newcastle Disease Virus is associated with activation of nuclear factor-κB. Int. Immunol. 8: 491-498 (1996).
32. Bai, L., Koopmann, J., Fiola, C., Fournier, P. and Schirrmacher V. Dendritic cells pulsed with viral oncolysates potently stimulate autologous T cells from cancer patients. Int. J. Oncol. 21: 685-694 (2002).
33. Lodolce I.P., Burkett P.R., Boone D.L., Chien M., Ma, A. T cell-independent interleukin 15R alpha signals are required for bystander proliferation. J. Exp. Med. 194: 1187-1194 (2001).
34. Kaech, S.M., Wherry, E.J. and Ahmed, R., Effector and memory T cell differentiation: implications for vaccine development. Nature Rev. 2: 251-262 (2002).
35. Schirrmacher V. T-cell immunity in the induction and maintenance of a tumor dormant state. Sem. Cancer Biol. 11: 285-295 (2001).
36. Müller M, Gounari, F., Prifti, S., Hacker, H.J., Schirrmacher V., Khazaie, K. Eb-lacZ tumor dormancy in bone marrow and lymph nodes: active control of proliferating tumor cells by CD8$^+$ immune T cells. Cancer Res. 58: 5439-5446 (1998).
37. Feuerer, M., Beckhove, P., Bai, L., Solomayer, E.-F., Bastert, G., Diel I.J., Heep J., Oberniedermayr M., Schirrmacher V. Umansky V. Therapy of human tumors in NOD/SCID mice with patient derived re-activated memory T cells from bone marrow. Nature Med. 7 (4): 452-458 (2001).
38. Beckhove, P., Schütz, F., I.J. Diel, E.-F. Solomayer, Bastert, G., Förster, J., Oberniedermayr, M., Feuerer, L., Bai, L., Umansky V. and Schirrmacher V. Efficient engraftment of human primary breast cancer transplants in NOD/SCID mice. Int. J. Cancer, in press (2002).
39. Schirrmacher V., and Von Hoegen P. Importance of tumor cell membrane integrity and viability for CTL activation by cancer vaccines. Vaccine Res. 2 No. 3, 183-196 (1993).

40. Schirrmacher V. Griesbach, A. Zangemeister U. γ-irradiated viable tumor cells as whole cell vaccines can stimulate in situ syngeneic anti-tumor CTL and DTH reactivity while tumor cell lysates elicit only DTH reactivity. Vaccine Res. Vol. 3 No. 1, 31-48 (1994).

41. Termeer, C.C., Schirrmacher, V., Bröcker, E.-B. and Becker J.C. Newcastle Disease Virus infection induces B7-1/B7-2-independent T-cell costimulatory activity in human melanoma cells. Cancer Gene Ther. 7: 316-323 (2000).

42. Schlag P., Manasterski, M., Gernerth T. et al. Active specific immunotherapy with Newcastle Disease Virus modified tumor cells following resection of liver metastases in colorectal cancer. First evaluation of clinical response of a phase II trial. Cancer Immunol. Immunother. 35 (3): 325-330 (1992).

43. Ockert D., Schirrmacher V. Beck N. et al. Newcastle Disease Virus-infected intact autologous tumor cell vaccine for active specific immunotherapy of resected colorectal carcinoma. Clin. Canc. Res. 2 (1): 21-28 (1996).

44. Ahlert, T. Sauerbrei W., Bastert G. et al. Tumor-cell number and viability as quality and efficacy parameters of autologous virus-modified cancer vaccine in patients with breast or ovarian cancer J. Clin. Oncol. 15 (4): 1354-1366 (1997).

45. Möbus, V, Horn, S., Stöck M. et al. Tumor cell vaccination for gynaecological tumors. Hybridoma 12 (5): 543-547 (1993).

46. Pomer S., Schirrmacher V., Thiele R., et al. Tumor response and 4 year survival data of patients with advanced renal carcinoma treated with autologous tumor vaccine and subcutaneous r-IL-2 and IFN-alpha2b. Int. J. Oncol. 6: 947-954 (1995).

47. Schirrmacher V., Ahlert, T., Pröbstle T. et al. Immunization with virus-modified tumor cells. Semi. in Oncol. 25: 677-696 (1998).

48. Steiner, H.H., Bonsanto, M.M., Beckhove P., Brysch, M. Schuele-Freyer R., Geletneky, K., Kremer, P., Golamrheza, R., Bauer, H., Kunze, S., Schirrmacher V., Herold-Mende C. Anti-tumor vaccination of patients with glioblastoma multiforme in a case-control study: Feasibility, safety and clinical benefit. Submitted.

CAUSATION AND PREVENTION OF SOLELY ESTROGEN-INDUCED ONCOGENESIS: SIMILARITIES TO HUMAN DUCTAL BREAST CANCER

Jonathan J. Li and Sara Antonia Li

Division of Etiology & Prevention of Hormonal Cancers, and Department of

Pharmacology, Toxicology and Therapeutics, University of Kansas Medical Center

Kansas City, KS 66160-7417

ABSTRACT

Estrogens are intimately involved in the causation of some of the most prevalent cancers afflicting women, particularly, breast, endometrial, cervico-vaginal, and possibly ovarian. Therefore, it has become particularly pertinent to elucidate the molecular changes and mechanisms whereby estrogens elicit their oncogenic actions so that better prevention strategies can be developed. The estrogen-induced Syrian hamster tumors of the kidney have emerged as one of the most intensively studied in-vivo models in solely estrogen-induced oncogenesis. An advantage of this model is that the tumors occur in the absence of any intervening morphologic changes, but rather they are the result of the continuous progression of a subset of interstitial stem cells in the kidney leading to tumor formation. Evidence is presented that the origin of these tumors is derived from ectopic "uterine" stem cells, which are responsive to estrogenic hormones. The other animal tumor model studied is the highly sensitive estrogen-induced mammary tumors of female ACI rats. Their steroid receptor and other gene alterations have been delineated. Importantly, a crucial early event in this solely estrogen-induced oncogenic process, common to both animal tumor models, is the overexpression and amplification of c-*myc* and its protein product. Chromosomal instability, in both early and large well-established frank tumors, is another important characteristic found during early E-induced oncogenesis. These features have been shown to be characteristic of human ductal carcinomas *in-situ* and in primary invasive ductal breast carcinomas. The molecular alterations seen are considered crucial in eliciting estrogen-induced oncogenesis and have established for the first time a direct causal link between estrogen and the induction of chromosomal instability and aneuploidy in these estrogen-associated neoplasms.

New Trends in Cancer for the 21st Century, edited by
Llombart-Bosch and Felipo, Kluwer Academic/Plenum Publishers, 2003

INTRODUCTION

Breast cancer (BC) comprises nearly 30% of all cancers occurring in women[1]. Approximately 90-95% of BCs are described as sporadic invasive ductal carcinomas[2]. Familial BC, although important, does not contribute substantially to the high overall BC frequency; that is, in developed countries it contributes only 5-7% of the reported BC cases[3]. Thus far, no single or group of environmental or dietary chemical carcinogenic agent(s) has been directly implicated in causing the high sporadic BC incidence seen[4-6]. In the past decade, it has become increasingly evident that both endogenous natural estrogens (Es) and exogenously ingested estrogenic agents are associated with increased BC risk (Table 1). Possibly the most compelling argument for a crucial role for E in BC is derived from the *Breast Cancer Prevention Trial* in which Tamoxifen (TAM) treatment was shown to decrease the risk of BC 44-55% in women considered at increased risk for the disease[7].

Table 1. Estrogen as the Major Risk Factor for Breast Cancer

Early Age of 1st Menses	Tissue Aromatase
Late Age Menopause	Obesity
Null Parity	Alcohol
Absence of Lactation	ERT/HRT
Lack of Exercise	Ovarian Tumors

While there is general agreement that Es are capable of promoting neoplastic processes, there is much less understanding of the role of Es in tumor induction, when they are the sole etiologic agents. Two seemingly disparate E-induced animal tumor models, the carcinomas arising in male hamster kidneys and those in female ACI rat mammary glands, remarkably exhibit very similar molecular changes driven by E. Moreover, the molecular alterations found in these E-induced animal models during oncogenesis and in established frank neoplasms closely resemble pertinent characteristics of human invasive ductal BCs.

SERUM AND TISSUE ESTRADIOL LEVELS

The maximum mean serum levels of 17β-estradiol (E_2) which elicited 100% tumor incidence in male hamster kidneys over a 6.0-month period was 2.28 ng/ml[8]. However, the minimal E_2 serum oncogenic concentration to induce tumors arising in the kidney remains to be determined. On the other hand, the mean E_2 serum levels which elicited 100% mammary tumor incidence in female ACI rats was only 132 pg/ml[9]. Moreover, we have shown that a mean E_2 serum concentration of 70 pg/ml also induced a similar mammary tumor incidence in this rat strain. Interestingly, the mean tissue E_2 concentration in the hamster kidney, 4.6 pg/mg protein during E_2 oncogenesis, is comparable to E_2 levels seen in breast tissues of cycling women, and in human BC tissues, 5.7 and 8.9 pg/mg protein, respectively. Therefore, to elicit E oncogenic processes, it is evident that only minute quantities of E are required.

CELL AND TISSUE CHARACTERISTICS

It has long been an enigma that neoplasms in the kidney are induced as a consequence of chronic E treatment. An initial clue to this puzzle may be obtained from histologic and electron microscopic findings which suggested an interstitial cell of origin for tumors arising in the hamster kidney[10-12]. We have recently proposed, based on accumulated evidence from our laboratory, that tumors of the kidney arise from germinal or multipotential interstitial "uterine" stem cells which are ectopically located in the kidney (Fig. 1). The basis for this contention is that the hamster reproductive and urinary tracts, as in most if not all mammalian species, are derived from a common germinal ridge of multi-potential cells. A subset of these ectopic "uterine" germinal cells in the kidney have migrated and established themselves in the corticomedullary region; the oldest section of the mature kidney. These ectopically located "uterine" germ cells remain dormant unless exposed to a sustained level of E_2. This contention is supported by the following findings: **1.** Resemblance of the early renal interstitial stem cell lesions to blastema, with positive staining of mesenchymal markers (vimentin, desmin), but only a trace of cytokeratin[13-14]. The cytokeratin expression, however, gradually increases during development to frank primary tumors residing in the kidney; **2.** Only a subset of interstitial stem cells in the kidney responded to E treatment by initially expressing progesterone receptor (**PR**) and E receptor (**ERα**)[15]; **3.** The absence of ERβ expression in E-induced tumors in the kidney is consistent with the known selective expression and proliferative role of ER□ in uterine tissue[16]; **4.** The initial detection and abundance of early tumorous foci in the corticomedullary region in the kidney after E treatment; **5.** The ability of either progesterone (**P**) or progestational agents to completely abolish the induction of tumors in the kidney when concomitantly administered with E_2[17,18]. This response is in contrast to the role of this hormone in the mammary gland where both E and P are mitogenic[19]; **6.** The essentially identical isoform profiles of ERα and PR seen in these tumors in the kidney compared to corresponding receptor profiles seen in the adult hamster uterus[15]; and **7.** Overexpression of E-responsive genes (c-*myc*, c-*fos*, c-*jun*) in tumor foci and frank tumors of the kidney[20]. On this basis, we have proposed that tumors in the hamster kidney arise from multi-potential interstitial "uterine" stem cells that ectopically reside in the kidney, and are now designated as ectopic uterine tumors in the kidney (**EUTK**).

During E-induced mammary tumor oncogenesis in female ACI rats, various tumor developmental stages have been detected[9,21]; that is hyperplasia, dysplasia, atypical dysplasia, and ductal carcinoma *in-situ* (**DCIS**). However, the progenitor cell(s) related to the origin of these E-induced mammary tumors, as is the case for human BC, has thus far remained elusive. Progress has been hampered by the absence of identifiable biomarkers for progenitor stem cells in the mammary gland. Nevertheless, small and large light cells, likely putative progenitor breast stem cells, have been identified in the mouse and rat mammary gland[22]. These putative breast stem cells exhibit distinctive morphologic characteristics, including either small or very large pale nucleoplasms, few organelles, and elevated mitotic activity, compared to mature mammary epithelial cells. This aspect is under intense study in our laboratory using the solely E-induced ACI rat mammary gland tumor model.

Figure 1. Schematic representation of the Syrian hamster germinal ridge. Germinal cells destined to the reproductive tract (round cells) and urinary tract (elongated cells) arise from the same germinal ridge of multi-potential stem cells. The reproductive germinal cells, normally destined to reside in uterus, migrate and establish themselves in the renal corticomedullary region[8].

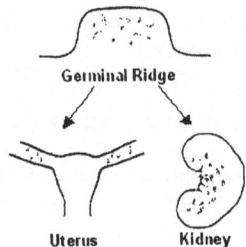

PREVENTION OF E-INDUCED ONCOGENESIS

Concomitant antiestrogen treatment, including TAM (Table 2), enclomiphene, or nafoxidine completely prevented the induction of EUTK by estrogen[17]. Additionally, concomitant treatment with P, androgen, or ethinyl estradiol also abolished E-induced EUTK oncogenesis[17, 18, 23]. Similarly, combined treatment of TAM and E completely inhibited the induction of mammary tumors in female ACI rats[9].

Taken together, these data provide strong evidence that the development of E-induced tumors in these animal models is an ERα-mediated processes. Furthermore, these findings are consistent with the substantial reduction in BC risk reported when TAM was administered to women who were susceptible to develop cancers at this tissue site[7].

Table 2. Prevention of Estrogen-induced Oncogenesis of Hamster Ectopic Uterine Tumors in the Kidney and ACI Rat Mammary Tumors by Tamoxifen

Species	Treatment	No. Animals	% Animals w/ Tumors	Tumor Multiplicity/ Animal
Hamster[1]	Untreated	8	0	0
	TAM	8	0	0
	E_2	10	100	16.7 ✕ 1.1
	E_2 + TAM	8	0	0
ACI Rat[2]	Untreated	10	0	0
	TAM	8	0	0
	E_2	12	100	15.6 ✕ 1.6
	E_2 + TAM	8	0	0

[1] Male hamsters were treated with pellets containing Tamoxifen citrate (TAM) (40 mg), E_2 (20 mg) each separately or in combination for 9.0 months.
[2] Female ACI rats were treated with pellets containing Tamoxifen citrate (TAM) (40 mg), E_2 (3 mg) each separately or in combination for 7.0 months.

ESTROGEN AND PROGESTERONE RECEPTORS

Both ER mRNA and protein expression was examined following different intervals of E-induced EUTK oncogenesis[15]. ER positive (ER$^+$) immunostaining was detected uniformly at modest levels in proximal tubular cells of the renal cortex of untreated castrated male hamsters. After E-treatment for 1.0-2.0 months, the nuclear ER$^+$ staining in the proximal tubules was uniformly down-regulated. Intense nuclear ER$^+$ staining was seen in individual and tiny clusters of renal interstitial stem cells (ISC) in the corticomedullary region after only 2.0-3.0 months of E-treatment. The ISC population was quite distinct from adult differentiated renal tubular cells. However, not all of the ISC in this region exhibited ER$^+$ expression. With continued E-treatment for 3.0-6.0 months, nascent tumorous foci, small and large tumor foci, and well-established EUTK displayed intense nuclear ER$^+$ staining[15].

While no detectable PR$^+$ staining was detected in untreated ISC in kidneys of untreated hamsters, PR$^+$ expression was seen after only two weeks of E-treatment in individual ISCs, largely confined to the corticomedullary region of the kidney[15]. The intense PR$^+$ staining in ISCs preceded the detection of ER$^+$ expression by at least a month. The pattern of PR$^+$ staining was similar to that of ER$^+$ expression in nascent and early tumorous foci and in large frank EUTK. Co-localization of ER$^+$ and PR$^+$ staining in all stages of EUTK development was ascertained by serial section.

Western blot analyses reveal that after 1.0-3.0 months of E-treatment, a marked rise in a 64-kDa ER$^+$ isoform was seen compared to untreated castrated hamsters (Fig. 2). It is suggested that the 64-kDa ER$^+$ isoform may affect the mitogenic responses of ISC by differentially affecting signaling pathways of early EUTK foci, thus supporting their growth advantage. With continued E-treatment, a 58-kDa ER$^+$ isoform was also evident. This is in contrast to a predominate 50-kDa truncated isoform seen in untreated castrated hamster kidneys. The primary EUTK ER$^+$ profile exhibited a 66-, 58-, and 50-kDa isoforms but the absence of the 64-kDa form. Interestingly, the ER$^+$ isoform profile in primary EUTK was essentially identical to that seen in adult hamster uteri[15]. Similarly, PR isoform profiles of established EUTK also resembled the pattern seen in adult hamster uteri (PR-B, PR-A, and PR-C). In contrast, only negligible to low levels of these PR forms were detected in untreated hamster kidneys (Fig. 2). E-treatment for 2.0-4.0 months resulted in a modest rise in PR-A expression and two PR-A1 and -A2 forms. After 5.0 months of E-treatment, PR-B was detected. The induction of PR found in all stages of EUTK development provides a PR based mechanism for its prevention when progestin is added in combination with E.

In mammary gland tissue from control untreated female ACI rats, a single ER 56-kDA isoform was detected (Fig. 3). After 6.0 months of E_2-treatment, a 47-kDa ER variant and the 66-kDa full-length ER form was evident. In primary E_2-induced mammary tumors, a 56-, 66-, and 54-kDa ER isoform was also seen in untreated adult ACI rat uteri[15]. This 54-kDa ER isoform in primary mammary tumors was predominant. Interestingly, when compared with E_2-treatment alone, both the 56-kDa and 47-kDa isoform expression declined markedly after TAM + E_2 treatment. TAM treatment alone suppressed the expression of the 56 kDa variant compared to untreated mammary glands. No positive signals for ER were observed in any of the mammary glands examined. Mammary glands from both untreated and TAM-treated female ACI rats exhibited the same level of PR-C expression (Fig. 3). After treatment with E_2 for 6.0 months, both PR-A and PR-B were induced, although the expression of the latter induced PR form was modest. In E_2-induced primary mammary tumors, PR-A expression was 6.0-10.0-fold higher than untreated mammary glands. Combined TAM + E_2 treatment resulted in PR expression profile that resembled those of either untreated or TAM-treated alone mammary glands. PR-A expression was extremely low in all of these groups. In E-induced primary mammary tumors, a prominent PR-B1 form was consistently found, which was less evident in mammary glands of E_2-treated group. Interestingly, the ER . and PR profiles of E-induced mammary tumors in female ACI rats did not closely resemble corresponding PR profiles seen in adult ACI rat uteri.

Figure 2. Western blot analysis of ER∀ and PR during estrogen-induced EUTK oncogenesis. Fifteen micrograms of total protein extract from hamster kidneys of intact males (IMK), castrated males (CMK), estrogen-treated for 1.0 m (E-1), 3.0 m (E-3), and 5.0 m (E-5), EUTK samples from estrogen-treated hamsters for 8.0-10.0 m (KT), uteri from intact female hamsters (HU), and kidneys from intact female hamsters (IFK) were separated by SDS-PAGE, transferred to nitrocellulose membrane, and immunoblotted with ER∀ and PR antibodies. The arrows at the left of the blot are molecular mass markers run beside the samples. Specific bands for ER∀ and PR are indicted by arrows on the right. Each slot contained three pooled samples from 2 or 3 individual kidneys, tumors, or uteri. The results are representative of three independent experiments. PR-A, 94kDa, PR-B, 120 kDa , PR-C, 64 kDa.

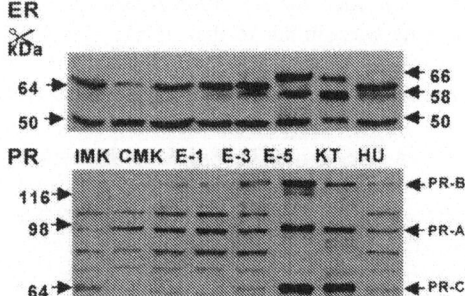

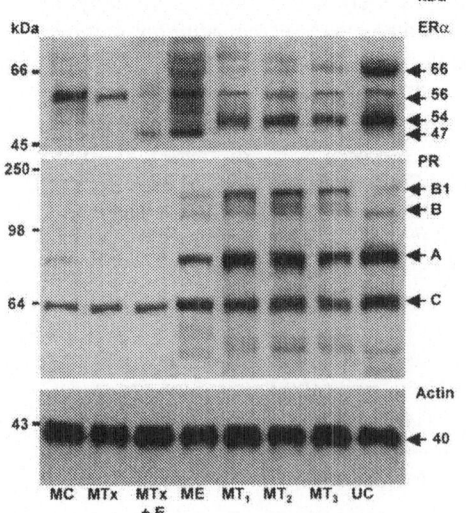

Figure 3. Representative ER and PR expression in MG and MGT samples. Western blot was performed on 20 μg protein aliquots after 6.0 months of treatment. MC, untreated, TAM-treated (MTx), TAM + E_2-treated (MTx + E), E_2-treated (ME), three individual E_2-induced MGT (MT$_1$ to MT$_3$), and untreated uterus (UC). The primary antibodies used were ER MC20, -actin C10, and PR MC19. The relative amount of protein was determined by densitometry. The figure is representative of three independent experiments.

ANEUPLOIDY AND CHROMOSOMAL INSTABILITY

Nuclear image cytometry (**NIC**) was employed to determine the ploidy status of EUTK foci from 3.0- and 4.0 month E-treated hamsters and large well-established primary EUTK from 6.0 to 8.0 month E-treated animals (Fig. 4) and compared to similar Feulgen stained sections of aged-matched untreated hamsters[15, 24]. Untreated renal sections exhibited a normal diploid frequency (n = 44) whereas early EUTK foci were all highly aneuploid (Fig. 4). Large well-established EUTK were also highly aneuploid. G-banded karyotype (Fig. 5) and comparative genomic hybridization confirmed and extended these NIC data. Primary EUTK contained nonrandom or consistent numerical gains (frequency ∃ 30% of the metaphases) in chromosomes 3, 6, 20, and 21. Recurrent gains (frequency # 25%) were observed in chromosomes 5, 11, 14, and 16[25]. These consistently gained chromosomes largely displayed trisomies but many exhibited tetrasomies. No consistent losses were seen employing this stringent criteria. However, recurrent chromosome losses occurred in chromosomes 7, 12, 17, and 19, with frequencies ranging from 23% to 26%. Monosomies were the most recurrent losses[25].

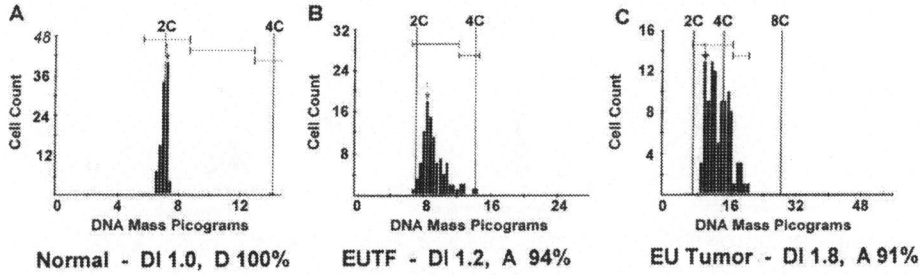

Figure 4. NIC of E-induced male hamster ectopic uterine stem cell tumors in the kidney.

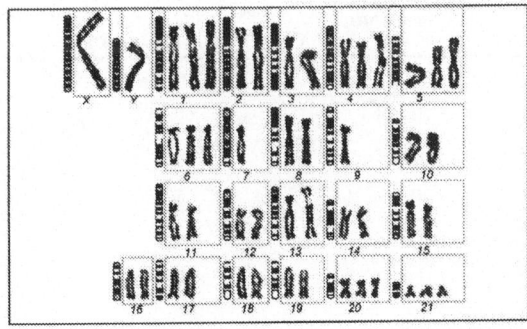

Figure 5. Representative karytotype of an E-induced ectopic uterine stem cell tumor of the kidney.

E-induced mammary tumors from two different rat strains, ACI and Noble, the latter promoted by androgen, were examined for their ploidy status using NIC on Feulgen-stained sections (Fig. 5, Table 3). When compared to normal untreated mammary glands in which both rat strains showed a normal diploid frequency, 2n = 42, the primary mammary tumors exhibited high aneuploid frequencies, ranging from 88-91%[21]. Of particular interest, the DCISs from each rat strain found after 3.5-5.0 months of E-treatment were also highly aneuploid, both showing 85% frequencies. In marked contrast, mammary tumors induced either by 7,12-dimethylbenz[a]anthracene (DMBA) or nitrosomethylurea (NMU), both synthetic chemical carcinogens not found in nature, in BuF/N and Sprague-Dawley (SD) female rat strains, exhibited high diploid frequencies (> 85%) (Fig. 6, Table 3). Moreover, an environmental chemical carcinogen, 6-nitrochrysene (6-NC), found in diesel exhaust, also showed high diploid frequencies (> 89%) in mammary tumors induced by this agent[21].

These data, taken together, clearly demonstrate that aneuploidy is a distinctive early event in E-induced oncogenesis. Moreover, it is evident that E-induced mammary tumorigenesis occurs via very different molecular pathways than mammary tumors induced by either synthetic or environmental chemical carcinogens.

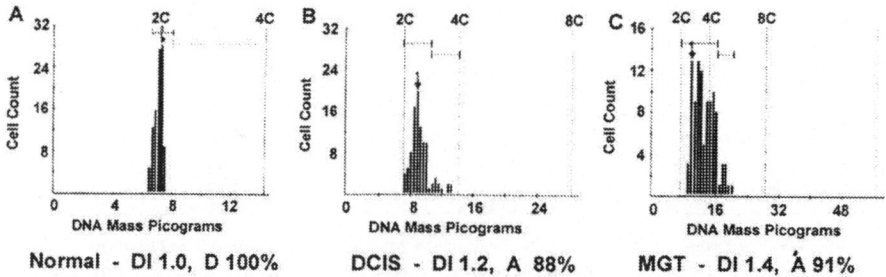

Figure 6. NIC of E-induced female ACI rat mammary gland tumors.

Table 3. NIC Aneuploid Frequency in Mammary Gland Tumors Induced by Estrogens or Chemical Carcinogens in Various Rat Strains

	Strain	% Diploid Normal MG cells	% Diploid cells		% Aneuploid cells	
			CIS	MGT	CIS	MGT
HORMONES						
None	ACI	99.8 (4)				
17α-E$_2$	ACI		15.5 (6)	9.2 (9)	84.5 (6)	90.8 (9)
None	Noble	99.7 (4)				
17ω-E$_2$ + TP	Noble		14.8 (5)	10.7 (5)	85.2 (5)	89.3 (5)
CHEMICAL CARCINOGENS						
None	BuF/N	98.5 (3)				
DMBA	BuF/N			85.4 (5)		14.6 (5)
NMU	BuF/N			87.2 (5)		12.8 (5)
None	SD	93.3 (3)				

Primary mammary tumors from female ACI rats were subjected to G-banded karyotype analysis. A representative E-induced mammary tumors karyotype from a female ACI rat is shown in Fig. 7. Employing the same stringent criteria used for EUTK, nonrandom gains were seen in chromosomes 7, 11, 12, 13, 19, and 20 and a consistent loss in chromosomes 12. Most frequent chromosome gains were seen as trisomies and chromosome losses as monosomies. In these consistently gained chromosomes, the frequency of tetrasomies ranged from 5-15%[21].

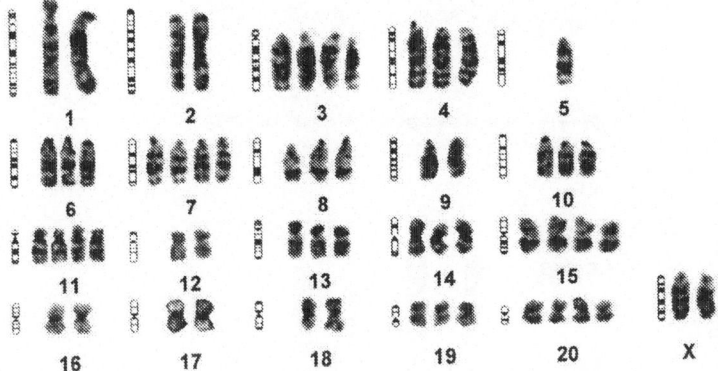

Figure 7. Representative karyotype of an E-induced mammary gland tumor from a female ACI rat.

C-MYC OVEREXPRESSION AND AMPLIFICATION

Early E-response genes, c-*myc*, c-*fos*, and c-*jun*, employing Northern blot analysis, were studied after various intervals of E-treatment during E-induced EUTK oncogenesis[20]. Compared to age-matched, untreated kidney samples, the expression of c-*myc* increased 2.8- and 4.1-fold, respectively. In primary EUTK c-*myc* expression rose 6.0-fold. Moreover, c-*fos* expression also rose 4.6-and 4.8-fold after 5.0 and 6.0 months, respectively, of E-treatment in hamster kidneys. Similarly, c-*jun* expression increased in the hamster kidney 2.8- and 5.1-fold at the same E-treatment intervals. In primary EUTK, c-*fos* and c-*jun* showed further elevation in the expression of these early E-response genes, 10.0- and 7.0-fold, respectively. Overexpression of MYC and FOS proteins was detected as early in hamster kidneys after 3.0 and 4.0 months of E-treatment[26]. The overexpression of c-*myc* RNA and c-*fos* RNA was largely confined to early EUTK foci as seen using *in-situ* hybridization of 4.0 and 5.0 month E-treated hamster kidneys[26]. The amplification of the c-*myc* gene in twelve primary EUTKs was determined by Southern blot analysis[26]. Eight of the 12 EUTK examined showed amplified copy numbers of the c-*myc* gene. The level of c-*myc* amplification ranged from 2.6 to 3.6. No gene amplification was seen when c-*fos* was similarly studied in the same EUTK specimens (Fig. 8). Employing fluorescent *in-situ* hybridization (FISH), the c-*myc* gene was localized to chromosome *6qb*. Previously, we have shown both by karyotype and CGH, that chromosome 6 is nonrandomly gained and exhibited a high frequency of trisomies and tetrasomies. These data strongly suggest that c-*myc* amplification occurs, at least in part, to a gain in chromosome number.

Similarly, Southern blot analysis of c-*myc* was performed on nine primary mammary tumors induced solely by E in female ACI rats[21]. It was shown that 66% of these mammary tumors exhibited amplified c-*myc* gene, ranging from 3.4- to 6.9-fold (Fig. 9). FISH and karyotype studies of c-*myc* reveal that c-*myc* is localized at chromosome *7q33* and this chromosome shows a high frequency of trisomies and tetrasomies[21]. These findings are remarkably similar to those seen in E-induced primary EUTK.

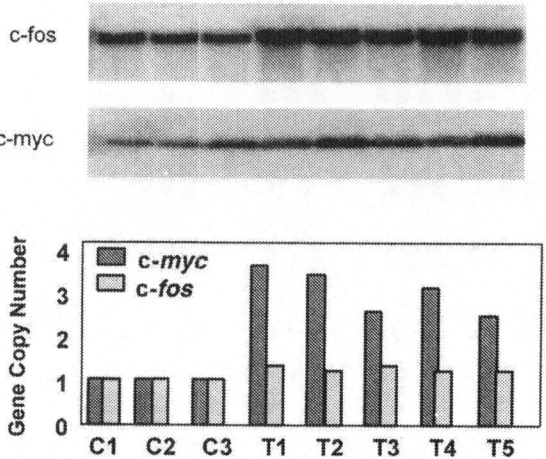

Figure 8. Southern blot analysis and densitometric quantitation of c-*myc* and c-*fos* expression in three age-matched (9.0-month) untreated control kidneys (C1-C3) and in five representative E-induced hamster renal tumors (T1-T5) isolated from individual 9.0- to 10.0-month E-treated hamsters. In samples from untreated normal kidney tissues, the mean densitometric levels of c-*myc* and c-*fos* was 1.29 ∀ 0.12.

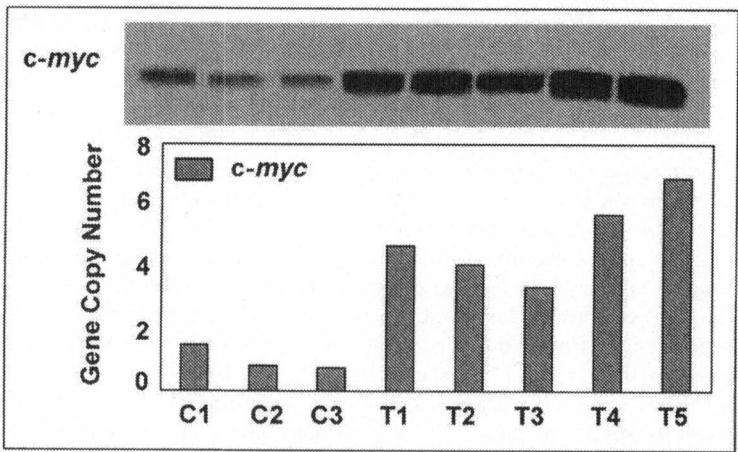

Figure 9. Southern blot of c-*myc* expression in E-induced ACI mammary gland.

SUMMARY

Results presented herein, using two seemingly disparate solely E-driven animal tumor models provide for the first time compelling evidence directly linking chromosomal instability (**CIN**) and aneuploidy to E and ER -mediated overexpression of c-*myc*/MYC. Invasive sporadic human ductal BCs have a number of highly pertinent characteristics which are similar to the molecular alterations seen in these E-induced animal tumor models. Two distinctive characteristics of human DCIS and primary invasive ductal BCs (Table 4), in addition to their shared pathology, are found in these E-induced animal tumor systems; a high frequency of ER positivity, as well as CIN and aneuploidy. Another pertinent characteristic seen in both DCIS and invasive ductal BC in common with these solely E-induced animal tumor models is the high frequency of c-*myc* overexpression, and, to a lesser extent, the amplification of this protooncogene. Present studies have directly related the overexpression of c-*myc* to eliciting CIN and aneuploidy[27-30]. Downstream molecular changes elicited by c-*myc* will be pivotal to our understanding of the relationship of BC causation to E mediation.

Table 4. Some Characteristics of DCIS and Invasive Ductal Breast Cancer

	Ductal Carcinoma in-situ (DCIS)	*Primary Invasive Ductal BC*
ER⁺	64%	60-65%
ER⁺ + PR⁺	66%	40%
Aneuploidy	65-78%	83-92%
c-*myc* Overexpression	-----	71%
c-*myc* Amplification	20%	32%

Acknowledgements

This work was supported by NIH grants R01 CA 58030 and R01 CA87591. We thank Dr. Dan Papa for performing the cytogenetic studies and Ms. Tandria Price for her assistance in the preparation of this manuscript.

References

1. Cancer statistics. Cancer J. Clin. 49:1-156 (1999).
2. Li, C.I., Weiss, N.S., Stanford, J.L., Daling J.R. Hormone replacement therapy in relation to risk of lobular and ductal breast carcinoma in middle-aged women. Cancer 88:2570-2577 (2000).
3. King, M.C., Rowell, S., Love, S.M. Inherited breast cancer and ovarian cancer. What are the choices? J. Am. Med. Assoc. 269:175-180 (1993).
4. Gammon, M.D., Santella, R.M., Neugut, A.I., Eng, S.M., Teitelbaum, S.L., Paykin, A., Levin, B., Terry, M.B., Young, T.L., Wang, L.W., et al. Environmental toxins and breast cancer on Long Island. I.

Polycyclic aromatic hydrocarbon DNA adducts. Cancer Epidem. Biomarkers & Prevent. 11:677-685 (2002).

5. Gammon, M.D., Wolff, M.S., Neugut, A.I., Eng, S.M., Teitelbaum, S.L., Britton, J.A., Terry, M.B., Levin, B., Sellman, S.D. Kabat, G.C., et al. Environmental toxins and breast cancer on Long Island. II. Organochlorine compound levels in blood. Cancer Epidem. Biomarkers & Prevent. 11:686-697 (2002).

6. Li, J.J., and S.A. Li. Breast cancer: Evidence for xenoestrogen involvement in altering its incidence and risk. In: Natural and Anthropogenic Environmental Oestrogens: The Scientific Basis for Risk Assessment. J. Pure & Appl. Chem. (IUPAC), 70:1713-1723 (1998).

7. Fisher B., Costantino, J.P., Wickerham, D.L., Redmond, C.K., Kavanah, M., Cronin, W.M., Vogel, V., Robidoux, A., Dimitrov, N., Atkins, J., Daly, M., Wieand, S., Tan-Chiu, E., Ford, L., Wolmark, N. Tamoxifen for prevention of breast cancer: Report of the National Surgical Adjuvant Breast and Bowel Project P-1 Study. J. Nat. Cancer Inst. 90:1371-1388 (1998).

8. Li, S.A., Xue, Y., Xie, Q., Li, C.I., Li, J.J. Serum and tissue levels of estradiol during estrogen-induced renal tumorigenesis in the Syrian hamster. J. Steroid Biochem. Molec. Biol. 48:283-286 (1994).

9. Li, S.A., Weroha, S.J., Tawfik, O., Li, J.J. Prevention of solely estrogen-induced mammary tumors by Tamoxifen: Evidence for estrogen receptor mediation. J. Endocrinol. 175:297-305 (2002).

10. Kirkman, H., Robbins, M. Histogenesis of estrogen-induced renal tumors in golden hamster. Anat. Res. 121:323 (1955).

11. Donten, W., Eder, M. Histogenese and biologische Verhaltenweise hormonell augeloster Geschwulste Beitr path. Anat. 120:270 (1959).

12. Llombart-Bosch, A., Peydro, A. Morphological, histochemical and ultrastructural observations of diethylstilbestrol-induced kidney tumors in the Syrian golden hamster. Europ. J. Cancer 11:403-412 (1975).

13. Gonzalez, A., Oberley, T.D., Li, J.J. Morphological and immunohistochemical studies of the estrogen-induced Syrian hamster renal tumor: Probable cell of origin. Cancer Res. 49:1020-1028 (1989).

14. Oberley, T.D., Gonzalez, A., Lauchner, L.J., Oberley, L.W., Li, J.J. Characterization of early lesions in estrogen-induced renal tumors in the Syrian hamster. Cancer Res. 51:1922-1929 (1991).

15. Li, J.J., Weroha, S.J., Davis, M.F., Hou, X., Tawfik, O., Li, S.A. Estrogen and progesterone receptors in renomedullary interstitial cells during Syrian hamster estrogen-induced tumorigenesis: Evidence for receptor-mediated oncogenesis. Endocrinology 142:4006-4014 (2001).

16. Pelletier, G., Labrie, C., Labrie, F. Localization of oestrogen receptor , oestrogen receptor , and androgen receptors in the rat reproductive organs. J. Endocrinology 165:359-370 (2000).

17. Li, J.J., Cuthbertson, T.L., Li, S.A. Inhibition of estrogen carcinogenesis in the Syrian golden hamster kidney by antiestrogens. J. Nat. Cancer Inst. 64:795-800 (1980).

18. Kirkman H. Estrogen-induced tumors of the kidney in Syrian hamsters. J. Natl. Cancer Inst. Monogr. 1:1-59 (1959).

19. Nandi, S., Guzman, R.C., Yang, J. Hormones and mammary carcinogenesis in mice, rats, and humans: A unifying hypothesis. Proc. Nat. Acad. Sci. USA 92:3650-3657 (1995).

20. Hou, X. Li, J.J., Chen, W.B., Li, S.A. Estrogen-induced protooncogene and suppressor gene expression in the hamster kidney: Significance for estrogen carcinogenesis. Cancer Res. 56:2616-2620 (1996).

21. Li, J.J., Papa, D., Davis, M.F., Weroha, S.J., Aldaz, M., El-Bayoumy, K, Ballenger, J., Tawfik, O., Li, S.A. Ploidy differences between hormone- and chemical carcinogen-induced mammary neoplasms: Relations to human breast cancer. Molec. Carcinogen. 33:56-65 (2002).

22. Chepko, G., Smith, G.H. Mammary epithelial stem cells: Our current understanding. J. Mammary Gland Biol. Neoplasia 4:35-52 (1999).

23. Li, J.J., Hou, X., Bentel, J.M., Yazlovitskaya, E.M., Li, S.A. Prevention of estrogen carcinogenesis in the hamster kidney by ethinylestradiol: Some unique properties of a synthetic estrogen. Carcinogenesis 19:471-477 (1998).

24. Li, J.J., Weroha, S.J., Cansler, M, Li, S.A. Estrogen receptor-mediated genomic instability in the Syrian hamster kidney: A critical event in hormonal carcinogenesis. In: Hormonal Carcinogenesis III (Eds. Li, J.J., Daling, J.R., Li, S.A.), Springer-Verlag, New York, pp. 149-157 (2000).

25. Li, J.J., Papa, D., Li, S.A. Ectopic uterine stem cell tumors in the hamster kidney: A unique model for estrogen-induced oncogenesis. Minerva Endocrinol., in press (2003).

26. Li, J.J., Hou, X., Banerjee, S.K., Liao, D.J., Maggouta, F., Norrris, J.S., Li, S.A. Overexpression and amplification of c-myc in the Syrian hamster kidney during estrogen carcinogenesis: A probable critical role in neoplastic transformation. Cancer Res. 59:2340-2346 (1999).

27. Felsher D.W., Bishop, J.M. Transient excess of MYC activity can elicit genomic instability and tumorigenesis. Proc. Nat. Acad. Sci. USA 96:3940-3944 (1999).
28. Eilers, M., Picard, D., Yammamoto, K.R., Bishop, J.M. Chimaeras of MYC oncoprotein and steroid receptors cause hormone-dependent transformation of cells. Nature 340:66-68 (1989).
29. Taylor, C., Jalava, A., Mai, S. c-Myc dependent initiation of genomic instability during neoplastic transformation. Curr. Top. Microbiol. Immunol. 224:201-207 (1997).
30. Yiu, X.Y., Grove L, Datta, N.S., Long, M.W., Prochownik, E.V. C-Myc overexpression and p53 loss cooperate to promote genomic instability. Oncogene 18:1177-1184 (1999).

CYCLOOXYGENASE-2 INHIBITORS IN CANCER PREVENTION AND TREATMENT

Jaime L. Masferrer

Science Fellow, Pharmacia Corporation, 700 Chesterfield parkway, St. Louis MO 63017

USA

COX-1 and COX-2

By inhibiting the cyclooxygenase (COX) enzyme, NSAIDs block the synthesis of prostaglandins, which are important mediators of multiple physiologic and pathophysiologic processes. There are 2 COX isoforms. COX-1 maintains physiologic processes, and its inhibition may be associated with undesirable effects. COX-2 is induced in response to growth factors, cytokines, and tumor promoters and is responsible for the therapeutic activity of NSAIDs. Epidemiologic, preclinical, and clinical evidence gathered over the last 15 years demonstrates that, in addition to their anti-inflammatory and analgesic properties, NSAIDs, particularly specific COX-2 inhibitors, such as celecoxib, also have a role in preventing tumor initiation and development.

The mechanisms by which COX-2 overexpression is involved in the biologic processes leading to cancer include promotion of angiogenesis, inhibition of apoptosis, and induction of proangiogenic factors, such as vascular endothelial growth factor (VEGF), inducible nitrogen oxide, synthetase promoter (iNOS), interleukin (IL-6), IL-8, and TIE-2.

COX-2 Expression

Using immunohistochemical techniques, we were able to demonstrate the up-regulation of COX-2 throughout the tumorigenic process in various tumor types. COX-2 expression was higher in cancerous than noncancerous tissue; in metastatic lesions than primary tumors; and in more differentiated cancers than less differentiated cancers.

COX-2 is found in noncancerous cells immediately adjacent to tumor cells, in angiogenic vasculature within tumors, and in pre-existing vasculature adjacent to tumors, but not in normal vasculature. Importantly, overexpression of COX-2 has been shown to be associated with increased invasiveness and poorer survival in patients with various types

New Trends in Cancer for the 21st Century, edited by
Llombart-Bosch and Felipo, Kluwer Academic/Plenum Publishers, 2003

209

of solid tumors. Collectively, these data support the theory that COX-2 activity is responsible for the increased prostaglandin levels found in cancer tissues

Role of COX-2 in disease process

COX-2 plays an important role during oncogenesis. This enzyme is expressed in cells involved in tumorigenesis, such as the neoplastic and surrounding stromal cells; including blood vessels, smooth muscle, and inflammatory cells. The scientific rationale for the use of COX-2 inhibitors in cancer is based on epidemiological studies, prominent COX-2 expression in tumor targets, and supportive pharmacology. Inhibition of COX-2 by Celecoxib results in anti-tumor and anti-metastatic activities by interrupting several processes during the pathophysiological progression to cancer.

Role of COX-2 in Cancer Prevention

Several epidemiologic studies have demonstrated that chronic NSAID use lead to reduced risk for developing many types of human tumors, including colon[1-10], lung[11], stomach[12, 13], and esophageal[14] neoplasias. For example, retrospective analyses suggest a 40-50% reduction in the relative risk of death by colon cancer in persons regularly taking aspirin or other NSAIDs[15, 16], indicating that inhibition of COX in humans has a chemopreventive effect. COX-2 expression and prostanoid levels[17-20] progressively increase as adenomatous polyps progress to adenocarcinomas in patients with familial adenomatous polyposis (FAP), suggesting COX-2 derived-prostaglandins may be directly correlated to adenoma size and stage. In rodent models of FAP, a genetic disease leading to colon carcinoma, blockade of COX-2, either by gene deletion[21] or by pharmacological inhibition of enzyme activity[22, 23] suppresses intestinal polyp formation. COX-2 inhibition by Celecoxib also demonstrated potent chemopreventive activity against colon carcinogenesis[24, 25]. Importantly, Celecoxib reduced the number and size of adenomatous polyps in FAP patients, the first validation of its clinical efficacy in cancer prevention in humans. Similarly, COX-2 is also expressed in premalignant lesions of the esophagus[26], lung[27-29], breast[27], bladder[30], skin[31], and prostate[32]. Further, Celecoxib potently inhibited tumor incidence in relevant animal models of these diseases. Taken together, the epidemiological data, COX-2 expression and the chemoprevention studies in animal models imply that COX-2 plays a critical role during initiation, proliferation, and/or transformation from normal to malignant disease.

Role of COX-2 in Cancer Therapy

Prostaglandin E_2 (PGE$_2$) is produced in large amounts by many animal and human tumors[33, 34], and is pro-tumorigenic. Prostaglandin levels have been positively associated with growth, metastatic potential[35], stage[36], recurrence[37], and negatively with survival[38]. Sheehan et al. also demonstrated that COX-2 levels are positively correlated to prognosis and survival in patients with colon cancer[39]. COX-2 is also markedly and consistently over expressed in all primary and metastatic epithelial cancers, including head and neck[40], pancreatic[41], prostate[42], breast[43, 44], lung[45, 46], esophageal[47], bladder[48, 49], and gastric[50] cancers. COX-2 is detected in ca. 40-80% of the total neoplastic cells in most tumors, and is also consistently detected in blood vessels, inflammatory cells, and fibroblasts. These observations indicated COX-2 significantly contributes to the maintenance and growth of the aberrant cell phenotype per se, as well as participate in the interaction between neoplastic nests and stromal components involved in angiogenesis, immunosuppression, and metastasis.

Based on the robust expression of COX-2 in human cancers, the effect of Celecoxib on tumor growth and metastasis was evaluated in multiple animal models of colon, lung, bladder, breast, melanoma, head & neck, and pancreatic cancer. Celecoxib consistently and dose-dependently inhibited tumor growth and the number and size of lung metastasis. The anti-cancer efficacy observed in the animal models with Celecoxib was devoid of any signs of gastrointestinal toxicity typically associated with non-selective NSAIDs that preclude their use in cancer therapy. One of the mechanisms by which Celecoxib exerts its anti-cancer activity is the inhibition of angiogenesis[51, 52]. Based on this mechanism of action, its potent efficacy and safety, Celecoxib was evaluated for its capacity to enhance the anti-tumor activity of conventional chemotherapeutics and radiation. The results indicate that Celecoxib potentiate radiation therapy by increasing cellular radiosensitivity and greatly enhance tumor response when administered in combination with radiation[53] without affecting the toxicity profile of radiation therapy[54]. Celecoxib also enhanced the efficacy of 5-fluorouracil, cyclophosphamide, and taxol in animal models.

In summary, the role of COX-2 in tumorigenesis, together with expression of the enzyme in human tumors, and the remarkable efficacy observed in animal models, indicate that inhibition of COX-2 should produce anti-angiogenic and anti-tumor results in the clinic. This is further supported by studies indicating a role for COX-2 in the production of angiogenic factors[55], increased cell proliferation[56], prevention of apoptosis[52], increased metastatic potential[57], and the inhibition of immune surveillance[58]. Taken together, these pre-clinical data strongly support the evaluation of Celecoxib in human clinical trials.

References

1. Gridley, G., McLaughlin, J.K., Ekbon, A, et al.: *Incidence of cancer among patients with rheumatoid arthritis. J. Natl. Cancer Inst.* (1993) **85**:307-311.
2. Sandler, RS: *Aspirin and other nonsteroidal anti-inflammatory agents in the prevention of colorectal cancer.* Lippincott-Raven Publishers (1996) Philadelphia, PA.
3. Suh, O, Mettlin, C, Petrelli, NJ: *Aspirin use, cancer, and polyps of the large bowel. Cancer* (1993) 72:1171-1177.
4. Marneit, LJ: *Aspirin and related nonsteroidal anti-inflammatory drugs as chemopreventive agents against colon cancer. Preventive Med.* (1995) 24:103-106.
5. Reeves, MJ, Newcomb, PA, Trentham-Dietz, A, Storer, BE, Remington, PL: *Nonsteroidal anti-inflammatory drug use and protection against colorectal cancer in women. Cancer Epidemiol. Biomark. Prev.* (1996) 5:955-960.
6. Rosenberg, L, Palmer, JR, Zauber, GA, Warshauer, ME, Stolley, PD, Shapiro, S: *A hypothesis: nonsteroidal anti-inflammatory drugs reduce the incidence of large bowel cancer. J. Natl. Cancer Inst.* (1991) **83**:355-358
7. Peleg, II, Maibach, HT, Brown, SH, Wilcox, CM: *Aspirin and nonsteroidal anti-inflammatory drug use and the risk of subsequent colorectal cancer. Arch. Intern. Med.* (1994) **121**:394-399.
8. Muscat, JE, Stellman, SD, Wynder, EL: *Nonsteroidal anti-inflammatory drugs and colorectal cancer. Cancer* (1994) 74:1847-1854.
9. Morgan, G: *Non-steroidal anti-inflammatory drugs and the chemoprevention of colorectal and oesophageal cancers. Gut* (1996) **38**:646-648.

10. Thun, MJ, Namboodiri, MM, Calle, EE, Flanders, WD, Heath, CW JR: *Aspirin use and risk of fatal cancer*. *Cancer Res.* (1993) **53**:1322-1327.

11. Schreinemachers, DM, Everson, RB: *Aspirin use and lung, colon, and breast cancer incidence in a prospective study*. *Epidemiology* (1994) **5**:138-146.

12. Thun, MJ: *NSAID use and decreased risk of gastrointestinal cancers*. *Gastroenterology Clinics of North America* (1996) **25**:333-348.

13. Farrow, DC, Vaughan, TL, Hansten, PD, *et al.*: *Use of aspirin and other nonsteroidal anti-inflammatory drugs and risk of esophageal and gastric cancer*. *Cancer Epid. Biom. & Prev.* (1998) 7:97-102.

14. Funkhouser, EM, Sharp, GB: *Aspirin and reduced risk of esophageal carcinoma*. *Cancer* (1995) **76**:1116-1119.

15. Giovannucci, E, Egan, KM, Hunter, DJ *et al.*: *Aspirin and the risk of colorectal cancer in women*. *N. Eng. J. Med.* (1995) **333**:609-614.

16. Rigas, B, Goldman Giovannucci, E, Rimm, EB, Stampfer, MJ, Coldtiz, GA; Ascherio, A, Willett, W C: *Aspirin use and the risk for colorectal cancer and adenoma in male health professionals*. *Ann. Intern. Med.* (1994) **121**:241-246.

17. Bennett, A, Berstock, DA, Raja, B, Stanford, IF: *Survival time after surgery is inversely related to amounts of prostaglandin extracted from human breast cancer*. *Br. J. Pharmacol.* (1979) **66**:451P.

18. Pugh, S, Thomas, GA: *Patients with adenomatous polyps and carcinomas have increased colonic mucosal prostaglandin E_2*. *Gut* (1994) **35**:675-678.

19. Rigas, B, Goldman, IS, Levine, L: *Altered eicosanoid levels in human colon cancer*. *J. Lab. Clin. Med.* (1993) **122**:518-523.

20. Yang, VW, Shields, JM, Hamilton, SR *et al.*: *Size-dependent increase in prostanoid levels in adenomas of patients with familial adenomatous polyposis*. *Cancer Res.* (1998) **58**:1750-1753.

21. O M, Dinchuk JE, Kargman SL et al.: *Suppression of intestinal polyposis in APC-delta-716 knockout mice by inhibition of cyclooxygenase 2 (COX-2)*. *Cell* (1996) **87**:803-809.

22. Labayle, D., Fisher, D., Vieln, P *et al.*: *Sulindac causes regression of rectal polyps in familial adenomatous polyposis*. *Gastroenterology* (1991) **101**:635-639.

23. Yoshimi, N, Kawabata, K, Hara, A: *Inhibitory effect of NS-398, a selective cyclooxygenase-2 inhibitor, on azoxymethane-induced aberrant crypt foci in colon carcinogenesis of F344 rats*. *Jpn. J. Cancer Res.* (1997) **88**:1044-1051.

24. Reddy BS, Rao, CV, Seibert,K: *Evaluation of cyclooxygenase-2 inhibito for potential chemopreventive properties in colon carcinogenesis*. *Cancer Res.* (1996) **56**:4566-4569.

25. Kawamori, T, Rao, CV, Seibert, K, Reddy, BS: *Chemopreventive activity of celecoxib, a specific cyclooxygenase-2 inhibitor, against colon carcinogenesis*. *Cancer Res.* (1998) **58**:409-412.

26. Wilson, KT, FU, S, Ramanujam, KS, Meltzer, SJ: *Increased expression of inducible nitric oxide and cyclooxygenase -2 in Barrett's esophagus and associated adenocarcinomas*. *Cancer Res.* (1998) **58**:2929-2934.

27. Soslow, RA, Dannenberg, AJ, Rush, D, *et al.*: *COX-2 is expressed in human pulmonary, colonic and mammary tumors*. *Cancer* (2000) in review.

28. Eeberhart, CE, Coffey, RJ, Radhika, A, *et al.*: *Upregulation of cyclooxygenase-2 gene expression in human colorectal adenomas and adenocarcinomas*. *Gastroenterology* (1994) **107**:1183-1188.

29. Hida, T, Tayabe, Y, Achiwa, H, *et al.*: *Increased expression of cyclooxygenase-2 occurs frequently in human lung cancers, specifically in adenocarcinomas*. *Cancer Res.* (1998) **58**:3761-3764.

30. Mohammed, SI, Knapp, DW, Bostwick, DG: *Expression of cyclooxygenase-2 in human invasive transitional cell carcinoma of the urinary bladder*. *Cancer Research Adv. In Brief* (1999) **59**:5647-5650.

31. Buckman, SY, Gresham, A, Hale, P, *et al.*: *COX-2 expression is induced by UVB exposure in human skin: implications for the development of skin cancer*. *Carcinogenesis* (1998) **19**(5):723-729.

32. Koki, AT, Leahy, KM, Masferrer, JL: *Potential utility of COX-2 inhibitors in chemoprevention and chemotherapy*. *Exp. Opin. Invest. Drugs* (1999) **8**(10):1623-1638.

33. Seed, MP:. *Angiogenesis inhibition as a drug target for disease: an update Exp. Opin. Invest. Drugs.* (1996) **5**(12):1617-1637.

34. Form, DM, Auerbach R: *PGE_2 and angiogenesis*. *Proc. Soc. Exp. Biol. Med.* (1983) **172**(2):214-218.

35. Rolland, PH, Martin, PM, Jacquemeier, J, Rolland, AM, Togs, M: *Prostaglandins in human breast cancer: evidence suggesting that an elevated prostaglandin production is a marker of high metastatic potential for neoplastic cells*. *J. Natl. Cancer Institute* (1980) **64**:1061-1070.

36. Karmali, RA, Welts, S, Thaler, HT, Lefevre, F: *Prostaglandins in breast cancer: relationship to disease stage and hormone status. Br. J. Cancer* (1983) **48**:689-696.
37. Fulton, AM, Ownby, HE, Frederick, J, Brennan, MJ: *Relationship of tumor prostaglandin levels to early recurrence in women with primary breast cancer: a clinical update. Invasion Metastasis* (1986) **6**:83-94.
38. Bennett, A, Berstock, DA, Raja, B, Stanford, IF: *Survival time after surgery is inversely related to amounts of prostaglandin extracted from human breast cancer. Br. J. Pharmacol.* (1979) **66**:451P.
39. Sheehan
40. C G, Boyle JO, Yang EK *et al.*: *Cyclooxygenase-2 expression is up-regulated in squamous cell carcinoma of the head and neck. Cancer Res.* (1999) **59**: 991-994.
41. Tucker ON, Dannenberg AJ, Yang EK *et al.*: *Cyclooxygenase-2 expression is up-regulated in human pancreatic cancer. Cancer Res.* (1999) **59**:987-990.
42. Gupta, S, Srivastava, M, Ahmad, N, Bostwick, DG, Mukhtar, H: *Over-expression of cyclooxygenase-2 in human prostate adenocarcinoma. Prostate* (2000) **42**:73-78.
43. Hwang, D, Scollard, D, Byrene, J, Levine. E: *Expression of cyclooxygenase-1 and cyclooxygenase-2 in human breast cancer. J. Natl. Cancer Insti.* (1998) **90**:455-460.
44. Parrett, ML, Harris, RE, Joarder, FS, Ross, MS, Clausen, KP, Robertson, FM: *Cyclooxygenase-2 gene expression in human breast cancer. Int. J. of Oncol.* (1997) **10**:503-507.
45. Wolff, H, Saukkonen, KL, Anttila, S, Karjalainen, A, Vainio, H, RISTIMAKI, A: *Expression of cyclooxygenase-2 in human lung carcinoma. Cancer Res.* (1998) **58**:4997 - 5001.
46. Toyoaki, H, Yatabe, Y, Achiva, H, *et al.*: *Increased cyclooxygenase-2 occurs frequently in human lung cancers, specifically in adenocarcinomas. Cancer Res.* (1998) **58**:3761-3764.
47. Zimmerman, KC, Sarbia, M, Weber, A, Borchard, F, Gabbert, H, Schror, K: *Cyclooxygenase-2 expression in human esophageal carcinoma. Cancer Res.* (1999) **59**:198-204.
48. Knapp, DW, Glickman, NW, Denicola, DB, Bonney, PL, Lin, TL, Glickman, LT: *Naturally-occurring canine transitional cell carcinoma of the urinary bladder, a relevant model of human invasive bladder cancer. Urologic Oncology* (1999) *(in press).*
49. Mohammed, S., Lafayette, W, Foster, R *et al.*: *Expression of cyclooxygenase COX-1 and COX-2 in human invasive transitional cell carcinoma of the urinary bladder. American Urological Association Meeting,* Dallas, TX (1999)
50. Lundholm, K, Gelin, J, Hyltander, A, Lonnroth, C, Sandstrom, R, Svaniger, G: *Anti-inflammatory treatment may prolong survival in undernourished patients with metastatic solid tumors. Cancer Res.,* (1994) **5**:5602-5606.
51. Masferrer, JL, Leahy, K, Koki, AT, Zweifel, BS, Settle, SL, Woerner, BM, Edwards, DA, Flickinger, AG, Moore, RJ, Seiebert, K: *Angiogenic and antitumor activities of cyclooxygenase-2 inhibitors.* (2000) *Cancer Res.* **60**(5):1306-1311.
52. Tsuji, M, Dubois, RN: *Alterations in cellular adehision and apoptosis in epithelial-cells overexpressing prostaglandin-endoperoxide synthase-2. Cell* (1995) **83**:493-501.
53. Milas, L, Kishi, K, Hunter, N, Masferrer, JL, Tofilon, PJ: *Enhancement of tumor response to g-irradiation by an inhibitor of cyclooxygenase-2 enzyme. J. Natl. Cancer Inst.* (1999) **91**:1501-1504.
54. Kishi, K, Petersen, S, Petersen, C, Hunter, N, Masferrer, JL, Tofilon, PJ, Milas, L: *Preferential enhancement of tumor radioresponse by a COX-2 inhibitor. Cancer Res.* (2000) **60**:1326-1331.
55. Tsuji, M, Kawano, S, Tsuji, S, Sawahoka, H, Hori, M, Duboise, RN: *Cyclooxygenase regulates angiogenesis induced by colon cancer cells.* (1998) *Cell* **93**:705-716.
56. Sheng, H, Williams, CS, Shao, J, Liang, P, Duboise, RN, Beauchamp, RD: *Induction of cyclooxygenase-2 by activated Ha-ras oncogene in Rat-1 fibroblasts and the role of mitogen-activated protein kinase pathway.* (1998) *J. Biol. Chem.* **273**:22120-22127.
57. Tsuji, M, Kawano, S, Duboise, RN: *Cyclooxgynase-2 expression in human colon cancer cells increases metastatic potential.* (1997) *Proc. Natl. Acad. Sci. USA* **94**:3336-3340.
58. Huang, M, Stolina, M, Sharma, S, Mao, JT, Zhu, L, Miller, PW, Wollman, J, Herschman, H, Dubinett, SM: *Non-small cell lung cancer cyclooxygenase-2 dependent regulation of interleukin-10 and down-regulation of interleukin-12 production.* (1998) *Cancer Res.* **58**:1208-1216.

EXOSOMES FOR IMMUNOTHERAPY OF CANCER

Nathalie Chaput[1], NEC Schartz[1,2], Fabrice Andre[1], and Laurence Zitvogel[1,*]

[1]ERIT-M 02-08 INSERM, Department of Clinical Biology, Institut Gustave Roussy (IGR), 39 rue Camille Desmoulins, 94805 Villejuif, France

[2] Department of Dermatology 2, AP-HP Hôpital Saint -Louis, Paris, France

ABSTRACT

Exosomes are 60 to 90 nm membrane vesicles originating from late endosomes and secreted from most hematopoietic and epithelial cells in vitro. B cell derived-exosome antigenicity was first reported in 1996 in MHC class II restricted CD4+ T lymphocytes. In 1998, we reported that dendritic cell derived-exosomes are immunogenic in mice leading to tumor rejection. These findings have renewed the interest in exosomes. The current challenge consists in understanding the mechanisms and the physiological relevance of exosomes that could contribute to the design of the optimal exosome based-vaccination. Here, we will focus on the biological features pertaining to dendritic cell- and tumor cell derived-exosomes and will discuss their potential clinical implementation.

INTRODUCTION

Recently, the study of the secretary compartment of antigen-presenting cells (APCs) called "exosomes"[1,3,4] has become an intense area of research due to the ability of exosomes to induce potent anti-tumor responses in vivo[5,6]. The origin of vesicle secretion was first described by Pan and Johnston[7] in differentiating red blood cells where multivesicular bodies (MVBs), containing intraluminal membrane-bound vesicles, were capable of fusing with the plasma membrane in an exocytic manner. This exocytic pathway was later shown to occur for a wide variety of cell types including

* Correspondence should be address to: Dr.Laurence Zitvogel, MD PhD., ERIT-M 02-08 INSERM, Unité d'Immunologie, Département de Biologie Clinique, (+12), Institut Gustave Roussy, 39 rue Camille Desmoulins, 94805 Villejuif, France. Phone : 33-1-42-11-50-41, Fax : 33-1-42-11-60-94, email : Zitvogel@igr.fr

Abbreviations: APC: Antigen presenting cells; ASI: Active specific immunotherapy; CT: Cytotoxique T lymphocytes; DC: Dendritic cells; EBV: Epstein-Barr virus; FDC: Follicular dendritic cells; GMP: Good manufacturing process; HLA: Human leukocyte antigen; HSP: Heat shock protein; MD-DC: Monocyte-derived dendritic cells; MHC: Major histocompatibility complex; MVB: Multivesicular body; Texas: Tumor ascitis-derived exosomes; Dex: DC derived-exosomes; Tex: Tumor cell derived-exosomes; TfR: transferring receptor.

New Trends in Cancer for the 21st Century, edited by
Llombart-Bosch and Felipo, Kluwer Academic/Plenum Publishers, 2003

215

hematopoietic and epithelial primary cells or established lines[6,8-15]. Vesicles (of 40-90 nm diameter) originating from late endosomes (MVBs) and released following fusion of such MVBs with plasma membarne are referred to as "exosomes".

Exosomes are unilamellar vesicles that can be studied in immunoelectron microscopy[9]. The protein composition of exosomes has been characterized using immuno-blotting[9], peptide mass spectroscopy mapping[16,17], and affinity extraction onto magnetic beads followed by phenotyping by flow cytometry[18]. These findings allowed to define the physical, biochemical and immunological features of exosomes, that distinguish them from vesicles originating from other cell compartments, such as plasma membrane or ER. Here, we will focus only on dendritic cell-derived exosomes (dexosomes), tumor cell-derived exosomes (texosomes) and tumor ascitis-derived exosomes (Texas).

PHYSICAL CHARACTERISTIC AND MOLECULAR COMPOSITION OF EXOSOMES

Exosomes are small unilamellar spherical vesicles with a diameter ranging between 60 to 100 nm. These vesicles float on sucrose gradient at a density ranging from 1,13 (for B Cell- derived exosomes) to 1,210 g/cm^3 (DEX/TEX/TEXAS)[4,6,11,16,19,22]. These exosomes are heat stable vesicles that can be frozen at $-80°C$ for at least 6 months (our unpublished data).

Exosomes are secreted by living cells and can be molecularly distinguished from apoptotic bodies[17]. The proteic composition of exosomes has been studied in mouse and human DC derived-exosomes using one D-electrophoresis and MALDI-TOF mass spectrometry (ref).

Both ubiquitous and cell-specific proteins are selectively targeted to exosomes. The former are most probably involved in exosomes biogenesis and/or alternate unknown common exosome functions. Some proteins are conserved between exosomes such as tetraspanins[18], and heat shock proteins[16]. Others differ as a function of the cell type from which exosome derive[4-9,15-23,25,26]: transferrin receptor TRf (reticulocytes), MHC and costimulatory molecules (B cells, DC, tumor cells, macrophages, enterocytes, T cells), integrines (DC, reticulocytes, macrophages, T cells), immunoglobulin-family members (B cells, DC, macrophages, platelets, enterocytes), cell-surface peptidases (enterocytes, macrophages), cytoskeleton related- proteins (DC, enterocytes, macrophages), membrane transport and fusion (DC, macrophages), signal transduction (DC, T cells), metabolic enzymes (enterocytes, DC), and whole cytosolic tumor antigens (tumor cells).

PRODUCTION AND CHARACTERIZACION OF EXOSOMES

As we will further elude to, exosomes were shown to mediate immunotherapeutic properties in mice[5] and to represent a suitable substitute to cellular therapies. Therefore, a GMP process allowing exosome harvesting has been set up. Exosomes derived from dendritic cells and tumor cells in culture can be quickly purified (e.g. 4-5 hrs of a 2-3 L culture) based on their unique size and density (Figure 1). Ultrafiltration of the clarified culture supernatant through a 500 kDa hollow fiber membrane and ultracentrifugation into a 30% sucrose/deuterium oxide cushion (density: 1,19 to 1.210 g/cm^3) reduced the volume and protein concentration approximately 200-fold and 1000-fold, respectively. The percentage recovery of exosomes ranged from 40-50% based on the exosome MHC class II concentration of the starting clarified supernatant. This methodology was extended to a mini-scale process with comparable results. Conversely, the classical sedimentation technique is a lengthy process resulting in exosomes being highly contaminated with media proteins, and containing only 5-15% of the starting exosome MHC class II concentration; hence, rendering this procedure difficult for clinical implementation. Furthermore, the development of quality control assays allowed the standardization of exosome preparations: quantity (concentration of MHC class II by an adsorption immunocapture assay, bioactivity based on reactivity of CD4+ T cells to GMP exosomes presenting superantigens) and protein patterns ((DC-derived exosomes are fixed on 4.5 micron beads that allows them to be identified by surface antigen-recognizing fluorescent antibodies). The combination of a rapid and reproducible purification method associated with quality control parameters for exosome bioactivity authorized exosome evaluation as a new device of cell free-peptide based-cancer vaccine in phase I clinical trials[24].

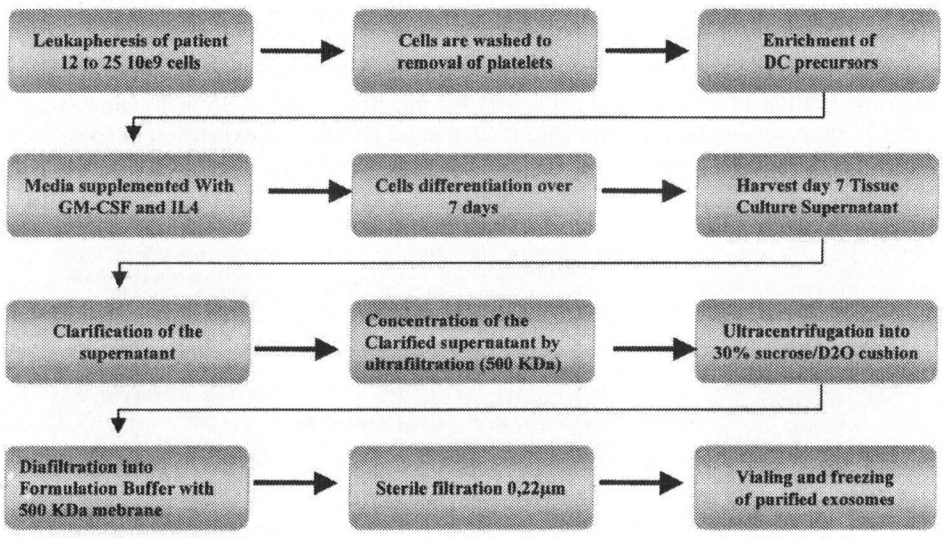

Figure 1. Schematic for the production and purification of dendritic cell derived exosomes by Ultrafiltration.

Based on the fact that tumor cells should secrete exosomes not only in culture dishes but also in human cavities, we examined the presence of exosomes in peritoneal or pleural effusions in cancer bearing patients[4]. To isolate exosomes, ascitis fluid was centrifuged to discard floating cells prior to high speed centrifugation. The pellet was then re-suspended in a sucrose gradient and ultra-centrifuged to pellet the exosomes[9,5,1]. Electronic microscopy of the pellet showed a high quantity of vesicles with a diameter ranging between 50-100 nm recalling exosomes and referred to as tumor ascitis-derived exosomes TEXAS (Figure 2A). No good manufacturing process is yet available to harvest the peritoneal cavity derived-exosomes (Figure 2B). TEXAS can also be characterized with electronic microscopy and measurement of the MHC class I concentration by immunocapture assays[4].

PRECLINICAL STUDIES OF DC DERIVED-EXOSOME IMMUNOGENICITY

The original observation was that exosomes secreted from bone marrow DC pulsed with acid eluted tumor peptides elicited T cell- dependent tumor rejection in P815 established tumors and significant tumor growth retardation in TS/A mammary tumors. Exosome-mediated tumor rejection was tumor peptide-specific and long term protection was tumor -specific. In tumor free mice, tumor- specific CTLs could be recovered after in vitro restimulation of splenocytes[5]. The precise mechanisms accounting for the immunogenicity of DC derived-exosomes remain to be studied.

Exosome MHC class I molecules can be efficiently loaded directly, after acid elution of purified exosomes (Dee Shu, unpublished data). In contrast, exosomal MHC class II molecules can present peptides that have been pulsed onto whole DC culture (27; Dee Shu, unpublished data). We demonstrated that exosomal MHC class I/peptide complexes trigger specific MHC class I restricted-CTL clones when pulsed onto DC *in vitro* (N. Chaput, submitted)). In the absence of DC, exosomes do not directly stimulate T cells *in vitro* (28; N.Chaput, submitted). In the HHD2 HLA-A2 transgenic mouse model, inoculation of DC derived-exosomes bearing functional A2/Mart1 complexes (up to 10^{10} class I molecules) pulsed onto H-2b mature DC, allows expansion of specific A2/Mart1 $_{26-35}$ tetramer positive CD8+ T cells in draining lymph nodes (N. Chaput, submitted).

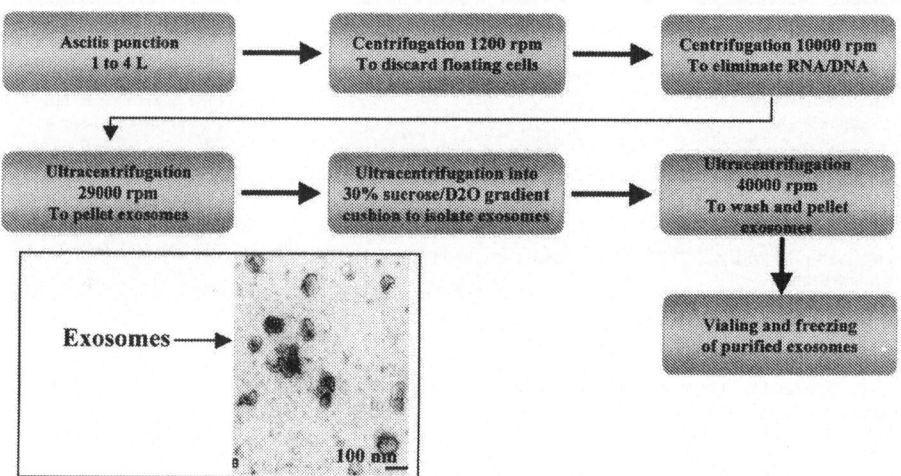

Figure 2. Schematic for the production of TEXAS by Ultracentrifugation. Electronic-microscopy image of Ascitis sample (in box). Exosomes-linked vesicles from the ascitis sample of patient of ovarian cancer.

PIONEERING CLINICAL TRIALS WITH DEX

Based on these results, vaccination with DC-derived exosomes in clinical trials has been undertaken. A Good Manufacturing Process (GMP) has been set up to harvest large amounts of MD-DC-derived exosomes (ultrafiltration followed by ultracentrifugation on a high density sucrose/D_2O cushion) and to load their MHC class I molecules with synthetic tumor peptides (Lamparski, Hsu) . The phenotypical analysis of these exosomes is possible with a FACS-beads-assay. An immunocapture assay determines the quantity of CMH class I and/or II molecules injected. After approval of regulatory agencies, a clinical grade manufacturing process of dexosomes has allowed to launch a feasibility phase I study in HLA-A1/B35 and –DP04 patients with stage III/IV melanoma expressing MAGE-3. Dexosomes were purified from the culture supernatant of day 7 autologous MD-DC. The MAGE-3 peptide was loaded onto MD-DCs (in the first 6 patients), or directly onto dexosomes (6 patients). Escalating doses of cryopreserved dexosomes were administrated by 4 weekly sc/id injections, then every 3 weeks in patients who achieved stable disease or a tumor regression. Fifteen patients have entered the study in progressive disease (metastatic sites including skin, nodes, lung and liver). The vaccine therapy was well tolerated, without any evidence of serious toxicity. One stage III patient achieved stabilization and received 8 additional vaccine injections with continual stable disease. A second patient achieved a mixed response with regression of subcutaneous sites and lung progression. A third patient had partial response. Three other patients are currently enrolled at a higher dose level of dexosomes. At this point, the study showed that administration of dexosomes is feasible and safe with encouraging clinical responses supporting a phase II study (29; Bamberg 2002, Angevin, Abstract 21, p28).

Another phase I study is ongoing in advanced non-small cell lung cancer. This trial enrolled 7 patients with unresectable stage III and IV non-small cell lung cancer who had previously been treated with up to 3 regimens. In addition, the patients' tumor cells express tumors antigens i.e MAGE-3,-4 and -10. Following purification, dexosomes were pulsed with MAGE-3,-4 and -10 tumor peptides and injected to the patients. 3 of the 7 immunized patients achieved prolonged disease stabilization (6, 9 and 10 months respectively), including one patient who had been progressing prior to therapy. The remaining four patients progressed. Administration of the vaccine was well tolerated and there was no evidence of serious toxicity (Valente, ASCO, 2002).

RATIONALE TO USE TUMOR DERIVED-EXOSOMES AS A SOURCE OF SHARED TUMOR ANTIGENS

Ideally, immunotherapy strategies aimed at immunizing the host should be able to elicit T cell based-immune responses directed against a broad repertoire of tumor rejection antigens. While mature DC appear to be the most potent natural adjuvants, suitable methods leading to efficient DC uptake, processing and cross presentation into MHC class I molecules are still awaited. Several approaches involving the use of whole tumor RNA, tumor lysates, apoptotic or necrotic debris, fusion is currently under investigation. Wolfers et al. reported that i) melanoma line derived-exosomes contain differentiation tumor antigens, ii) those tumor exosomes loaded onto dendritic cells transfer shared tumor antigens triggering MHC class I restricted- T clones *in vitro*, and iii) tumor exosomes are a source of rejection tumor antigens since tumor exosomes promote T cell dependent -cross protection against syngeneic and allogeneic tumors in mice[6].

Tumor-derived exosomes are not simply released in vitro by tumor cell lines in culture supernatants. We went on examining malignant effusions for the presence of tumor derived-exosomes and analysed exosome immunogenicity on autologous peripheral T lymphocytes. Ultracentrifugation on sucrose and D2O gradients of 11 malignant effusions allowed isolation of abundant amounts of exosomes. Malignant effusions accumulate high amounts of membrane vesicles with a mean diameter of 60-90nm. These vesicles bear antigen presenting molecules (MHC class I ± MHC class

II, heat shock proteins), tetraspanins (CD81) and contain tumor antigens (Her2/Neu, Mart1, TRP, gp100) . Up to $2x10^{14}$ exosome associated-MHC class I molecules are recovered from malignant ascitis. Exosomes from melanoma patients vehicle Mart1 tumor antigen to MD-DC for cross presentation to Mart1 specific CTL clones. In 7/9 cancer patients, tumor specific lymphocytes could be efficiently expanded from peripheral blood cells using autologous MD-DC pulsed with autologous ascitis-derived exosomes[4]. Therefore, tumor-derived exosomes accumulate abundantly in cancer patients. Ascitis exosomes represent a natural and novel source of tumor rejection antigens, opening up novel immunization avenues in advanced ovarian cancers or mesothelioma. The clinical implementations of ascitis derived-exosomes should require the demonstration that exosomes from ascitis fluids can be immunogenic in mice leading to tumor rejection and safe in preclinical GMP settings in mice. We are also currently developing a clinical grade process for purification of ascitis exosomes. This strategy opens up new therapeutic avenues in mesothelioma or ovarian tumors.

CONCLUSION

Exosomes represent a new approach to cell free-immunotherapy of cancer. Exosomes produced by DC are highly stable, display a molecularly defined characterization. This rationale prompted us to set up a reproducible GMP process validating exosome implementation into the clinic. The interest in exosomes arose because of their unique proteomic profile and their in vitro and in vivo functions. Indeed, exosomes play a role in the transfer of antigens to APCs, eliciting initiation and amplification of antigen-specific immune responses. This rationale allowed implementation of exosomes in a phase I clinical trial currently ongoing in France. The comprehensive molecular characterization and the understanding of the mechanisms underlying exosome immunogenicity might unravel their relevance and their potential biotechnological future.

References

1. Denzer, K., et al. Exosome: from internal vesicle of the multivesicular body to intercellular signaling device. J Cell Sci 2000; 113: 3365-74.
2. Denzer, K. et al. Follicular dendritic cells carry MHC class II-expressing microvesicles at their surface. J Immunol 2000; 165: 1259-65.
3. Quah, B. and O'Neill, H.C. The application of dendritic cell-derived exosomes in tumour immunotherapy. Cancer Biotherapy and Radiopharm 2000; 15: 185-194.
4. André, F. et al. Malignant effusions and immunogenic tumor derived-exosomes. The Lancet 2002; 360: 295-305.
5. Zitvogel, L. et al. Eradication of established murine tumors using a novel cell-free vaccine: dendritic cell-derived exosomes. Nat Med 1998;4 : 594-600.
6. Wolfers, J. et al. Tumor-derived exosomes are a source of shared tumor rejection antigens for CTL cross-priming. Nat Med 2001;7 : 297-303.
7. Johnstone, R. M.et al. Vesicle formation during reticulocyte maturation. Association of plasma membrane activities with released vesicles (exosomes). J. Biol. Chem 1987; 262: 9412-9420.
8. Raposo, G. et al. Accumulation ofmajor histocompatibility complex class II molecules in mast cell secretory granules and their release upon degranulation. Molec. Biol. Cell 1997; 8: 2631-2645.
9. Escola, J. M. et al. Selective enrichment of tetraspan proteins on the internal vesicles of multivesicular endosomes and on exosomes secreted by human B-lymphocytes. Journal of Biological Chemistry 1998;273;20121-7.
10. Arnold, P.Y. and Mannie, M.D. Vesicles bearing MHC class II molecules mediate transfer of antigen-presenting cells to CD4+ cells. Eur. J. Immunol 1999;29 :1363-1373.

11. Heijnen, I. A. et al. Antigen targeting to myeloid-specific human Fc gamma RI/CD64 triggers enhanced antibody responses in transgenic mice. Journal of Clinical Investigation 1996; 97: 331-8.

12. Hess, C. et al. Ectosomes released by human neutrophils are specialized functional units. J Immunol 1999;163 : 4564-73.

13. Patel, D. et al. Class II MHC/peptide complexes are released from APC and are acquired by T cell responders during specific antigen recognition. J Immunol 1999;163 : 5201-10.

14. Geminard, C. et al. Characteristics of the Interaction between Hsc70 and the transferrin receptor in exosomes released during reticulocyte maturation. J. Biol. Chem. 2001;276 : 9910-9916.

15. Skokos, D. et al. Mast cell-dependent B and T lymphocyte activation is mediated by the secretion of immunologically active exosomes. J Immunol 2001;166 : 868-76.

16. .Thery, C. et al. Molecular characterization of dendritic cell-derived exosomes. Selective accumulation of the heat shock protein hsc73. J Cell Biol 1999;147 : 599-610.

17. Thery, C. et al. Proteomic analysis of dendritic cell-derived exosomes: a secreted subcellular compartment distinct from apoptotic vesicles. J Immunol 2001;166 : 7309-18.

18. Clayton, A. et al. Analysis of antigen presenting cell derived exosomes, based on immuno- magnetic isolation and flow cytometry. J Immunol Methods 2001;247 : 163-74.

19. Raposo, G. et al. B lymphocytes secrete antigen-presenting vesicles. J. Exp. Med. 1996;183 : 1161-1172.

20. Blanchard, N. et al. TCR activation of human T cells induces the production of exosomes bearing the TCR/CD3/z complex. J. Immunol 2002;168 : 3235-3242.

21. Hanayama, R. et al. Identification of a factor that links apoptotic cells to phagocytes. Nature 2002 May 9;417 :182-7.

22. van Niel, G. et al. Intestinal epithelial cells secrete exosome-like vesicles. Gastroenterology 2001;121 : 337-49.

23. Heijnen, H. F., Schiel, A. E., Fijnheer, R., Geuze, H. J. & Sixma, J. J. Activated platelets release two types of membrane vesicles: microvesicles by surface shedding and exosomes derived from exocytosis of multivesicular bodies and alpha-granules. *Blood* 1999; 94, 3791-9.

24. Lamparski H. et al. Production and characterization of clinical grade exosomes derived from dendritic cells. *J. Immunol. Methods*, 2002; 270 : 211 .

25. Pan, B.T. et al. Electron microscopic evidence for externalization of the transferrin receptor in vesicular form in sheep reticulocytes. J. Cell Biol. 1985;101 : 942-948.

26. Théry C, Zitvogel L, Amigorena S. Exosomes : composition, biogenesis and function. *Nature Review Immunol.* 2002; 2 : 569-579.

27. Théry C, Duban L, Segura E, Véron P, Lantz O, Amigorena S. Exosomes activate naive CD4+ T cells by transfer of MHC/peptide complexes to dendritic cells. *Nat. Immunol.* In press.

28. Vincent-Schneider H., Stumptner-Cuvelette P., Lanka D., Pain S., Raposo G., Benaroch P., and Bonnerot C. Exosomes bearing HLA-DR1 molecules need dendritic cells to efficiently stimulate specific T cells. *Int Immunol.* 2002; 14, 713-722.

29. Escudier B, Dorval T, Angevin E, Boccaccio C, Robert C, Avril MF, Lantz O, Bonnerot C, Tursz T, Dhellin O, Serra V, Valente N, Le-Pecq JB, Zitvogel L. Novel approach to immunotherapy of cancer: Phase I trial of dexosome vaccine for patients with advanced melanoma. *Proc. Am. Soc. Clin. Oncol.* 2002; A1857.

BREAST CANCER GENE EXPRESSION ANALYSIS
The Case For Dynamic Profiling

Matthew J. Ellis

Duke University Breast Cancer Program, Duke University Medical Center
DUMC PO Box 3446, Durham, NC 27710

ABSTRACT

Cancer is a complicated disease with each individual tumor exhibiting to a variable degree a set of overlapping phenotypes that include abnormal proliferation and cell survival, genetic instability, tissue invasion, metastasis and angiogenesis. Each of these pathophysiological functions requires abnormal signaling that fails to respect the normal restraints imposed on healthy cells through homeostatic regulation. Understanding of deregulated gene expression is therefore an essential goal for cancer research because unraveling this problem will provide insights into the fundamental nature of cancer as well as provide opportunities for therapeutic intervention. Gene expression profiling is a remarkable technique that addresses this complexity by documenting the expression of thousands of genes at the level of mRNA abundance. From the standpoint of clinical investigation, the initial focus of gene profiling experiments has been on screening primary tumors for markers of poor prognosis. However this is only a first step in demonstrating the utility of this technique. Future advances will focus on understanding the evolution of an organ confined primary cancer to a treatment resistant lethal systemic disease through repeated tumor sampling and analysis, an approach termed in this paper "dynamic profiling". Using breast cancer endocrine therapy as an example our initial approaches to dynamic profiling will be described.

GENE EXPRESSION PROFILING AND BREAST CANCER

With the completion of the first maps of the human genome, together with new technologies to screen tumors for gene expression and somatic mutations, the number of biomarkers and therapeutic targets to translate into clinical practice is increasing dramatically. Recent publications on gene expression profiling in breast cancer have underscored the considerable potential of this technology[1]. There are, in a broad sense, two

New Trends in Cancer for the 21st Century, edited by
Llombart-Bosch and Felipo, Kluwer Academic/Plenum Publishers, 2003

223

approaches to the statistical analysis of the huge data sets generated by gene expression profiling termed "unsupervised" analysis and "supervised" analysis. An unsupervised analysis aims to compare the profile of each tumor to identify "relatedness" to other tumors to create a molecular-based classification of the disease that is distinct from traditional clinical classification systems. The objective of this analysis is to identify tumors with similar molecular etiologies that may exhibit characteristic clinical behaviors and also share therapeutic targets. On this basis Sorlie *et al* have recently suggested that breast cancer can be sub-classified into five groups of tumors with clinical implications. Of note, they propose that ER+ breast cancers are composed of 3 subgroups, a luminal ER+ subtype A with a relatively good prognosis and luminal subtypes B and C that carry a worse prognosis and express a novel set of genes whose coordinated functions are unknown, a feature they share with the poor prognosis (ER-) basal subtype and the HER2+ subtype[2]. This classification clearly relates to the approach to biomarker analysis already used in routine clinical practice that relies on ER and HER2 analysis but further suggests that the ER+ group can be sub-classified into good and poor prognostic groups.

In contrast to the unsupervised approach, a "supervised" analysis compares the gene expression profiles of tumors that have been classified on the basis of a clinical characteristic, for example the patients is alive or dead from disease, the tumor responded to treatment versus not or node positive and node negative. This approach is termed binary supervised analysis. Once a gene expression "cluster" has been identified that cleanly distinguishes one group from the other (usually a set of genes that numbers between 10 and 100) its predictive properties must be subsequently validated in a prospective manner in an independent data set. The supervised approach has been successful in, for example, identifying a signature of 75 genes whose absence is characteristic of tumors from women who are free from recurrence after local treatment of breast cancer[1]. Until recently it was not clear how many patients were required for supervised analysis. The obvious concern was that, like "traditional" single predictive biomarker studies, hundreds of patient samples would be required in order to develop robust predictive models. However the power generated by the large number of genes examined (and presumably their complex interactions) appears to overcome statistical weaknesses associated with relatively small patient data sets. Recent investigations in lymphoma and breast cancer suggest that binary supervised analysis can generate statistically significant prognostic models in studies of between 50 to 100 patients[2,3].

CAN GENE EXPRESSION PROFILING TO OPTIMIZE ENDOCRINE TREATMENT FOR BREAST CANCER?

Estrogen receptor (ER) measurements are essential to the management of breast cancer, despite the fact that ER has significant limitations as a predictive biomarker. The absence of ER expression indicates of a low chance of responding to endocrine therapy with about 95% certainty. However the presence of ER is a relatively poor predictor of therapeutic benefit, with only one third to about one half of ER+ tumors responding to endocrine therapy in the metastatic or adjuvant disease settings. A number of studies have attempted to improve upon the positive predictive value of ER expression by assessing the expression of estrogen-regulated genes such as PgR and TTF1 (trefoil factor 1 or "PS2") - both considered surrogates for the "functional" status of ER[4-6]. These studies have met with only limited success, however, because ER+ tumors that do not express PgR or TFF1 still have a reasonable chance of responding to treatment. On this basis it can be argued that the principle value of PgR measurement is to improve upon the negative predictive value of ER- status by identifying rare, endocrine therapy responsive ER-, PgR+ tumors. The tyrosine kinase growth factor receptor HER2 has also been investigated as a predictive biomarker for tamoxifen resistance but the evidence to date on the clinical behavior of ER+, HER+ tumors remains contradictory[7,8].

The inability to distinguish ER+ endocrine therapy resistant breast cancer from ER+ endocrine therapy sensitive disease at diagnosis leads to considerable over-treatment. Endocrine therapy with adjuvant tamoxifen provides considerably more protection from relapse and death from breast cancer than chemotherapy for postmenopausal women with ER+ disease[9,10]. Yet many of these women still receive adjuvant chemotherapy because randomized trials have demonstrated a small but significant benefit for adding chemotherapy to tamoxifen, presumably because chemotherapy improves outcomes for the subgroup of patients destined to develop endocrine therapy resistant advanced disease[11,12]. An ability to prospectively identify patients with endocrine therapy sensitive disease who can safely forego treatment with chemotherapy would be a major advance in breast cancer management and is, therefore, a major long-term goal for our biomarker research program. Furthermore, the identification of resistance genes may pinpoint the molecular basis for endocrine therapy failure and promote therapeutic trials of agents that may enhance efficacy. Gene expression profiling has recently been shown to distinguish between hitherto indistinguishable disease states. This may lead to more rational, molecularly defined approaches to treatment. We have therefore set out to identify a gene expression profile that can be identified at the time of diagnosis to differentiate between ER+ estrogen-therapy responsive forms of breast cancer from ER+ tumors that are endocrine therapy resistant.

THE IDENTIFICATION ESTROGEN RECEPTOR GENE CLUSTERS

Several initial breast cancer gene expression studies have focused on identifying gene clusters that either associate with or predict ER status. In an investigation lead by West, Nevins and Marks at Duke, gene expression profiles were compared between ER+ and ER- breast cancers using Affymetrix Human FL 6800 gene arrays. These data lead to a statistical model that could discriminate ER+ tumors from ER- tumors with a high degree of certainty through a cluster of ER associated genes, about half of which had previously been linked to ER function[13]. By studying a relatively small number of tumors (25 ER positive and 24 ER negative) a set of 50 biomarkers was selected from 6800 potential genes (Table 1). These data underscore the point that a successful supervised analysis can be the conducted with relatively small number of tumor samples. However, fifty potential biomarkers still represent a considerable challenge for the development of single gene techniques since a diagnostic reagent needs to be developed and validated for each gene/protein before predictive properties can be prospectively investigated in existing paraffin embedded tumor banks.

Another group focused on obtaining gene expression profiles from 14 gauge core needle biopsy samples obtained during the execution of a neoadjuvant endocrine therapy study[14]. Affymetrix analyses were successfully completed both before and after the initiation of treatment although the overall numbers were small. To gain statistical power for ER cluster analysis, the needle biopsy set was supplemented with 30 biopsies from a Swedish tumor bank (representing a total 59 breast tumors and 8 cell lines). A subset comprised of 1156 genes on the Human FL 6800 array was used as the input for cluster analysis. This subset was comprised of those genes called "present" by Affymetrix software in at least one of the 59 samples examined and also exhibited at least a 20-fold difference in expression (average difference) between a normal pooled breast tissue sample and at least one of the 59 samples. In other words, criteria were set for an "interesting gene" on the basis of marked increase in expression with respect to normal breast epithelium. Gene expression values were used to cluster genes and samples using Gene-Spring 3.2.8 (Silicon Genetics, Redwood City, CA) with the average difference measurement for each gene normalized across samples to a median of one. Gene expression similarity was measured by standard correlation with a minimum distance of 0.001 and a separation ratio of 0.5. The list of genes co-clustering with ER was compiled from the branch of the dendrogram that contained ER (Table 2). A comparison between ER clusters generated with different tumor sets reveals the presence of a large number of genes that were not known to be estrogen-regulated and relatively few genes are common to both lists. Each novel cluster member may, therefore, be present due to random association, because of a true association with ER without direct estrogen regulation, or finally, regulation by estrogen is not a previously described property of the gene in question.

ER Rank	ER Weight	Acc. #	Unigene Cluster	Symbol	Estrogen Relation
1	0.08	x52003	Trefoil Factor 1 (pS2)	TFF1	Estrogen induced
2	0.079	x03635	Estrogen Receptor 1	ESR1	ER
3	0.067	m29874	Cytochrome P450, Subfamily IIB	CYP2B	
4	0.064	l08044	Trefoil Factor 3	TFF3	Estrogen induced
5	0.061	s37730	(Insulin-Like Growth Factor)	IGFBP2	Estrogen induced
6	0.057	u79293	Human Clone 23948 mRNA Sequence	N/A	
7	0.055	j03778	Microtubule-Assoc'd Protein Tau	MAPT	Estrogen induced
8	0.055	x07732	Hepsin	HPN	
9	0.048	x58072	GATA-binding protein 3	GATA3	Co-expressed with ER
10	0.047	u22376	v-myb Avian Myeloblastosis Viral Oncogene Homolog	MYB	Estrogen induced
11	-0.043	u04313	Serine Proteinase Inhibitor, Clade B, Member 5	SERPINB5	Induced by tamoxifen; inverse with ER
12	0.041	x17059	N-Acetyl transferase 1	NAT1	
13	-0.041	m26311	S100 Calcium Binding Protein A9	S100A9	
14	-0.041	u27185	Retinoic Acid Receptor Responder 1	RARRES1	
15	-0.039	u84487	Small Inducible Cytokine Subfamily D, Member 1	SCYD1	
16	0.039	u39840	Hepatocyte Nuclear Factor 3 Alpha	HNF3A	Synergistic with ER
17	0.038	u32907	37 kDa Leucine-Rich Repeat (LRR) Protein	P37NB	
18	0.038	m35851	(Androgen Receptor)	AR	Physical interaction with ER
19	-0.038	x87212	Cathepsin C	CTSC	
20	0.037	u96922	Inositol Polyphosphate-4-Phosphatase, Type II, 105 kD	INPP4B	
21	0.036	a000234	Purinergic Receptor P2X, Ligand-Gated Ion Channel, 4	P2RX4	Estrogen biosynthesis
22	-0.036	d50915	KIAA0125 Gene Product	KIAA0125	
23	0.035	l07615	(Neuropeptide Y Receptor Y1)	NPY1R	
24	0.035	u68385	Meis (Mouse) Homolog 3	MEIS3	
25	0.035	u41060	LIV-1 Protein, Estrogen-Regulated	LIV-1	Estrogen induced

Table 2. A series of genes that cluster in ER positive breast cancers (14) (Reproduced with permission from The Pharmacogenomics Journal)

Gene	GenBank Accession Number
sodium channel, nonvoltage-gated 1 alpha (SCNN1A)	X76180
serine or cysteine proteinase inhibitor, member 3 (SERPINA3)	X68733
N-acylsphingosine amidohydrolase (acid ceramidase) (ASAH)	U70063
lipocalin 1 (LCN1)	L14927
transforming growth factor-beta type III receptor (TGFBR3)	L07594
glutamate receptor precursor 2 (GRIA2)	L20814
cytochrome P450-IIB, phenobarbital-inducible (CYP2B)	M29874
carcinoembryonic antigen mRNA (CEACAM5)	M29540
mammaglobin 1 (MGB1)	U33147
estrogen regulated LIV-1 protein (LIV1)	U41060
prolactin induced protein (PIP)	HG1763
matrix Gla protein (MGP)	X53331
trefoil factor 3 (TFF3)	L08044
trefoil factor 1 (TFF1)	X52003
hepatocyte nuclear factor-3 alpha (HNF3A)	U39840
serine protease hepsin (HPN)	X07732
X box binding protein-1 (XBP1)	M31627
Zn-alpha2-glycoprotein (AZGP1)	X59766
estrogen receptor alpha (ESR1)	X03635

Figure 1 illustrates the complexity of a typical ER cluster analysis. Individual gene expression patterns vary in terms of the degree of up-regulation of expression from a pooled sample of RNA from normal breast epithelium, the degree of variation from tumor to tumor and the level of expression in ER- breast cancer (different shades of grey correlate with different levels of expression, in reality this is a blue to red scale). All these factors may alter the utility of an individual gene as a predictive biomarker for endocrine therapy. For example prolactin-induced protein is occasionally expressed in ER- breast cancer and is also expressed at intermediate levels in normal tissue. There was also a relatively narrow range of expression in ER+ tumors. These features may limit the value of baseline measurement of prolactin-induced protein as it cannot be considered to be either a tumor marker (strong distinction between normal and malignant tissue) or as a unique marker for ER+ disease (since ER- tumors express the gene). Similarly a surprising member of the ER cluster "Sodium Channel, non-voltage gated alpha" also does not meet these *a priori* criteria for a useful tumor marker because there is expression in both ER- breast cancer and pooled normal breast epithelial cell mRNA. In contrast, both cytochrome P450-IIB, phenobarbital inducible and serine protease hepsin show promising biomarker characteristics, i.e. clear up-regulation in ER+ breast cancer in comparison with ER- breast cancer and normal tissue. Further more one can clearly see that ER+ tumors do show a marked difference in the degree to which these two genes are expressed. A high degree of variation from tumor to tumor is obviously a critical feature for a potential biomarker because tumors must be cleanly divided into those exhibiting high or low levels of expression in order to be designated positive or negative for the purposes of outcome prediction.

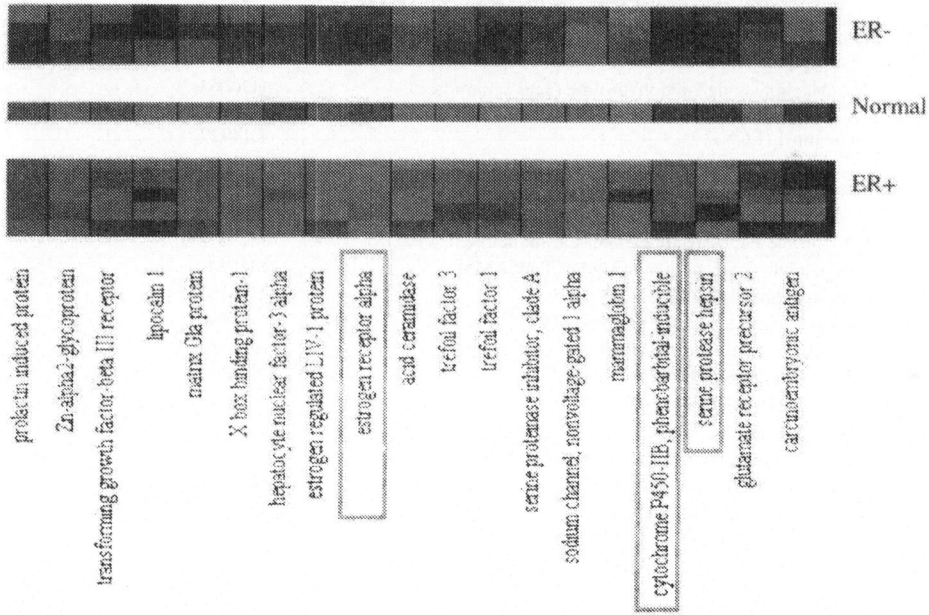

Figure 1. This is a detail from an ER alpha gene cluster published by Dressman *et Al[14]*. Individual tumor profiles of these genes in ER negative cases, normal pooled breast RNA and ER+ cases are presented[14] (Reproduced with permission from The Pharmacogenomics Journal).

USING ER CLUSTER ANALYSIS AS A PROBE FOR THE FUNCTIONAL STATUS OF ER BY DYNAMIC PROFILING

It is unproven at this point that ER cluster analysis carried any prognostic information. The worry is that ER cluster analysis may turn out to be similar to PgR and TFF1 i.e. not definitive in terms of predicting that tumor in question is sensitive or resistant to endocrine treatment. After all, key predictive biomarkers for endocrine therapy may not, in fact, be associated with ER status. This possibility was hinted at by the unsupervised analyses by Sorlie *et al*, who defined poor prognosis ER+ luminal subtypes B and C with gene expression features typical of the basal subtype tumors that were ER-[1]. Rather than consider ER cluster analysis as a classic predictive marker, conducted on a tumor sample taken at diagnosis, it might be more informative to repeat the profiling after a period of endocrine therapy to look at dynamic changes in ER function with treatment. Comparing treatment induced changes in the ER cluster with changes in other cellular programs associated with proliferation, apoptosis and tissue invasion one might get closer to making a definitive distinction between responsive and non-responsive tumors. In Figure 2 a series of simple models are presented to argue this point. In the hormone receptor positive endocrine therapy sensitive tumor presented in model one, the baseline gene expression profiling indicates that the ER is active because multiple ER cluster members are expressed and the tumor is progressing because the proliferation, invasion and apoptosis suppression clusters are also present. Treatment with estrogen deprivation will turn off ER with subsequent suppression of the clusters for ER, proliferation, invasion, and apoptosis suppression in concert. Model two considers a situation where the ER pathway is constitutively activated by mutation (s) *upstream* of ER or within the ER complex itself to generate an ER dependent but ligand-independent growth pattern (Class one mutation). This mechanism of endocrine therapy resistance has been proposed to occur though a number of mechanisms including activation of peptide growth factor receptor pathways though receptor gene (HER2) or transcription coactivator gene amplification (AIB1), mutations in signal transduction pathways (RAS) or even through mutations in ER itself. Thus in model two the ER cluster is not switched off by estrogen deprivation because the pathway is ligand-independent and all four clusters remain active in the post treatment sample. Model three represents the possibility of a lesion (mutation) in one or more *downstream* effector pathways that prevents estrogen deprivation inducing its therapeutic effect (Class 2 mutation). A mutation in a G1/S checkpoint gene such as p21 and p27, or constitutive over expression of a G1 cyclin (such as cyclin D1 or E), might have this phenotype. In this case one might see a mixed picture in the post treatment sample. Expression from the ER cluster might be inhibited because the transcriptional functions of ER are switched off, but the proliferation cluster remains active because of the checkpoint lesion. The phenotype in these tumors might be mixed – the estrogen dependent apoptosis program may be intact and so an initial reduction in cell number may occur with perhaps a minor response, however subsequent tumor progression seems likely without an effect on the cell cycle.

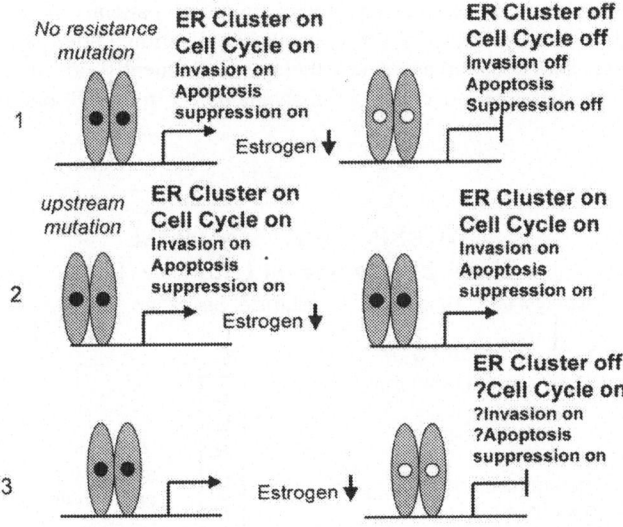

Figure 2. A series of models to illustrate how dynamic gene expression profiling may distinguish different mechanisms of resistance to estrogen deprivation therapy (for details see discussion in manuscript).

THE RATIONALE FOR A PHASE 2 TRIAL OF NEOADJUVANT AROMATASE INHIBITOR THERAPY WITH DYNAMIC GENE EXPRESSION PROFILING

In order to pursue the hypotheses laid out in Figure 2, a clinical trial was designed in which post treatment tumor sampling was possible. The study incorporated multiple opportunities for post-treatment sampling in order to address both primary endocrine therapy resistance and secondary resistance mechanisms that may take months or years to become evident. A neoadjuvant endocrine therapy design was decided upon on the basis of recent data concerning the use of aromatase inhibitors in the treatment of postmenopausal women with locally advanced ER+ disease (Figure 3). The oral aromatase inhibitor letrozole, 2.5 mg daily, administered for 4 months before surgery, had been shown to be an effective and well-tolerated neoadjuvant therapy[8,15]. These findings are an important breakthrough for research on the endocrine treatment of early stage breast cancer because data on primary tumor responsiveness are available after only a short period of treatment[16]. Predictive biomarker studies can therefore be carried out prospectively and efficiently with remarkable insights into the molecular basis for response to endocrine agents in prospect[8]. The use of neoadjuvant endocrine therapy in place of neoadjuvant chemotherapy can be justified on the basis that the patients under study (older postmenopausal women with ER+ tumors) are receiving a form of systemic treatment that is as least twice as effective as chemotherapy in providing protection from relapse and death from the disease[9,10]. While a randomized clinical trial of neoadjuvant chemotherapy versus neoadjuvant endocrine therapy will ultimately be required to unequivocally establish a role for neoadjuvant endocrine therapy as a routine treatment option, well conducted phase II and phase III studies of this treatment modality are justified on the basis of the precedent set by the numerous phase II studies of preoperative chemotherapy that were conducted before it was definitively demonstrated that delaying surgery to administer preoperative chemotherapy did not affect long-term outcomes. The focus on older patients in the application of neoadjuvant endocrine therapy is another relevant consideration. Older patients are a poorly studied population and neoadjuvant chemotherapy is frequently not an option for these individuals on the basis of poor performance status, co-morbid conditions or patient refusal[17].

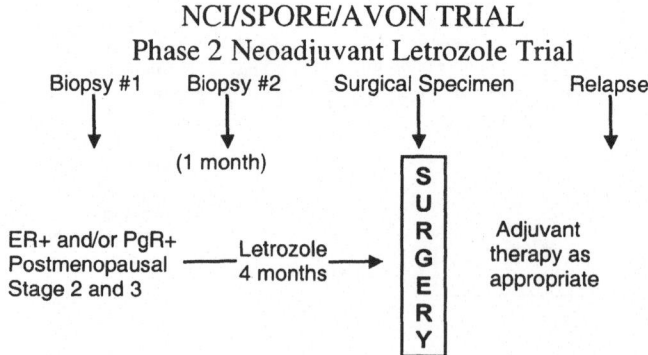

NCI/SPORE/AVON TRIAL
Phase 2 Neoadjuvant Letrozole Trial

Figure 3. Schema for a Phase 2 clinical trial incorporating dynamic gene expression profiling.

PRELIMINARY DATA FROM THE PHASE 2 NEOADJUVANT AROMATASE INHIBITOR TRIAL WITH DYNAMIC GENE EXPRESSION PROFILING

The principle objective of the clinical trial was to develop a baseline gene expression signature that will increase the value of ER in predicting response to neoadjuvant therapy. Since the anticipated response rates are in the range of 60 to 80%, a relatively large number of cases must be treated in order to document the expression profiles of the resistant cases. At this point we can present some limited information[18] on cases in which a baseline expression array has been compared with the expression array in the sample taken at one month (Table 1). The samples used to generate the data in Table 3 were taken from a postmenopausal women with a T4 (skin edema) N2, M0 locally advanced, strongly ER+ tumor. The patient had a remarkable response, all evidence of skin edema had resolved at the time of surgery at 24 weeks and the lesion size upon mastectomy was 3.5 cm. Baseline estimates of size based on an MRI were over 14 cm. The pair-wise array comparison at one month illustrated in Table 3 shows genes showing the greatest changes between the two samples on a log base 2 scale i.e. 2, 4, 8, 16 fold changes are represented by 1, 2, 3 and 4. On the basis of the changes observed this tumor fits into the proposed responding model (model 1) in Figure 2. The proliferation cluster has been switched off (topoisomerase (DNA) II alpha (170kD), ribonucleotide reductase M2 polypeptide, 5-methyltetrahydrofolate-homocysteine methyltransferase reductase and Cell division cycle 2, G1 to S and G2 to M), likewise the invasion cluster (matrix metalloproteinase 1 [interstitial collagenase], carboxypeptidase B1 (tissue), CD36 antigen [collagen type I receptor, thrombospondin receptor] and protein regulator of cytokinesis 1) and the apoptosis suppression cluster (baculoviral IAP repeat-containing 5 (survivin) and nucleolar protein 3 apoptosis repressor w/CARD domain).

SUPPLEMENTING RESPONSE DEFINITIONS FOR BINARY SUPERVISED ANALYSIS WITH DYNAMIC PROFILING

An interesting aspect of a dynamic gene expression analysis is that it may help classifying responders and non-responders for a supervised analysis of the baseline sample - the ultimate goal of the study. Binary supervised analysis is very sensitive to the accuracy of the clinical classification. For example a supervised analysis of "alive and no evidence of relapse" versus "relapsed from cancer and dead from disease" sounds definitive, but of course the classification is sensitive to the duration of follow up, otherwise cases with tumors destined to relapse are miss-classified because not enough time has elapsed for the relapse to occur. This problem is, of course, overcome by focusing on tumor banks that have long follow up. However relying on long term follow up studies presents a major problem because in order to make rapid progress we cannot solely rely on such a distant outcome to assess the effectiveness of treatment. The most common intermediate marker for outcomes in oncology is response. Unfortunately trials that demonstrate improvements in response rates do not always show prolongations in cancer survival. Furthermore response is defined by radiological means with arbitrary definitions. Some tumors may be responding but the response is slow, or an extensive stromal reaction may mask a major decline in the population of malignant cells in the lesion. Thus dynamic profiling to show therapeutic changes in proliferation, apoptosis and invasion may supplement radiological information so that responders and non responders are not misclassified.

Table 3. Genes showing the greatest decline in expression in a single tumor responding to neoadjuvant endocrine therapy with an aromatase inhibitor

Log base 2 scale	Genes decreased one month
-4.5	topoisomerase (DNA) II alpha (170kD) (proliferation)
-3.3	ataxin 2 related protein
-4.1	ribonucleotide reductase M2 polypeptide (proliferation)
-3.5	baculoviral IAP repeat-containing 5 (survivin) (apoptosis suppression)
-3.8	forkhead box M1
-3.6	interferon-induced protein with tetratricopeptide repeats 1
-3.3	5-methyltetrahydrofolate-homocysteine methyltransferase reductase (proliferation)
-3.7	Cell division cycle 2, G1 to S and G2 to M (proliferation)
-4.0	S100 calcium-binding protein P
-6.5	matrix metalloproteinase 1 (interstitial collagenase) (invasion)
-3.8	orosomucoid 1
-4.4	carboxypeptidase B1 (tissue) (invasion)
-3.5	CD36 antigen (collagen type I receptor, thrombospondin receptor) (invasion)
-4.5	prolactin-induced protein (ER cluster)
-3.7	CGI-142
-3.5	H2A histone family, member A
-4.1	protein regulator of cytokinesis 1 (invasion)
-4.2	hypothetical protein MGC4309
-4.1	nucleolar protein 3 apoptosis repressor w/CARD domain (Apoptosis suppression)
-4.1	WD40 repeat domain 11 protein
-4.6	hemoglobin, alpha 1 (Angiogenesis)

CONCLUSIONS

It seems clear to most clinical investigators at this point that they should attempt to incorporate molecular endpoints into their study designs. Most of our therapies for common solid malignancies are only partially effective and so efforts to understand resistance and treatment failure are key to making progress. Dynamic gene expression profiling requires considerable resources but is a promising technology that is available for this effort (Figure 4). Potential advantages include the generation of rapid surrogate markers of tumor responsiveness, documenting response within individual cellular programs such as the cell cycle, cell death and invasion to help pin point resistance mechanisms and finally the ability to relate "early" profiles with "late" profiles to understand the nature of acquired resistance and relapse after adjuvant therapy.

Potential advantages of dynamic gene expression profiling
•Surrogate markers for response
•Defining response by individual cellular programs to classify resistance mechanisms
•Binary supervised analysis within the context of the array data alone.
•Predicting the long term outcome of therapy though brief drug exposure and dynamic profiling.
•Can compare "early" profiles with late "profiles" to determine the nature of secondary resistance

Figure 4. A list of genes exhibiting a marked decrease in mRNA expression with neoadjuvant aromatase inhibitor therapy from samples taken at baseline and one month

Acknowledgements

I would like to acknowledge my collaborators in this project, including Drs William Miller, Antonio Llombert-Cussac, Dean Evans, Marlene Dressman, Micheal Polymeropoulos, Jeffery Marks, Holly Dressman, Baljit Singh and Andrew Coop.

References

1. van't Veer, L. J., Dal, H., van de Vijver, M. J., He, Y. D., Hart, A. A. M., Mao, M., Peterse, H. L., van de Kooy, K., Marton, M. J., Witteveen, A. T., Schreber, G. J., Kerkhoven, R. M., Roberts, C., Linsley, P. S., Bernards, R., and Friend, S. F. Gene expression profiling predicts clinical outcome of breast cancer, Nature. 415: 530-536, 2002.
2. Sorlie, T., Perou, C. M., Tibshirani, R., Aas, T., Geisler, S., Johnsen, H., Hastie, T., Eisen, M. B., van de Rijn, M., Jeffrey, S. S., Thorsen, T., Quist, H., Matese, J. C., Brown, P. O., Botstein, D., Eystein Lonning, P., and Borresen-Dale, A. L. Gene expression patterns of breast carcinomas distinguish tumor subclasses with clinical implications, Proc Natl Acad Sci U S A. 98: 10869-74., 2001.
3. Shipp, M. A., Ross, K. N., Tamayo, P., Weng, A. P., Kutok, J. L., Aguiar, R. C., Gaasenbeek, M., Angelo, M., Reich, M., Pinkus, G. S., Ray, T. S., Koval, M. A., Last, K. W., Norton, A., Lister, T. A., Mesirov, J., Neuberg, D. S., Lander, E. S., Aster, J. C., and Golub, T. R. Diffuse large B-cell lymphoma outcome prediction by gene-expression profiling and supervised machine learning, Nat Med. 8: 68-74., 2002.
4. Clark, G. M. and McGuire, W. L. Steroid receptors and other prognostic factors in primary breast cancer, Semin Oncol. 15: 20-5, 1988.
5. Foekens, J. A., Portengen, H., Look, M. P., van Putten, W. L., Thirion, B., Bontenbal, M., and Klijn, J. G. Relationship of PS2 with response to tamoxifen therapy in patients with recurrent breast cancer, Br J Cancer. 70: 1217-23, 1994.
6. Schwartz, L. H., Koerner, F. C., Edgerton, S. M., Sawicka, J. M., Rio, M. C., Bellocq, J. P., Chambon, P., and Thor, A. D. pS2 expression and response to hormonal therapy in patients with advanced breast cancer, Cancer Res. 51: 624-8, 1991.
7. Hu, J. C. C. and Mokbel, K. Does c-erbB2/HER2 overexpression predict adjuvant tamoxifen failure in patients with early breast cancer?, Eur J Surg Oncol. 27: 335-337, 2001.
8. Ellis, M. J., Coop, A., Singh, B., Mauriac, L., Llombert-Cussac, A., Janicke, F., Miller, W. R., Evans, D. B., Dugan, M., Brady, C., Quebe-Fehling, E., and Borgs, M. Letrozole is more effective neoadjuvant endocrine therapy than tamoxifen for ErbB-1- and/or ErbB-2-positive, estrogen receptor- positive primary breast cancer: evidence from a phase III randomized trial, J Clin Oncol. 19: 3808-16., 2001.
9. Polychemotherapy for early breast cancer: an overview of the randomised trials. Early Breast Cancer Trialists' Collaborative Group, Lancet. 352: 930-42, 1998.
10. Tamoxifen for early breast cancer: an overview of the randomised trials. Early Breast Cancer Trialists' Collaborative Group, Lancet. 351: 1451-67, 1998.
11. Fisher, B., Dignam, J., Wolmark, N., DeCillis, A., Emir, B., Wickerham, D. L., Bryant, J., Dimitrov, N. V., Abramson, N., Atkins, J. N., Shibata, H., Deschenes, L., and Margolese, R. G. Tamoxifen and chemotherapy for lymph node-negative, estrogen receptor- positive breast cancer, J Natl Cancer Inst. 89: 1673-82, 1997.
12. Albain, K. S., Green, S., Ravdin, P., Cobau, C., Levine, J. E., Ingle, J. N., Pritchard, K., Schneider, M., Abeloff, M. D., Norton, L., Lew, D., Martino, S., and Osborne, C. K. Overall survival after cyclophosphamide, Adriamycin, 5FU and Tamoxifen (CAFT) is superiour to T alone in postmenopausal, receptor (+), Node (+) Breast cancer: New findings from Phase III Southwest Oncology Group Intergroup Trial S8814 (INT-0100) (Abstract 94), Proc ASCO. 20: 24a, 2001.
13. West, M., Blanchette, C., Dressman, H., Huang, E., Ishida, S., Spang, R., Zuzan, H., Olson, J. A., Jr., Marks, J. R., and Nevins, J. R. Predicting the clinical status of human breast cancer by using gene expression profiles, Proc Natl Acad Sci U S A. 98: 11462-7., 2001.
14. Dressman, M. A., Walz, T. M., Barnes, L., Buchholtz, S., Kwon, I., Lavedan, C., Ellis, M. J., and M.H., P. Genes that co-cluster with estrogen receptor alpha in microarray analysis of breast biopsies, The Pharmacogenomics Journal. 1: 135-141, 2001.

15. Eiermann, W., Paepke, S., Appffelstaedt, J., Llombard-Cussac, A., Eremin, J., Vinholes, J., Mauriac, L., Ellis, M., Lassus, M., Chaudrai, H. A., Dugan, M., Borgs, M., and Semiglazov, V. Preoperative treatment of postmenopausal breast cancer patients with letrozole: A randomized double-blind multicenter study., Annals Oncol. *12:* 1-6, 2001.

16. Ellis, M. J. Neoadjuvant endocrine therapy for Breast Cancer: Medical perspectives., Clin Cancer Res. *7:* 4388s-4391s, 2001.

17. Ellis, M. J. Preoperative endocrine therapy for older women with breast cancer: renewed interest in an old idea., Cancer Control. *7:* 557-62, 2000.

18. Ellis. M.J., Rosen, E, Dressman H and Marks J. Neoadjuvant comparisons of aromatase inhibitors and tamoxifen: Pretreatment determinants of response and on-treatment effect. J Steroid Chemistry and Mol Biol. In Press.

DEVELOPMENT OF THE EPIDERMAL GROWTH FACTOR RECEPTOR INHIBITOR TARCEVA™ (OSI-774)

Viktor Grünwald and Manuel Hidalgo[*]

The Sidney Kimmel Comprehensive Cancer Center at Johns Hopkins, Baltimore, MD

ABSTRACT

The epidermal growth factor receptor (EGFR) is a transmembrane receptor involved in the regulation of a complex array of essential biological processes such as cell proliferation and survival. Dysregulation of EGFR signaling network has been frequently reported in multiple human cancers and has been associated with the processes of tumor development, growth, proliferation, metastasis and angiogenesis. Inhibition of the EGFR was associated with antitumor effects in preclinical models. On the bases of these data, therapeutics targeting the EGFR were explore in clinical trials. Tarceva™ (OSI-774, OSI Pharmaceuticals, Uniondale, NY) is a small molecule selective inhibitor of the EGFR tyrosine kinase (TK). In preclinical studies, Tarceva™ inhibited the phosphorylation of the EGFR in a dose and concentration dependent manner resulting in cell cycle arrest and induction of apoptosis. In *in vivo* studies, the agent caused tumor growth inhibition and shoved synergistic effects when combined with conventional chemotherapy. Subsequent single agent phase I studies and phase I studies in combination with chemotherapy demonstrated that the agent has a good safety profile and induced tumor growth inhibition in a substantial number of patients with a variety of different solid tumor. Preliminary report from phase II studies confirmed the excellent tolerability of Tarceva™ as well as showed encouraging preliminary activity. Phase III studies have either been completed or are ongoing in several tumor types such as lung cancer and pancreatic cancer. In summary, Tarceva™ is a novel inhibitor of the EGFR TK which has shown promising activity in initial studies and is currently undergoing full development as an anticancer drug.

---

[*] **Corresponding author:** Manuel Hidalgo, M.D. The Sidney Kimmel Comprehensive Cancer Center at Johns Hopkins, The Bunting-Blaustein Cancer Research Building 1M86, 1650 Orleans Street, Baltimore, MD 21231-1000, Phone: 410 502-7149; Fax: 410 614-9006; e-mail: mhidalg1@jhmi.edu

New Trends in Cancer for the 21st Century, edited by
Llombart-Bosch and Felipo, Kluwer Academic/Plenum Publishers, 2003

INTRODUCTION

The epidermal growth factor (EGF) receptor, also know as HER-1 or Erb-1, is a member of the EGF family of receptors which is formed by a total of four members (HER-2, -3, -4)[1]. Structurally, these receptors are transmembrane molecules composed of an extracellular ligand binding domain, a transmembrane membrane-anchoring domain and an intracellular domain with intrinsic tyrosine (TK) kinase activity. Binding of activating ligands to the extracellular domain of the receptor initiates a process of receptor homo or heterodimerization that activates the intracellular TK domain of the receptor and results in phosphorylation of the receptor. The phosphorylated receptor serves as a docking domain for binding and activation of several downstream signaling mediators that ultimately result in cell proliferation (Figure 1)[1, 2].

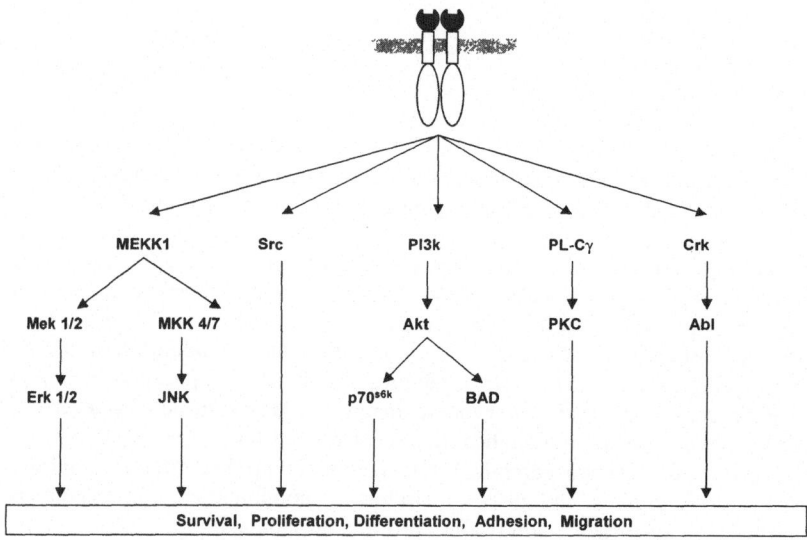

Figure 1. Summary structural and biochemical features of Tarceva[TM].

A substantial number of preclinical studies have indicated that dysregulation of the EGFR functioning by either overexpression, paracrine or autocrine secretion of activating ligands, and mutations that result in constitutive activation of the receptor is a key process in malignant transformation and has been is involved in cell growth and proliferation, survival, angiogenesis, and the development of metastasis. Parallel studies using tumor tissues from patients with cancer have demonstrated that the EGFR is dysregulated in the vast majority of human epithelial neoplasm with frequencies ranging from 15% to as high as 90 %. On the bases of these findings, the EGFR became a target for the development of novel cancer therapeutics. Pharmacologically, two main strategies have been used to inhibit the EGFR consisting of either monoclonal antibodies against the extracellular domain of the receptor that compete with the binding of activating ligands to the extracellular domain of the receptor and small molecules that inhibit the intracellular TK domain. An increasing number of these agents targeting the EGFR are currently in clinical development. This review article summarizes the current status in the clinical development of small molecule inhibitor of the EGFR OSI-774 (Tarceva™; OSI Pharmaceuticals, Uniondale, NY)[3].

MECHANISM OF ACTION AND PRECLINICAL DEVELOPMENT

Tarceva™ ([6,7-bis (2-methoxy-ethoxy)-quinazolin-4-yl]-[3-ethylphenyl] amine is a low-molecular weight (MW 393.4) quinazoline derivative that binds competitively to the adenosine trisphosphate (ATP) binding site at the EGFR intracellular TK domain and therefore inhibits EGFR autophosphorylation. Figure 2 summarizes the structural and biochemical features of Tarceva.™ The inhibitory concentrations for the EGFR TK ranged from 2 to 20 nM in either purified *in vitro* kinase or in cell culture respectively, whereas other tyrosine kinases were blocked with 1000-fold higher concentrations. In preclinical models, exposure of cancer cells to OSI-774 resulted in up-regulation of p27, G_0/G_1 cell cycle arrest and induction of apoptosis[4].

OSI-774 PROPERTIES

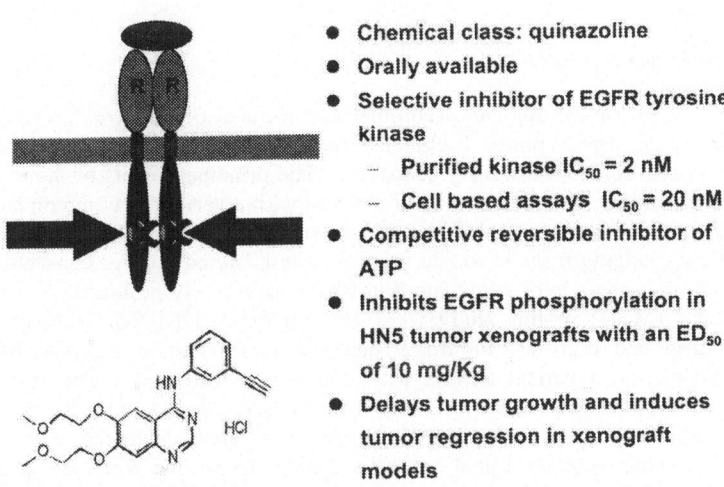

- Chemical class: quinazoline
- Orally available
- Selective inhibitor of EGFR tyrosine kinase
  - Purified kinase IC_{50} = 2 nM
  - Cell based assays IC_{50} = 20 nM
- Competitive reversible inhibitor of ATP
- Inhibits EGFR phosphorylation in HN5 tumor xenografts with an ED_{50} of 10 mg/Kg
- Delays tumor growth and induces tumor regression in xenograft models

Figure 2. Representative cutaneous toxicity in a petient treated with 200 mg/day of Tarceva™.

In *in vivo* studies, Tarceva™ exerted a dose dependant tumor growth inhibition in the HN5 EGFR rich head and neck carcinoma model with significant antitumor effects noted at dose above 12.5 mg/kg per day for 20 consecutive days. In these studies, the agent exerted a dose dependant inhibition of the EGFR phosphorylation with maximum inhibitory effects of 80 % one hour after treatment and remained inhibited in the 70-80 % range or approximately 12 hours and recovered to baseline in 24 hours. The ED_{50} for inhibition of the EGFR was ≈ 10 mg/Kg and did not differ between oral and intraperitoneal route of administration. In preclinical pharmacokinetic studies in mice, plasma concentration ranged from 2.9 to 100 μM at doses ranging from of 2.9 to 92 mg/kg which is equivalent to 400 nM-600 nM of free, non-protein bound, Tarceva™, a concentration well above the IC_{50} for inhibition of the EGFR activation. An important observation in the preclinical studies with Tarceva™ is the linear relationship between inhibition of the target and antitumor effects in *in vivo* studies suggesting that assessment of target inhibition could aid in the clinical development of this compound. Finally, in *in vivo* studies, the combination of Tarceva™ with chemotherapy exerted synergistic antitumor effects suggesting that combinations of Tarceva™ with conventional chemotherapy should be pursued in the clinic[5].

CLINICAL STUDIES WITH TARCEVA™

Based on the strong rationale supporting the notion that the EGFR is an attractive target for cancer therapeutics and the fact the significant activity of Tarceva™ in preclinical studies, the agent entered clinical development. A large number of clinical trials ranging from single agent phase I studies to larger randomized clinical trials have been completed in record time. This section summarize the results of the principal trials conducted with Tarceva™

Single Agent Phase I Studies

The toxicity, pharmacology and preliminary assessment of Tarceva™ was explored in two parallel single agent phase I clinical studies utilizing a continuous oral dosing administration schedule and a weekly schedule. The principal results of those studies are summarized in Table 1. A total of 40 adult patients with a variety of common solid tumors were treated in the first phase I dose escalation schedule finding phase I clinical trial of Tareva.™ Doses ranging from 25 to 200 mg were administered in three consecutive studies parts in which the schedule of administration was progressively prolonged. The maximum tolerated doses (MTD) in this study were 150 mg/day. DLT consisted of cutaneous acneiforme rash and diarrhea. Figure 3 shows a representative example of a severe cutaneous toxicity in a patient treated with 200 mg of Tarceva.™ The rash was dose dependant and limited the dose escalation above 150 mg/day. Clinically, the cutaneous toxicity preferentially affected the face and upper trunk areas, appeared at the end of the first week of dosing, reached a peak intensity during the second week and progressively recovered even in patients who continue taking the same dose of Tarceva,™ and was in general minimally or asymptomatic causing only a cosmetic problem. Treatment with topical or systemic tetracycline-type antibiotics appears to accelerate the resolution of the rash in non-controlled studies. The second principal toxicity with Tarceva ™ was the development of watery diarrhea in patients treated at doses above 150 mg that was controllable with the aggressive used of Loperamide treatment. Other toxicities were mild to moderate and consisted of nausea and vomiting, elevation in bilirubine, headaches, and mucositis. In contrast, the MTD was not reached in the weekly administration schedule at doses up to 1600 mg/week. An objective tumor response was observed in a patient with renal cell cancer and minor responses or prolonged stable diseases were observed in patients with other common solid tumors including squamous carcinoma of the head and neck, colon cancer, non-small cell lung cancer, and prostate cancer.

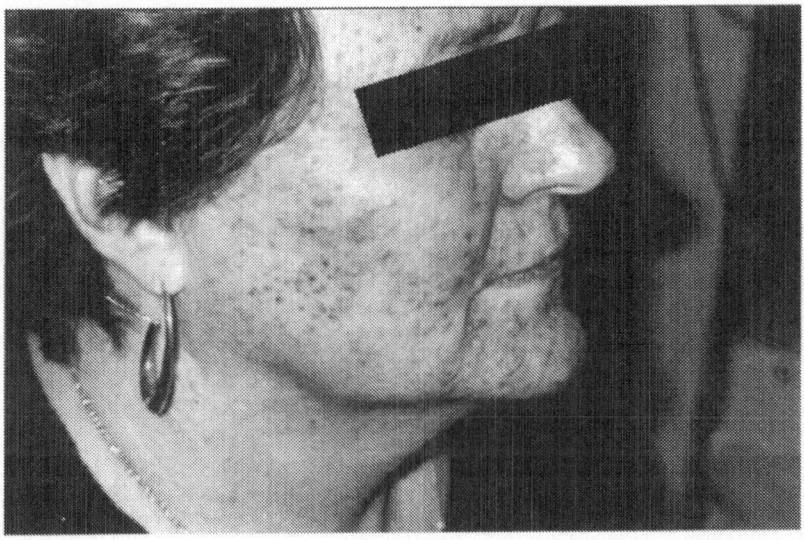

Figure 3. Representative example of a severe cutaneous toxicity in a patient treated with 200mg of Tarceva™.

Concomitant pharmacokinetic studies demonstrated a linear pharmacokinetics with proportional increment in peak plasma concentration and area under the concentration versus time curve, a moderate interpatient variability, no drug accumulation by day 28, a large volume of distribution after oral dosing and a plasma half life of 31 hours. At the recommended phase II dose of 150 mg day, the steady state concentration average 1.168 µg/mL. which is above the concentration deemed to e necessary for antitumor effects based on preclinical models. In these phase I clinical trials, patients with cutaneous toxicity had higher area under the concentration versus time curve in the first 24 hours after dosing but similar peak plasma and steady state concentration. There were no differences with regard to any parameter of exposure in patients with different degrees of diarrhea. In addition, no differences were observed between patients outcome and exposure to the drug in this study. In addition, the early clinical studies with Tarceva ™ assessed the pharmacodynamic effects of the agent in normal epidermis (Figure 4 and 5)[7]. In these studies, a total of 27 patients treated with increasing doses of Tarceva ™ underwent a biopsy of normal skin at baseline prior to treatment and at the conclusion of the first cycle of therapy. Using a quantitative immunohistochemistry method, there was a statistically significant difference in the ratio of activated EGFR in the post-treatment biopsy versus pre-treatment (64 vs 49 %, p = 0.02). Furthemore, the average number of epidermal cells with nuclear staining for p27 increased from 185 ± 101 pre-treatment to 253 ± 111 after treatment (p = 0.002). Interestingly, there was a correlation between the effects on p27 upregulation and the administered dose of Tarceva[TM] with effects noticed at doses above 100 mg/day.

Combination Phase I Clinical Studies

Based on the preclinical data indicating synergistic effects of Tarceva[TM] in combination with chemotherapy, several phase I clinical trials exploring the tolerability and pharmacokinetic interactions of Tarceva[TM] in combination with chemotherapy have been conducted or are currently ongoing. Preliminary data from three of these studies has been presented including combination of Tarceva[TM] with paclitaxel-carboplatin, gemcitabine-cisplatin, and docetaxel and are summarized in (Table 2)[8-10]. The standard dose of chemotherapy needed to be decreased in two of these studies due to increase toxicity but, in general, the combinations have been very well tolerated with no evidence of increase toxicity above the expected toxicities based on the nature of the chemotherapy regimen. No major pharmacokinetic interaction has been observed in these studies which served as the bases for subsequent randomize trials.

Phase II-III Studies with Tarceva[TM]

Three disease oriented phase II clinical trials explored the antitumor activity of Tarceva[TM] at its recommended dose of 150 mg/d in patients with previously treated non-small cell lung, ovarian, and head-and-neck cancers have been reported (Table 3)[11-13]. Generally, these trials demonstrated antitumor activity, albeit modest, in patients with chemoresistant diseases. The principal toxicities were skin rash and diarrhea consistent with the results observed in phase I studies. In patients with overexpressing EGFR, chemotherapy refractory NSCLC, one of 57 total patients achieved a complete response (1.8 %), eight attained a partial response (14 %) and 15 (26 %) had disease stabilization. The median survival was 37 weeks and the 1-year survival was 48 %. In addition, responses in the range 5-6 % were observed in patients with EGFR + ovarian cancer and un-selected patients with head and neck cancer. In this last study, there was not a correlation between the expression level of the EGFR and outcome.

Subsequently, a number of phase III studies were designed and initiated. The status of these trials is summarized in Table 4. These randomized clinical trials used the general design of comparing the overall survival of Tarceva[TM] in combination with conventional chemotherapy versus placebo in combination with chemotherapy in patients with advanced disease. This strategy is based on the tremendous synergism observed in preclinical models between EGFR inhibitors and chemotherapy. The two phase III studies in lung cancer have already completed enrollment and the results will hopefully be available soon.

Table 1. Single Agent Phase I Studies with Tarceva™

Authors	Tumor type	No. of Pts.	Dose	Regimen	MTD (mg/d)	DLT Toxicities	Activity
Hidalgo et al	All	40	25-200 mg/d	Part A: 3d/week x 3 q4wk Part B: weekly x 3 q 4wk Part C: continuous	150	Diarrhea Skin rash	11% PR 22% MR 22% SD
Karp et al	All	28	100-1600 mg/week	Day 1, 8, 15 q 4 wk	Not reached	Diarrhea	30% MR 30% SD

Table 2. Phase I Studies of Tarceva™ in Combination with Chemotherapy

Author	Tumor type	No. of Pts.	Tarceva Dose (mg/d)	Regimen	MTD (mg/d)	Toxicities	Activity
Forero Et al	All	9	100-150	paclitaxel + carboplatin$	NA	Neutropenia*, diarrhea*, rash*	
Ratain Et al	All	7	100	gemcitabine + cisplatin||	NA	Neutropenia*, renal toxicity, increased prothrombin time	
onouzesh et al	All	22	100-150	+ docetaxel **	NA	Febrile neutropenia*	5% CR 5% MR 23% SD

CR: complete response; PR: partial response; MR: minor response; SD: stable disease
* DLT: Dose Limiting Toxicity
** docetaxel 75 mg/m² was reduced to 60 mg/m² q3wk after reaching DLT
$ paclitaxel 225 mg/m², carboplatin AUC 6 i.v. q3wk
|| gemcitabine 1000 mg/m² d1, 8, 15 and cisplatin 100 mg/m² d1 q28d; regimen was reduced to gemcitabine 1000 mg/m² d1, 8 and cisplatin 60 mg/m² d1 q21

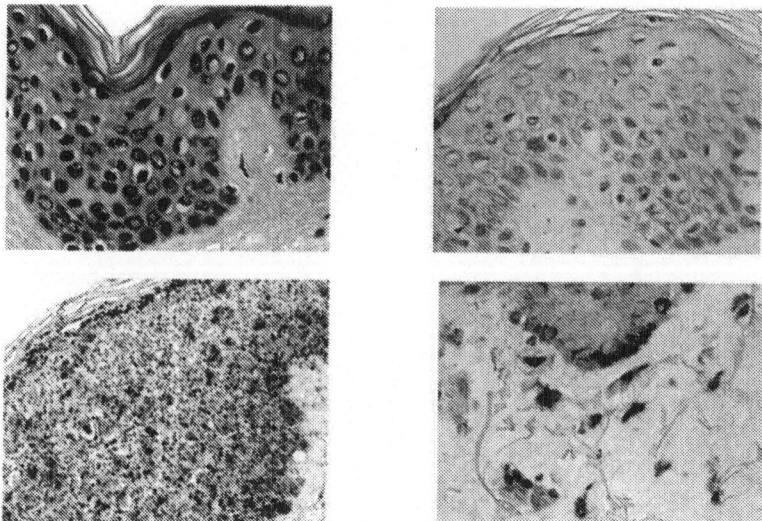

Figure 4. Immunoperoxidase staining for p27: a) Normal skin , H + E staining; b) The same specimen stained with an isotypic mouse IgG (negative control); c) Immunoperoxidase staining for p27 in the pre-treatment specimen showing scattered staining in the basal epidermal layer and d) immunoperoxidase staining for p27 post-treatment showing marked increment in the number of + cells staining. X 400.

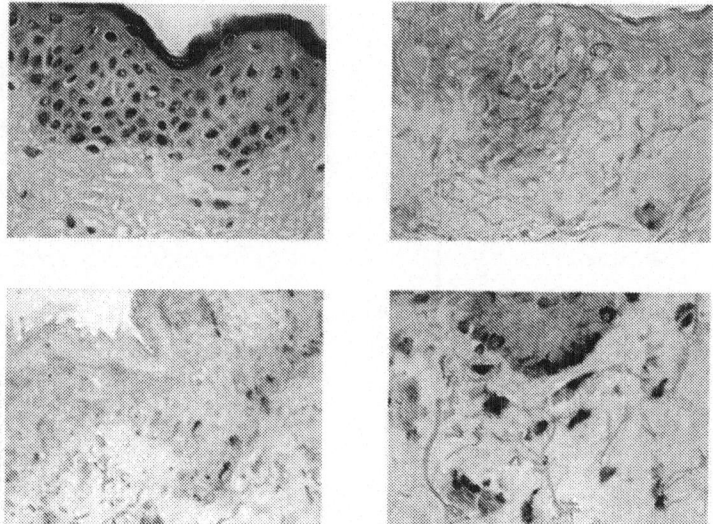

Figure 5. Immunoperoxidase staining for phospho-EGFR (Y1173): a) Normal skin , H + E staining; b) The same specimen stained with an isotypic mouse IgG (negative control); c) Immunoperoxidase staining for phospho-EGFR in the pre-treatment specimen showing strong staining in the basal epidermal layer (3+) and d) immunoperoxidase staining for phospho-EGFR in the post-treatment specimen showing marked decrement in staining (1 +). X 400.

Table 3. Phase II Studies with Tarceva[TM]

Authors	Tumor type	No. of Pts.	Toxicities	Activity	Median Survival	Comments
Perez-Soler et al	Non-small cell lung	57	Skin Rash 91 % Diarrhea 32 %	2% CR 14% PR 26% SD	9.3 months	Chemorefractory EGFR positive
Senzer et al	Head-and-Neck	124	Skin Rash 74 % Diarrhea 31 %	6%PR 40% SD	5. 8 months	Chemorefractory EGFR positive and negative
Finkler et al	Ovarian	34	Skin Rash 88 % Diarrhea 35 %	6% PR 50% SD	8 months	Chemorefractory EGFR positive

Table 4. Phase III Studies with Tarceva[TM]

Indication	Regimen	Status
Non Small Cell Lung Cancer	1st line with cisplatin and gemcitabine (TALENT)	Enrollment complete
	1st line with carboplatin and paclitaxel (TRIBUTE)	Enrollment complete
	2nd/3rd-line monotherapy	Enrolling
	2nd line with docetaxel	Imminent start
Pancreas	1st line with gemcitabine	Enrolling
CRC	1st line with Xeloda[®]	Imminent start
Ovarian	2nd line with paclitaxel and carboplatin	Imminent start
	1st line with carboplatin	Imminent start

CHALLENGES IN THE DEVELOPMENT OF TARCEVA[TM]

The clinical development of Tarceva[TM] represents a genuine example of the potential difficulties and challenges in the development of a argeted agent. Despite the fact that this agent has already completed phase III clinical studies using, in general, classic developmental strategies as employed in the development of classic agent, and that many of initial considerations were theoretical more than practical, a significant number of questions, which response would optimize the development of these agents, are still answered. This section of the article summarizes some of the most relevant issues that are pertinent to the Tarceva[TM] including the selection of patients more likely to benefit from this agent, the selection of the most appropriate dose and schedule of administration, incorporation of pharmacodynamic markers and surrogates of patients outcome.

Most debate has been generated with the selection of appropriate population of patients for participation in clinical studies with these compounds. The predominant hypothesis was that only patients with overexpression of the receptor would benefit from treatment with these agents. Though the analysis of preclinical data is complicated because in general the majority of studies have been conducted in artificial EGFR-rich models, there appears to be a relationship between the expression of the receptor and the susceptibility to the inhibitors. However, the mere expression of the receptor is not sufficient to predict the response of cell lines to these agents in vitro. Other factors such as the activation of downstream signaling pathways, the dependence of cell growth and proliferation on EGF- regulated pathways, the presence of activating growth factors, and the relative expression of the EGFR versus other receptors members of the family, has been demonstrated in preclinical models to influence the cellular response to these inhibitors[14-16]. These data would suggest that a useful pharmacodiagnostic marker should incorporate a broader analysis of various elements of in the EGFR signaling such as downstream signaling pathways. In this regard, the development and validation of immunohistochemical methods to measure the activation of signaling pathways with phospho-specific antibodies could be of importance[17]. In addition, tumors with vIII mutations could be classified as EGFR depending on the method used to measure the expression of the receptor, when indeed, cells with vIII mutations are inhibited by some of these compounds. An additional complicating factor derives from the lack of properly validated assays to measure the expression and activation of the EGFR and the semi-quantitative and subjective nature of the most commonly used immunohistochemical methods. At this juncture, the majority of clinical trials conducted with Tarceva have not selected patients based on any molecular feature. This decision appears appropriate based on the lack of data to support the selection of a specific subset of patients and the availability of adequate assays. However, this should not decrease the interest to investigate this question in future clinical studies.

The second relevant aspect is the selection of appropriate dose and schedule of administration. The selection of the dose and schedule of administration of Tarceva™ has been based on toxicity as well as pharmacokinetic parameters indicating either plasma concentrations above a biologically relevant level. Subsequent disease oriented studies have been conducted utilizing the optimal dose as determined in phase I evaluations. Two pieces of data from the laboratory are relevant to this discussion. First, there is a linear relationship between target inhibition and antitumor activity and; second, only tumors in which inhibition of the receptor result in inhibition of downstream signaling pathways are growth arrested. This information would suggest that the optimal dose is the dose at which the target is inhibited[7]. The definition of pharmacological active-dose is, however, difficult. The approach that has been employed is the collection of tumor biopsies pre-treatment and after treatment. However, the implementation of these correlative studies in large scale clinical trials is non-realistic given the technical difficulties and paucity of patients with biopsiable tumors.

To overcome this barrier, investigators have focused in the used of normal tissues and, in the case of inhibitors of the EGFR, the use of normal skin, to develop pharmacodynamic surrogates. In fact, these studies have demonstrated that treatment of patients with Tarceva™ inhibits the activation and signaling of the EGFR in normal epidermis (Figure 4 and 5). There are however, several limitations with these studies the principal one being that the relationship between inhibition of the EGFR in skin and tumor tissues does not need to be a parallel phenomenon. In addition, it is possible that the downstream effects of inhibiting the EGFR in skin tissues and tumor tissues are different because tumors tend to have mutations and alterations of downstream signaling elements that could result in constitutive activation of these pathways.

Another important question is the definition of activity in phase II studies. Based on preclinical data, it was expected that the principal effect of Tarceva™ would be the induction of tumor stabilization rather that tumor response. The phase II studies however demonstrated that these agents indeed are capable of inducing tumor response though the meaninfull response rate for this class of agents is not known. Innovative methods to determine activity in phase II studies included the incorporation of functional imaging techniques such as positron emission tomography and the development of novel clinical trials methods such as the randomized discontinuation method and the multinomial method. In addition, the pharmacodynamic markers of biological activity mentioned in the prior paragraph should also be explored as surrogates of activity in phase II disease oriented studies.

SUMMARY

The EGFR is an attractive target for cancer therapeutics. Tarceva™ is a small molecule inhibitor of the EGFR. In preclinical studies Tarceva™ demonstrated mechanistic-based antitumor effects in relevant cancer models. Subsequent phase I studies demonstrated an adequate tolerability profile, favorable pharmacokinetics, evidence of target inhibition and antitumor effects. Enrollment has been completed for some of the randomized phase III studies while other definitive studies are currently underway. The results of these eagerly awaited clinical studies will determining the role of Tarceva™ in cancer treatment.

References

1. Schlessinger J. Cell signaling by receptor tyrosine kinases. Cell 2000;103:211-25.
2. Yarden Y. The EGFR family and its ligands in human cancer. signalling mechanisms and therapeutic opportunities. Eur J Cancer 2001;37 Suppl 4:S3-8.
3. Grunwald V, Hidalgo M. The epidermal growth factor receptor: a new target for anticancer therapy. Curr Probl Cancer 2002;26:109-64.
4. Moyer JD, Barbacci EG, Iwata KK, Arnold L, Boman B, Cunningham A, et al. Induction of apoptosis and cell cycle arrest by CP-358,774, an inhibitor of epidermal growth factor receptor tyrosine kinase. Cancer Res 1997;57:4838-48.
5. Pollack VA, Savage DM, Baker DA, Tsaparikos KE, Sloan DE, Moyer JD, et al. Inhibition of epidermal growth factor receptor-associated tyrosine phosphorylation in human carcinomas with CP-358,774: dynamics of receptor inhibition in situ and antitumor effects in athymic mice. J Pharmacol Exp Ther 1999;291:739-48.
6. Karp D FK, Tensfeldt TG, Thurer RL, LoCiecero J, Huberman M, et al. A phase I dose escalation study of epidermal growth factor receptor (EGFR) tyrosine kinase (TK) inhibitor CP-358,774 in patients (pts) with advanced solid tumors. Lung Cancer 2000:29.
7. Manuel Hidalgo SM, Eric Rowinsky, Alexander Miller, Dianne Duffey, Linda de'Grafenried, Lillian Siu, Cecelia Simmons, Jeffrey Kreisberg, Michael Brattain. Inhibition of the Epidermal Growth Factor Receptor (EGFR) by OSI-774, a Specific EGFR Inhibitor in Malignant and Normal Tissues of Cancer Patients. Proceedings of the American Society of Medical Oncology 2001;20.

8. Forouzesh B HM, Takimoto C, DeBono JS, Forero L, Beeram M, et. Phase I, pharmacokinetic (PK), and biological studies of the epidermal growth factor-tyrosine kinase (EGFR-TK) inhibitor OSI-774 in combination with docetaxel. Proc. Am. Soc. Clin. Oncol 2002.

9. Forero L PA, Hammond LA, Tolcher A, Schwartz G, Hidalgo M, et al. Phase I, pharmacokinetic (PK) and biologic study of OSI-774, a selective epidermal factor receptor (EGFR) tyrosine kinase (TK) inhibitor in combination with paclitaxel and carboplatin. Proc. Am. Soc. Clin. Oncol 2002.

10. Ratain MJ GC, Janisch L, Kindler HL, Ryan C, Wood DL, et al. Phase I trial of elotinib (OSI-774) in combination with gemcitabine (G) and cisplatin (P) in patients with advanced solid tumors. Proc. Am. Soc. Clin. Oncol 2002.

11. Neil Finkler AG, Mark Crozier, Robert Edwards, Jose Figueroa, Agustin Garcia, John Hainsworth, David Irwin, Sandra Silberman, Lee Allen, Karen Ferrante, Douglas Fisher, Paul Nadler. Phase 2 Evaluation of OSI-774, a Potent Oral Antagonist of the EGFR-TK in Patients with Advanced Ovarian Carcinoma. Proceedings of the American Society of Medical Oncology 2001.

12. Neil N. Senzer DS, L Siu, S Agarwala, E Vokes, M Hidalgo, S Silberman, L Allen, K Ferrante, D Fisher, C Marsolais, P Nadler. Phase 2 Evaluation of OSI-774, a Potent Oral Antagonist of the EGFR-TK in Patients with Advanced Squamous Cell Carcinoma of the Head and Neck. Proceedings of the American Society of Medical Oncology 2001;20.

13. Roman Perez-Soler AC, Mark Huberman, Daniel Karp, James Rigas, Lisa Hammond, Eric Rowinsky, G Preston, Karen J Ferrante, Lee F Allen, Paul I Nadler, Philip Bonomi. A Phase II Trial of the Epidermal Growth Factor Receptor (EGFR) Tyrosine Kinase Inhibitor OSI-774, Following Platinum-Based Chemotherapy, in Patients (pts) with Advanced, EGFR-Expressing, Non-Small Cell Lung Cancer (NSCLC). Proceedings of the American Society of Medical Oncology 2001;20.

14. Bishop PC, Myers T, Robey R, Fry DW, Liu ET, Blagosklonny MV, et al. Differential sensitivity of cancer cells to inhibitors of the epidermal growth factor receptor family. Oncogene 2002;21:119-27.

15. Moulder SL, Yakes FM, Muthuswamy SK, Bianco R, Simpson JF, Arteaga CL. Epidermal growth factor receptor (HER1) tyrosine kinase inhibitor ZD1839 (Iressa) inhibits HER2/neu (erbB2)-overexpressing breast cancer cells in vitro and in vivo. Cancer Res 2001;61:8887-95.

16. Motoyama AB, Hynes NE, Lane HA. The efficacy of ErbB receptor-targeted anticancer therapeutics is influenced by the availability of epidermal growth factor-related peptides. Cancer Res 2002;62:3151-8.

17. Malik SN, Brattain M, Ghosh PM, Troyer DA, Prihoda T, Bedolla R, et al. Immunohistochemical demonstration of phospho-akt in high Gleason grade prostate cancer. Clin Cancer Res 2002;8:1168-71.

GEFITINIB (IRESSA, ZD 1839) FOR NON-SMALL CELL LUNG CANCER (NSCLC): RECENTS RESULTS AND FURTHER STRATEGIES

C. Manegold

Thoraxklinik-Heidelberg gGmbH, Amalienstraße 5, 69126 Heidelberg Germany

INTRODUCTION

Chemotherapy for the first-line treatment of Non-Small Cell Lung Cancer (NSCLC) is widely perceived to have reached a plateau in terms of efficacy. A recent study of several platinum-based dublet chemotherapy regimens for the treatment of advanced NSCLC failed to show a survival advantage for any of the regimens when compared with each other (Schiller et al. 2002). Therefore, it appears that the potential for improving current treatments is limited, and novel targeted therapies are urgently needed. One promising therapeutic target is the epidermal growth factor receptor (EGFR), whose activation has a major involvement in processes essential for tumor growth, including proliferation, metastasis, and angiogenesis. Expression of EGFR has been shown to correlate with a poor prognosis, disease progression and resistance to chemotherapy (Wells 2000). EGFR is targeted by the novel agent gefitinib (Iressa, ZD 1839), a small-molecule EGFR tyrosine kinase inhibitor (EGFR-TKI). Gefitinib is an orally active agent, which blocks signal transduction pathways implicated in the proliferation and survival of cancer-cells, in addition to host-dependent processes promoting cancer-cell growth. Several clinical trials of gefitinib in NSCLC have been carried out or are underway.

PHASE I STUDIES

The efficacy and tolerability of gefitinib have been investigated in 4 phase I dose-escalation studies involving a variety of solid tumors, including 100 patients with the diagnosis of advanced NSCLC (Kris et al 2000; Negoro et al 2001, Ranson et al 2002).

Here, gefitinib was well tolerated. The maximum tolerated dose was >= 700 mg/day. The most common adverse events seen in this trial where diarrhea, nausea, rash/acne, vomiting, and asthenia. Most of these adverse events where transient and mild in severity (CTC grade I or II). The incidence and severity of gifitinib-related adverse events generally increased as the dose increased.

New Trends in Cancer for the 21st Century, edited by
Llombart-Bosch and Felipo, Kluwer Academic/Plenum Publishers, 2003

Gefitinib exhibited encouraging antitumor activity at a rage of dose levels. Responses were seen across the dose range 150-700 mg/day, with no clear dose-response relationship. Despite inter-patient variability in exposure, biologically relevant plasma concentrations (exposure levels well above the inhibitory concentration that causes 90% inhibition [IC90] for KB oral carcinoma cells) were maintained at the doses of 150mg/day and above. Fixed doses of 250 and 500 mg/day were therefore selected for subsequent phase II and III studies; 250mg/day is higher than the lowest dose level at which objective tumor regression was seen, while 500 mg/day is the highest dose that was well tolerated when taken chronically in phase I trials.

Two phase I studies were undertaken to examen the effect of adding gifitinib (250 mg and 500 mg once daily) to two different standard cytotoxic chemotherapy regimens commonly used in the first-line treatment of advanced NSCLC. In a study that combined gefitinib with carboplatin and paclitaxel in 24 chemotherapy-naïve patients it was shown that this combination was well tolerated, with no new, increased, or cumulative toxicity (Miller et al, 2001). After having received two courses of cytotoxic chemotherapy plus either 2 or 8 weeks of gefitinib, approximately three out of every five patients received clinical benefit; six (25 %) patients showed a partial response and a further eight (33 %) showed disease stabilization.

A second study of gefitinib combined with cisplatin and gemcitabine in 18 chemotherapy-naïve patients (Gonzalez-Larriba et al, 2002). In this study gefitinib did not appear to increase the overall toxicity of cytotoxic agents. The pharmacokinetic data showed that the combination had not clinically significant effect on the exposure to gefitinib, cisplatin, or gemcitabine. The acticity data were promising of 17 evaluable patients, nine (five NSCLC) had a partial response and seven (four NSCLC) had disease stabilization.

RANDOMIZED PHASE II STUDIES

So far gefitinib's clinical development has concentrated on advanced NSCLC and efficacy and toxicity data for second and first-line therapy using gefitinib as single agent or in combination with standard chemotherapy have recently been released.

Gefitinib for chemotherapy pretreated patients having advanced NSCLC ($2^{nd}/3^{rd}$-line) (IDEAL-trials: IRESSA Dose Evaluation in Advanced Lung cancer): Two randomized, double-blind phase II trials investigated tumor response, disease related symptom response, and safety of daily oral gefitinib (250 versus 500 mg/day) (Kris et al. 2002, Fukuoka et al 2002) (fig.1). Patients treated had locally advanced or metastatic NSCLC and had failed two or more prior chemotherapy regimens containing platinum and/or docetaxel. More than 400 patients were randomized. The median age was 61 years. Most of the patients had a performance status of 0-1, histologically an adeno-carcinoma and no tumor induced symptoms at entry. Tumor response rates for the 250 mg (18,4 %; 11,8 %) and 500 mg (19,0 %; 8,8 %) were similar and did not show any statistical difference in both studies (fig. 2). Symptom response rates were about 40 % with no difference between 250 and 500 mg/day. Approximately 60 % of patients who experienced symptom response did so by the second week of treatment. Improvement in disease-related symptoms was associated with objective tumor responses and an increase in median progression-free and overall survival. Medium survival was about 7 months in both studies for the two doses. Adverse events were generally mild, most common were grade 1/2 rash, diarrhea, puritus and dry skin. Fewer patients on 250 mg experienced drug related toxicity grade 3/4 or withdrawals compared with 500 mg. Therefore it can be concluded that gefitinib single agent used for $2^{nd}/3^{rd}$-line therapy provides durable clinically meaningful antitumor activity, rapid significant and clinically meaningful symptom relief and improvement in quality of life (Natale et al. 2002, Douillard et al 2002). Gefitinib 250 mg has comparable efficacy but a more favourable safety profile and better tolerability than 500 mg/day. The data support gefitinib 250 mg as an important novel treatment option for patients with chemotherapy-pretreated advanced NSCLC.

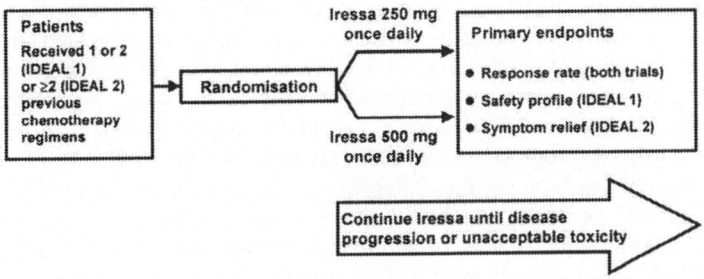

Fig. 1 Iressa as 2nd/3rd – Line Therapy for advanced NSCLC: Phase II-Study results (Fukuoka, 2002; Kris, 2002).

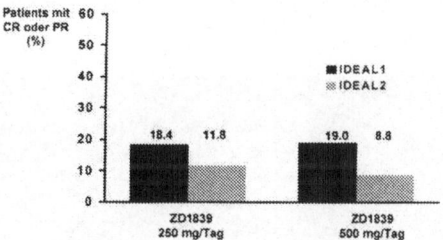

Fig. 2 Iressa as 2nd/3rd – Line Therapy for advanced NSCLC: Phase II-Study results (Fukuoka, 2002; Kris, 2002).

Gefitinib in combination with standard chemotherapy in chemotherapy-naive patients (1st-line) (INTACT-trials: IRESSA NSCLC Trial Assessing Combination Therapy): Because of encouraging phase I data, gemcitabine/cisplatin and taxol/carboplatin were assest in two randomized, double-blind, placebo-controlled, multicenter trials (fig.3).

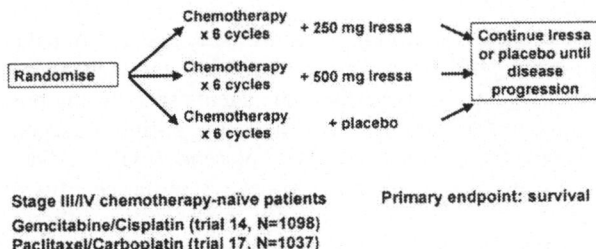

Fig. 3 Gefitinib (Iressa, ZD1839) combination therapy in NSCLC: Phase III trials (Johnson, 2002; Giaccone 2002).

Chemotherapy-naive patients with stage III/IV disease, performance status 0-2 and, age ≥ 18 years were randomized to chemotherapy plus placebo, chemotherapy plus 250 mg/day or chemotherapy plus 500 mg/day gefitinib. Chemotherapy consisted of six cycles. Treatment with gefitinib or placebo could be continued until disease progression. The primary endpoint was overall survival, secondary endpoints were progression-free survival and time to worsening of symptoms as assessed by the lung cancer subscale (LCS) of the FACT-L questionnaire. Other endpoints included symptom improvement, objective tumor response, disease control rate (CR/PR/SD), quality of life, and safety. A total of more than 2000 patients were recruited (median age 61 years, performance status of 0-1 in about 2/3 of the patients, stage IV disease in about 70 %). The three treatment groups were well balanced across all disease and demographic characteristics. There were no statistically significant differences in overall survival (fig.4), progression-free survival and time to worsening of symptoms across the three arms in both studies (Giaccone et al. 2002, Johnson et al 2002). The toxicity profile of gefitinib combined with chemotherapy was comparable to chemotherapy alone, with exception of additive, dose dependent diarrhea and skin-rash. From the INTACT-data presented it can, therefore, be concluded that gefitinib in combination with platin-based doublet chemotherapy for advanced NSCLC did not improved treatment outcome. These results are not unique. Other novel combinations with "gold standard" chemotherapy regimens have also failed to show additive survival benefits.

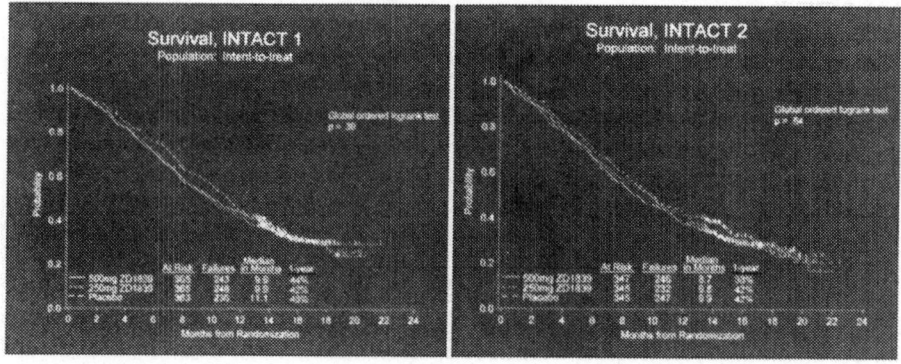

Fig. 4 Gefitinib (Iressa, ZD1839): NSCLC Trial Assessing, Combination Treatment (Johnson, 2002; Giaccone 2002).

FUTURE PROJECTS

As NSCLC is a heterogeneous disease, it seems likely that additional clinical benefit will be derived from using gefitinib in combination with other anticancer agents, either the traditional cytotoxic agents, or newer biologic agents such as angionesis inhibitors. Trials are under way/planned to compare the activity of gefitinib as second-line therapy in combination with docetaxel versus docetaxel/placebo (EORTC 08011) (fig.5). A number of further trials are ongoing/planned to determine the benefits of single-agent gefitinib in different clinical settings: as maintenance therapy following chemoradiotherapy and consolidatory docetaxel in patients with inoperable stage III NSCLC (SWOG 0023) as adjuvant therapy after complete resection of stage IB, II and IIIA NSCLC (fig.6) and as a chemopreventive agent in former or current smokers with a previous specified smoking-related cancer (SPORE-trial). Biologically targeted agents, such as those that selectively inhibit the EGFR, have the potential to provide antitumor activity while being better tolerated than conventional cytotoxic drugs.

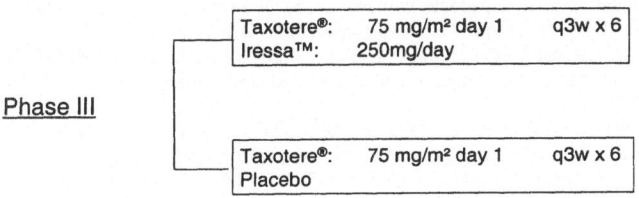

Primary endpoint: survival

Fig. 5 Gefitinib (Iressa, ZD1839) combination therapy in NSCLC: Phase III trials. EORTC 08011: Second line Chemotherapy

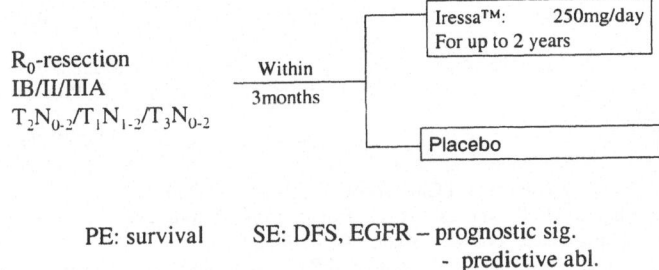

PE: survival   SE: DFS, EGFR – prognostic sig.
                              - predictive abl.

Fig. 6 NCIC CGT BR 19: operable Stage NSCLC; Phase III – Adjuvant Iressa vs Placebo.

Summary

Phase I and II clinical studies demonstrated that gefinitib single agent therapy is well tolerated and provides clinically significant antitumor activity in patients with advanced NSCLC who have previously received prior treatment with cytotoxic chemotherapy. Large-scale studies to assess the clinical benefit of gefitinib versus placebo when combined with cisplatin/gemcitabine and carboplatin/paclitaxel as first-line treatment, however, did not prove that the three drug combinations be able to improve survival and compared to "standard"-doubled chemotherapy. Therefore it can be summarized that gefinitib may provide evaluable addition to the therapeutic options available for the treatment of advanced NSCLC and may also have potential for use in early NSCLC.

References

Douillard JY, Giaccone G, Horai T et al: Improvement in disease-related symptoms and quality of life in patients with advanced non-small cell lung cancer treated with ZD1839 (IRESSA) (IDEAL 1). Proc ASCO 299a (abstr. 1195), 2002

Fukuoka M, Yano S, Giaccone G et al: Final results from a phase II trial of ZD1839 (IRESSA) for patients with advanced non-small cell lung cancer (IDEAL 1). Proc ASCO 21, 298a (abstr. 1188), 2002

Giaccone G, Johnson DH, Manegold C et al: A phase III clinical trial of ZD1839 (IRESSA) in combination with gemcitabine and cisplatin in chemotherapy-naive patients with advanced non-small cell lung cancer (INTACT 1). Ann Oncol 13 (suppl. 5), 2 (abstr. 4 O), 2002

Gonzalez-Larriba J, Giaccone G, van oosterom AT et al. ZD 1839 ("Iressa") in combination with gemcitabine in chemonaive patients with advanced solid tumors: final results of a phase I trial. Proc Am Soc Clin Oncol; 21:95a (A376), 2002.

Johnson DH, Herbst R, Giaccone G et al: ZD1839 (IRESSA) in combination mit paclitaxel and carboplatin in chemotherapy-naive patients with advanced non-small cell lung cancer: results from a phase III clinical trial (INTACT 2). Ann Oncol 13 (suppl. 5), 127 (abstr. 468 O), 2002

Kris M, Natale RB, Herbst T et al: A phase II trial of ZD1839 (IRESSA) in advanced non-small cell lung cancer patients who had failed platinum- and docetaxel-based regimens (IDEAL 2). Proc ASCO 21, 292a (abstr. 1166), 2002

Kris M, Herbst R, Rischin D et al. Objective regressions in non-small cell lung cancer patients treated in phase I trials of oral ZD 1839 („Iressa"), a selective tyrosine kinase inhibitor that blocks the epidermal growth factor receptor (EGFR). Lung Cancer; 29 (suppl 1): 72 (A233), 2000.

Manegold C, Gatzemeier U, Averbuch S, et al. An open label pilot trial of two doses of ZD 1839 ("Iressa") in combination with docetaxel in patients with advanced or metastatic non-small cell lung cancer (NSCLC); Preliminary results. Ann Oncol 2002; 13 (Suppl 5): 149a (Abstract 545)

Miller VA, Johnson D, Heelan RT et al. A pilot trial demonstrates the safety of ZD 1839 (« Iressa ») an oral epidermal growth factor receptor tyrosine kinase inhibitor (EGFR-TKI), in combination with carboplatin © and paclitaxel (P) in previously untreated advanced non-small cell lung cancer (NSCLC). Proc Am Soc Clin Oncol 20326a (A1301), 2001.

Natale RB, Skarin A, Maddaox AM et al: Improvement in symptoms and quality of life for advanced non-small cell lung cancer patients receiving ZD1839 (IRESSA) in IDEAL 2. Proc ASCO 21, 292a (abstr. 1167), 2002

Negoro S, Nakagawa K, Fukuoka M et al. Final results of a phase I intermittent dose –escalation trial of ZD 1839 ("Iresssa") in Japanese patients with various solid tumors. Proc Am Soc Clin Oncol;20:324 (A1292), 2001.

Ranson M, Hammond L, Ferry D et al. ZD 1839 ("Iressa"), a selective oral EGFR-TKI (epidermal growth factor receptor tyrosine kinase inhibitor) is well tolerated and active in patients with solid. Malignant tumors:results pf a phase I trial. J Clin Oncol; 20:2240-2250, 2002.

Schiller JH, Harrington D, Belani CP, et al. Comparison of four chemotherapy regimens for advanced non-small cell lung cancer. N Engl J Med., 346:92-98, 2002

Wells A. The epidermal growth factor receptor (EGFR) – a new target in cancer therapy. Signal 1:4-11, 2000

MECHANISM OF ACTION OF ANTI-HER2 MONOCLONAL ANTIBODIES: SCIENTIFIC UPDATE ON TRASTUZUMAB AND 2C4

Joan Albanell[*], Jordi Codony, Ana Rovira, Begoña Mellado, Pere Gascón

ICMHO, Laboratory of Oncology Research, Medical Oncology Service (J.A., J.C., A.R., B.M., P.G.) & IDIBAPS (J.A., P.G.), Hospital Clínic i Provincial de Barcelona

This work has been supported by Spanish Ministry FIS grant 00/0679 (J.A., B.M., P.G.). A.R. is the recipient of a post-doctoral fellowship grant of the Asociación Española Contra el Cáncer (AECC 2002).

ABSTRACT

The HER family of transmembrane tyrosine kinase receptors is composed of four members, HER1 to HER4. HER2 is a ligand-orphan receptor expressed in many human tumors and overexpressed in 25-30% of breast cancers. HER2 amplifies the signal provided by other receptors of the HER family by forming heterodimers. The essential role of HER2 in the HER signaling network led to the development of anti-HER2 monoclonal antibodies (MAbs) for cancer therapy. In particular, the humanized MAb trastuzumab (Herceptin) has antitumor activity against HER2-overexpressing human breast tumor cells and is widely used for the treatment of women with HER2 overexpressing breast cancers. Trastuzumab induces HER2 receptor downmodulation and, as a result, inhibits critical signalling pathways (i.e. ras-Raf-MAPK and PI3K/Akt) and blocks cell cycle progression by inducing the formation of p27/Cdk2 complexes. Trastuzumab also inhibits HER2 cleavage, preceding antibody-induced receptor downmodulation, and this effect might contribute to its antitumor activity in some cancers. *In vivo*, trastuzumab inhibits angiogenesis and induces antibody-dependent cellular cytotoxicity. A limitation of trastuzumab is that its activity is largely restricted to breast cancers with the highest level of HER2 overexpression or HER2 gene amplification. However, there is a large population of breast cancers and of many other tumors that have low or moderate HER2 expression. In such tumors, HER2 functions as a preferred coreceptor to form heterodimers with HER1 (EGFR), HER3 or HER4. For this reason, a humanized monoclonal antibody, called 2C4, that targets the role of HER2

[*] Correspondence to: Dr. Joan Albanell, ICMHO, Medical Oncology Service,Hospital Clínic i Provincial de Barcelona, C/ Villarroel 170, Barcelona 08036, Phone and Fax: +34 93 2275402, email: albanell@clinic.ub.es

New Trends in Cancer for the 21st Century, edited by
Llombart-Bosch and Felipo, Kluwer Academic/Plenum Publishers, 2003

as a coreceptor is under active development. 2C4 binds to a different epitope of HER2 ectodomain than trastuzumab and sterically hinders HER2 recruitment in heterodimers with other HER receptors. This results in the inhibition of signalling by HER2-based heterodimers both in cells with low and high HER2 expression. *In vitro* and *in vivo* antitumor activity has been reported in a range of breast and prostate tumor models. Therefore, 2C4 may have potential against a wide variety of solid tumors. Phase I trials are underway.

INTRODUCTION

The ErbB family signaling network is dysregulated in a broad range of human tumors[1]. Within this signaling network, the HER2 receptor plays a critical role and has been used as a target of therapeutic monoclonal antibodies[2]. Trastuzumab (Herceptin), a recombinant humanized anti-HER2 antibody[3], is effective for the treatment of women with advanced breast cancers that express high levels of HER2[4, 5, 6]. Trastuzumab is the only anti-HER2 antibody that has been approved for cancer therapy. However, trastuzumab activity relies on the presence of HER2 overexpression while it is not active against tumors that express moderate or normal levels of HER2.

While overt HER2 overexpression occurs only in ≈ 25% of human breast tumors and very rarely in other cancers, HER2 is present at moderate or normal amounts in many tumors[7-10]. The importance of this observation is that in tumors that do not overexpress HER2, this receptor has a critical role as a coreceptor with other ErbB family members. Therefore, monoclonal antibodies, such as 2C4, that can disrupt HER2 association with other ErbB receptors have been produced and might have broader clinical applications than trastuzumab[11].

To put in perspective how diverse antibodies targeting a single receptor, HER2, exert distinct anti-tumor effects, it is necessary to review the biology of the ErbB network and the mechanisms of HER2 activation.

ErbB Receptor Family

HER2 belongs to the ErbB tyrosine kinase receptors (also known as type I receptor tyrosine kinases). This receptor family is comprised of four homolog receptors; the epidermal growth factor receptor (ErbB1/EGFR/HER1), HER2 (ErbB2), HER3 (ErbB3), and HER4 (ErbB4)[1]. These receptors share a common structure that consists of an extracellular ligand binding domain, a transmembrane lipophilic segment, and an intracellular protein tyrosine kinase domain with a regulatory carboxyl terminal segment (Figure 1). There are two receptors within the family that have distinctive features. One is HER2, the only ligand orphan receptor. The other three members have multiple ligands (growth factors) that can bind to their extracellular domain and result in receptor activation. The other receptor that has a distinct feature is HER3, since is the only one that has a deficient tyrosine kinase domain. The physiologic functions of the ErbB signaling network are the regulation of normal cell growth and differentiation by means of their role in mesenchyme-epithelial crosstalk and in the interactions between neurons and muscle, glia and Schwan cells. However, the overexpression of certain receptors of the family or their ligands confer an oncogenic role to them[12].

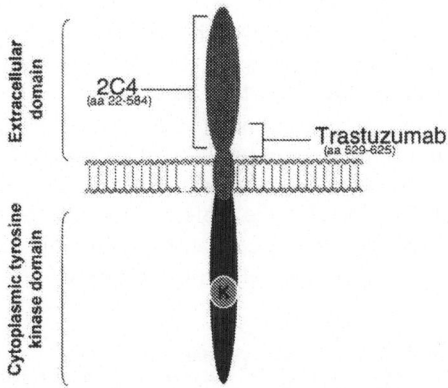

Figure 1. HER2 and binding regions for monoclonal antibodies. HER2 is composed of an extracellular domain and an intracellular domain that has tyrosine kinase activity (K). The epitopes to which the anti-HER2 monoclonal antibodies 2C4 and trastuzumab bind are schematically represented (from Ref. 2).

Mechanisms of HER2 Activation

HER2, like the other receptors of the family, is inactive when is present in a monomeric state. The activation of HER2 requires the formation of dimers or oligomers[13]. There are two mechanisms that might drive the formation of HER2-based dimers, and hence, result in receptor activation (Figure 2).

One mechanism is though to be due to HER2 overexpression (Figure 2). Some tumor cells in culture and from clinical samples have extremely high levels of receptor in the surface, in the order of thousands times more than normal cells, and HER2 is constitutively activated/phosphorylated[14]. Studies with wild-type neu, the rat homologue of human HER2, have shown that when present at high concentrations, neu exists as dimers or multimers[15]. According to this, it is though that when human HER2 is overexpressed, the receptors also form dimers or oligomers of HER2 (homodimerization). This process would be dependent upon the high concentration of receptor at the cell surface and occurs without the need of a receptor ligand. In support of the role of HER2 overexpression in tumorigenesis, it was shown that the introduction of HER2 into non-neoplastic cells causes their malignant transformation[16]. Also, transgenic mice expressing neu develop mammary tumors[17]. From a clinical point of view, HER2 overexpression and activation also occurs in a proportion of human tumors [14]. The most comprehensive studies have been conducted in breast cancer showing that HER2 is overexpressed, most commonly by gene amplification, in 25% to 30% of human breast cancers and predicts for a worse prognosis in patients with primary disease [8]. HER2 overexpression has been also reported in other tumor types such as ovarian, gastric, colon, and non-small cell lung carcinoma, but the results are less consistent to what has been reported in breast cancer[7].

A second mechanism of HER2 activation is the formation of ligand-dependent HER2-based heterodimers (Figure 2). The formation of HER2-based heterodimers relies initially on the binding of a ligand to the HER2 receptor partner[1, 18-20]. Once a ligand binds to EGFR, HER3 or HER4, then the receptor can dimerize with HER2. There is a multiplicity of ErbB receptor ligands that drive the formation of homo- or heterodimeric complexes among the four ErbB receptors. At least six different ligands, known as EGF-like ligands, bind to the EGFR (HER1). These ligands include epidermal growth factor (EGF), transforming growth factor alpha (TGF-α), amphiregulin, heparin binding EGF (HB-EGF), betacellulin, and epiregulin. A second class of ligands, collectively termed neuregulins (also known as neu differentiation factors and neuregulins) bind directly to HER3 and/or HER4. HER2 is the preferred co-receptor for the EGFR, HER3 and HER4. This preference for heterodimerization within the ErbB receptor family explains how HER2 signals in the absence of a cognate ligand [21].

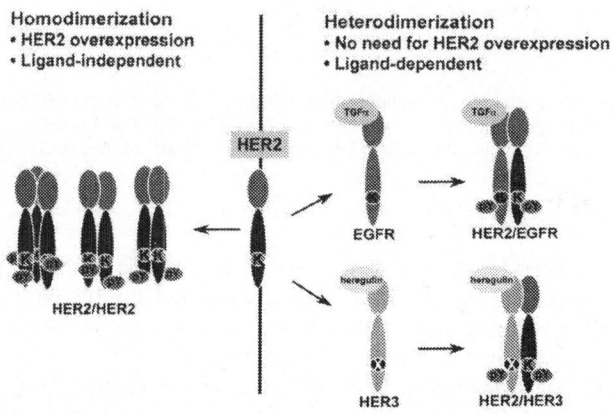

Figure 2. Ligand-independent and ligand-dependent mechanisms of HER2 activation. K = tyrosine kinase; pY denotes the phosphorylation of tyrosine residues that are indicative of receptor activation; X = kinase death domain of HER3. See text for further details.

HER2 is considered the preferred hererodimerization partner of all ErbB receptors[21]. The heterodimers between HER2 and the other ErbB receptors have relatively high ligand affinity, potent signaling activity and are synergistic for cell transformation[22-24]. These features may be related to the ability of HER2 to decelerate the rate of ligand dissociation that would imply a prolonged signaling by all ErbB family ligands. The best example of the ability of HER2 to transactivate signaling initiated by ligands that bind to other ErbB receptors is that the HER2/HER3 heterodimers exhibit an extremely potent mitogenic activity, while HER3 homodimers are inactive[25]. Overall, HER2 is proposed as the master coordinator of the signaling network that functions as a shared co-receptor for ErbB ligands rather than as a receptor that mediates the action of a specific (unidentified) ligand. This mechanism of ligand-dependent HER2 activation could be more general in tumors compared to the one related to HER2 overexpression. Many studies have confirmed the expression of HER2 and other ErbB receptors and their ligands in many tumor types[7]. For instance, HER2 and the EGFR are frequently co-expressed in breast cancer and their overexpression is associated with a more aggressive clinical behaviour. HER3 is overexpressed in about 20% of breast cancers and the frequent co-expression of HER2 and HER3 suggests a role for the heterodimer in carcinogenesis *in vivo*[25].

HER2 Signaling Pathways

Following receptor dimerization, activation of the intrinsic protein tyrosine kinase activity, and tyrosine autophosphorylation occurs[13]. These events lead to activation of a cascade of biochemical and physiological responses that are involved in the regulation of essential cellular functions such as proliferation, survival, angiogenesis and invasion (Figure 3). Each receptor complex may activate different signaling pathways that elicit specific cellular responses, resulting in an enormous signaling diversity. The formation of specific dimeric complexes of ErbB receptors and the consequent stimulation of differential intracellular signaling pathways is viewed as the result of the cellular expression of each receptor and the availability of ligands in each individual cell[22 1].

There are many signaling pathways activated by HER-based dimers, such as Ras-Raf-MAPK, PI3K-Akt, PLC-γ1, Src, STATs and others (Figure 3). One of the best caractherized is the Ras-Raf-MAPK pathway[1]. Activation of Ras initiates a multistep phosphorylation cascade that leads to the activation of MAPKs. The MAPKs ERK1 and ERK2 are activated by dual phosphorylation on a tyrosine and a threonine residue by dual specificity kinases. MAPK subsequently regulates cell transcription and have been linked to cell proliferation, survival and transformation in laboratory studies and more recently in studies in human tumors[26, 27].

Another signaling transduction pathway activated by the HER2 network is the PI3K/Akt pathway that plays an important role in cell survival (Figure 3). Phosphatydilinositol-3 kinase (PI3K) is lipid kinase activated by HER2/HER3 dimers and other receptor complexes that generates phosphorylated phosphoinositides. These phosphorylated lipids then bind and recruit to the cell membrane the proto-oncogene Akt via its pleckstrin homology domain. These events result in activation of Akt kinase activity upon phosphorylation at Thr 308 and Ser 473. Recent evidence indicates that its role in promoting cell survival is critical *in vivo* for tumor development. Akt may also have a role in the control of cell proliferation. As an example, Akt phosphorylates and inhibits glycogen synthase kinase 3, resulting in an increase in cyclin D1 and entry into the cell cycle. HER2 is also an important regulator of CDK inhibitors such as p21[28] and p27[29]. Several studies have also shown that Akt phosphorylates p27 and redirects it to the cytoplasm, thus preventing p27 from acting as a brake to the cell cycle[30-32].

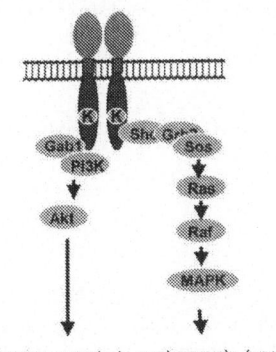

proliferation survival angiogenesis invasion

Figure 3. ErbB receptor activation triggers a series of intracellular signaling pathways that regulate essential cellular processes. Additional pathways not shown in the schema are also regulated by these receptors.

ANTI-HER2 MONOCLONAL ANTIBODIES TARGETING HER2 OVEREXPRESSING CANCER CELLS: FOCUS ON TRASTUZUMAB

Trastuzumab (Herceptin) is a recombinant humanized anti-HER2 MAb directed at the HER2 ectodomain that is active against tumor cells that overexpress HER2[3] (Figure 1). The parental murine version of trastuzumab, the antibody 4D5, was among the most potent antibodies that inhibited the proliferation of cultured breast and ovarion tumor cells overexpressing HER2[2][33]. 4D5 exhibited a clear relationship between the level of HER2 receptor expression and sensitivity to the growth inhibitory effects of the MAb 4D5[33]. In cells with moderate or low expression of HER2, both trastuzumab and 4D5, display little or no antitumor activity. In contrast, these antibodies display a potent antiproliferative effect against tumor cells with high expression of HER2. Trastuzumab has mainly a cytostatic effect in cell culture experiments[3]. However, *in vivo* studies showed that trastuzumab can induce tumor regressions and cures in animals. For instance, trastuzumab has *in vivo* antitumor activity against human breast cancer BT-474 xenografts, that overexpress HER2. Repeated administrations of the antibody given at doses equal to or greater than 1 mg/kg resulted in strong growth suppression and eradication of tumors in a significant proportion of animals[34]. This observation points to the importance of mechanisms of action that only work *in vivo*, such as the induction of antibody-dependent cellular cytotoxicity or by antiangiogenic effects[35,36] (Figure 4).

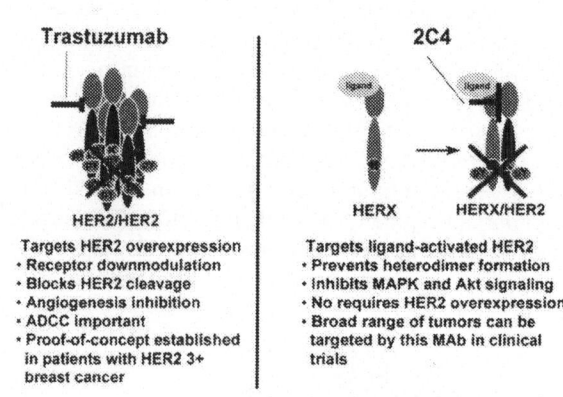

HER2: single target, multiple antibodies

Figure 4. Summary of the mechanism of action of anti-HER2 antibodies trastuzumab and 2C4. HERX = EGFR, HER3 or HER4.

HER2 Downmodulation

A clue for the selective anti-tumor activity of murine 4D5 and trastuzumab against HER2 overexpressing cells seems to be their ability to downmodulate the levels of HER2 at the cell surface. This effect parallels the downmodulation that occurs in other receptor-ligand complexes, which is a major attenuation mechanism for receptor-induced signaling[37]. Although the rate of HER2 downmodulation during exposure to 4D5 or trastuzumab is slow when compared to other receptors such as EGFR[37], a significant removal of HER2 from the plasma membrane takes place during treatment with any of these two antibodies[35,38]. This effect is consistent with the view that trastuzumab or 4D5 lead to the formation of HER2 dimers, especially in cells that overexpress HER2. Such dimers would have a limited capacity for transphosphorylation, resulting in receptor downmodulation but in the absence of effective downstream signaling[35]. The efficiency of HER2 downmodulation by trastuzumab varies among cell lines overexpressing HER2[39], which may relate to the multiple steps that are required for this process[40].

There are two observations that support the importance of HER2 downmodulation in the activity of anti-HER2 MAbs. One is that antibody-induced downregulation of HER2 has been shown to induce reversion of the transformed phenotype in HER2-transformed cells[41]. In another study using a large battery of anti-HER2 antibodies, a relationship between receptor degradation and antitumor effects of anti-HER2 antibodies was observed[42]. The same group showed that a specific ubiquitin ligase involved in this process is c-Cbl, a major substrate of many tyrosine kinases. In their study, an anti-HER2 antibody that inhibits the growth of HER2 overexpressing cells, enhances a Cbl-mediated process of ubiquitination and degradation of HER2[43]. This Cbl-mediated mechanism of receptor downmodulation is similar to the accelerated degradation of EGFR following ligand binding.

Taken together, it is presumed that the removal of HER2 from the plasma membrane reduces the availability of receptor for dimerization, which in turn diminishes the HER2-initiated growth signals. A series of events downstream of the receptor would then follow the antibody-induced HER2 downmodulation (Figure 4).

HER2 Downstream Effects

A series of receptor downstream effects have been reported in cells treated with trastuzumab or 4D5. A recent paper has established that trastuzumab treatment in SKBR3 or BT474 cells, that greatly overexpress HER2 and have HER2 gene amplification, result in the blockade of the two major signaling transduction pathways of HER2, as shown by the inhibition of MAPK and Akt phosphorylation[44]. Interestingly, it takes several hours of exposure to trastuzumab to see these effects and varies among different cell lines. This observation points to the view that it is likely necessary to induce receptor downregulation before the signaling pathways are affected by trastuzumab and supports the notion that trastuzumab does not directly block receptor activation and signaling transduction.

The inhibition of Akt was due to the ability of trastuzumab to uncouple the constitutive association of HER2 with HER3 that occurs in cells that overexpress HER2 and co-express HER3[44]. Akt played a major role in trastuzumab activity since when cells were genetically manipulated to have an activated form of Akt, trastuzumab was without effect[44]. In the same study, cyclin D1 protein levels declined and p27 protein levels increased when cells were exposed to trastuzumab for several hours or days, again depending on the cell line. The increase of p27 levels was predominantly nuclear, thus allowing p27 to inhibit cdk2 activity and cell proliferation. When cells were modified to have low levels of p27, trastuzumab could not inhibit cell growth. In another study, trastuzumab also inhibited p21 activation in breast tumor cell lines that overexpress HER2[39].

Altogether, the effect of trastuzumab on receptor downnmodulation and the resulting consequences on signaling pathways and cell cycle regulatory molecules, causes a cytostatic effect in cultures of tumor cells that overexpress HER2[35, 45]. The sensitivity to the growth inhibitory effects of trastuzumab is highly dependent not only to the presence of HER2 protein overexpression but also to HER2 gene amplification[44]. Cell cycle analysis of cells treated with trastuzumab reveal a partial block in G1 and a reduction of cells undergoing S phase. The induction of apoptosis varies among cell lines[45, 44].

Inhibition of Angiogenesis

Several studies have confirmed that anti-HER2 MAbs have antiangiogenic effects *in vitro* and *in vivo*[46, 47]. The most comprehensive study addressing the effects of trastuzumab on angiogenesis has been recently published[47]. The authors showed in an experimental human breast tumor xenograft model that overexpresses HER2 that trastuzumab induces normalization and regression of the vasculature. Notably, these effects were not dependent on trastuzumab effects on tumor size. By studying the expression of a large number of angiogenesis-related genes using a gene array, it was shown that trastuzumab acted as an anti-angiogenic cocktail. In tumors treated with trastuzumab, there was a reduction in the expression of pro-angiogenic factors such as VEGF (vascular-endothelial growth factor), TGF-α, angiopoitein-1 and plasminogen-activator inhibitor-1, when compared with the expression in control tumors. The expression of the anti-angiogenic factor thrombospondin-1 was increased. These effects are consistent with the role of HER2 on controlling the expression of pro-angiogenic factors, suggesting that the anti-angiogenic effect of trastuzumab is related to the blockade of HER2 signaling pathways.

Inhibition of HER2 Cleavage

An additional property of trastuzumab is the prevention of HER2 cleavage. Cleavage of the HER2 receptor is a regulated, metalloprotease dependent, process in breast cancer cells that results in the production of a soluble fragment that contains the extracellular domain (ECD) and a truncated intracellular fragment with the kinase domain (HER2 p95)[48, 49]. A series of studies indicate that breast cancer cells have the HER2 cleavage machinery ready to act on HER2 well beyond their basal activity and that diverse mechanisms that can have a role *in vivo* (i.e. phosphorylation/dephosphory-lation, metalloprotease activity levels and possibly expression of ErbB ligands) can activate this machinery[38, 48, 50]. A recent study has indicated that trastuzumab inhibits HER2 cleavage. In breast cancer cells, trastuzumab appears to have a direct inhibitory effect on basal and induced HER2 cleavage, likely due to antibody binding to the receptor ectodomain in a way that may hide the cleavage site from the protease responsible for HER2 shedding (Figure 1). Interestingly, the inhibition of HER2 cleavage preceded receptor downmodulation, thus uncoupling the effects of trastuzumab on cleavage from the well characterized effect on receptor plasma levels[38]. It is attractive to hypothesize that this inhibition of HER2 cleavage by trastuzumab may have therapeutic value by preventing the formation of the potentially deletereous truncated HER2 p95 fragments. The potential clinical relevance of this finding is that a HER2 p95 fragment is phosphorylated in human breast cancer tumors. The presence of this fragment is linked to an increase rate of lymph node metastasis[51] and a worse prognosis (manuscript in preparation), further suggesting a role of truncated HER2 in the aggressiveness of breast cancer. A complementary observation is that high serum levels of HER2 ECD, presumably due in part to a high rate of receptor cleavage, correlate with a poor prognosis and decreased responsiveness to endocrine therapy and chemotherapy in patients with advanced breast cancer.

Immunological mechanisms

Trastuzumab triggers antibody-dependent cellular cytotoxicity (ADCC)[3]. ADCC takes place when antibody-coated (opsonized) target cells interact with the Fc receptors that are present on effector immune cells. The activated effector cells destroy they targets by release of cytoplasmic granules that contain perforin and granozymes. As predicted from the IgG1 Fc region of trastuzumab, it was shown in HER2 overexpressing cancer cells that antibody-dependent ADCC was mediated by Fcγ receptors, which are present in effector magrophages, monocytes and natural killer cells[35]. Considering that trastuzumab is bivalent and the concentration of HER2 protein at the cell surface of HER2 overexpressing cells is very high, an avidity component also likely contributes to the near-irreversible binding of trastuzumab to cells that overexpress HER2. Based on this observation, it has been proposed that the trigger of ADCC might be an additional explanation for the selective antitumor action of trastuzumab towards HER2 overexpressing cells compared to cells with low or moderate HER2 expression[35]. Recent evidence has provided support for a substantial role of ADCC in the *in vivo* antitumor activity of trastuzumab[52]. The activity of these antibodies was reduced human breast tumors xenografted in mice lacking Fcγ receptors when compared to wild-type animals. The anti-tumor activity observed in this model showed that trastuzumab retained about 40% of its antitumor activity in mice lacking activating Fcγ receptors, indicating that some of the anti-tumor effect of the antibody *in vivo* is due to biological effects that are independent of Fc receptor, such as the ones that have been described previously[53].

Because trastuzumab contains a human immunoglobulin G1 (IgG1) Fc region, it also activates the human complement cascade. In fact, it has been shown that the binding of trastuzumab to HER2 results in activation of the complement in many human breast cancer cell lines and in *in vitro* systems[35]. Despite this, trastuzumab-induced complement-mediates tumor cell lysis was not observed, possibly due to the presence of membrane-associated complement regulatory proteins[54]. However, neutralization of these proteins sensitized cells to trastuzumab-mediated cell lysis. It was concluded that humanized antibodies like trastuzumab promote complement activation leading to tumor cell phagocytosis and cell- mediated cytotoxicity[54].

Enhancement of chemotherapy activity

Extensive studies showed in the laboratory that anti-HER2 antibodies can markedly enhance or promote sensitivity to the antitumor effects of chemotherapeutic agents such as doxorubicin, paclitaxel, docetaxel, etoposide, cisplatin, to cite a few examples[34, 55]. In *in vivo* models, the combination of various chemotherapeutic agents with trastuzumab has resulted in an enhancement of the tumoricidal effects of chemotherapy and in a striking rate of tumor eradication. Many of these combinations have been tested in the clinic and one of them, trastuzumab plus paclitaxel, has been approved for the treatment of advanced breast cancers that overexpress HER2[56]. The simplest explanation for the enhanced activity of chemotherapy and trastuzumab is that it is the result of the summation of effects of two anticancer drugs that act on different targets; trastuzumab acts on the HER2 receptor signaling pathway and chemotherapy acts on other targest (DNA, tubulin, topoisomerases, etc). However, the magnitude of the enhanced antitumor activity with certain combinations may be well beyond a simple summation of effects. A particular case is the combination of trastuzumab and the anti-tubulin agent paclitaxel. The combination of these two agents was extremely active in human breast tumor xenografts models overexpressing HER2 and, importantly, when trastuzumab and paclitaxel are used in combination in patients with breast cancer it results in increased antitumor activity and prolongs the survival of the patients whose tumors overexpress HER2 [57]. Searching for mechanisms, it has been shown that overexpression of HER2 activates the cyclin dependent kinase inhibitor p21, which inhibits p34^{cdc2} kinase. p34^{cdc2} kinase activation is required for paclitaxel induced apoptosis and overexpression of HER2 blocks paclitaxel-induced apoptosis by inhibiting p34^{cdc2} activation. This finding provides a mechanistic link between HER2 overexpression and paclitaxel resistance[28]. Recently it has been shown that trastuzumab, by downregulating HER2, reduced the inhibitory phosphorylation of Cdc2, and down-regulated the expression of p21(Cip1), a Cdc2 inhibitor. The treatment with trastuzumab thus prevents p21 activation and sensitizes breast cancer cells that overexpress HER2 to paclitaxel-induced apoptosis[39].

Resistance to Trastuzumab

The clinical benefit of trastuzumab is mainly seen in patients whose breast tumors have the highest level of protein expression (i.e. HER2 3+ by immunohistochemistry) or HER2 gene amplification, the mechanism underlying protein overexpression. In such selected patients the response rate to trastuzumab given as a single agent ranges from 18% to 41%, depending on whether trastuzumab was applied in first or second line of treatment and the method (FISH or IHC) used for the analysis. This observation lends to the issue of what are the mechanisms of clinical sensitivity versus resistance in trastuzumab-treated patients with a well defined overexpression/amplification of HER2. Unraveling such mechanisms is of fundamental importance since it would provide clues for specific strategies to prevent or reverse resistance and additional predictive factors for trastuzumab response resulting in an improved selection of patients[58].

Recent studies have started to address this issue. In one study, it was shown a critical role for insulin-like growth factor- I (IGF-I) receptor signaling in trastuzumab response. The IGF-I receptor is a transmembrane tyrosine kinase receptor that is activated by binding of the IGF ligands. The authors elegantly showed that an increased level of IGF-I receptor signaling adversely interferes with trastuzumab action on cell growth[59]. In another study, activation of Akt by gene transfection resulted in resistance to trastuzumab[44]. There are, obviously, many other mechanisms that may interfere with trastuzumab response, such as co-expression of EGF receptor, mutations of downstream molecules (i.e. ras activation, PTEN deletion), HER2 mutations[60], or a low level of p27[11, 44]. As an example, it has been shown that transactivation of HER2 by the closely related EGFR is critical for the growth of HER2 overexpressing breast cancer cells and, as a result, a combined treatment with trastuzumab and inhibitor of the EGFR tyrosine kinase results in enhanced growth inhibition and apoptosis[45]. Another potential marker of resistance is a high serum level of HER2 ectodomain (ECD). As reviewed above, HER2 ECD arises by a regulated metalloprotease-dependent cleavage of the HER2 receptor and soluble HER2 ECDs have the capability to bind to anti-HER2 monoclonal antibodies preventing their binding to full length HER2 at the cell surface. It is plausible that an excess rate of cleavage would result in the sequestering of trastuzumab by HER2 ECD in the serum, thus preventing the antibody to reach the full-length HER2. In this scenario, metalloprotease inhibitors that can prevent HER2 cleavage are envisioned as a possible strategy to reduce HER2 ECD and let trastuzumab to act on cell surface HER2. Finally, *in vivo* resistance to trastuzumab might be also related to a decreased immune function in advanced breast cancer[53].

It is evident that trastuzumab development has been a model of a rationally designed targeted treatment where laboratory predictions have been followed by remarkably successful clinical studies. There are, however, many outstanding biological questions regarding mechanisms of action of trastuzumab and causes of resistance to this antibody. Additional preclinical and clinical studies are clearly warranted in this area. An alternative approach is the development of anti-HER2 antibodies that act differently to trastuzumab against tumor cells that express HER2.

ANTI-HER2 MONOCLONAL ANTIBODIES TARGETING LIGAND-ACTIVATED HER2: FOCUS ON 2C4

Trastuzumab is effective in the treatment of breast cancers with the highest levels of HER2 protein expression or with HER2 gene amplification. However, more that 75% of breast cancers and the majority of many other malignancies, have moderate or low HER2 expression. Many tumors also co-express other receptors of the ErbB family such as the EGFR or HER3, or their ligands. Ligands are commonly produced by stromal cells leading to paracrine mechanisms of receptor activation. In such tumors, HER2 may be activated due to the formation of ligand-dependent heterodimers. While trastuzumab has a poor ability to disrupt the formation of ligand dependent HER2-heterodimers, other anti-HER2 MAbs are useful to block the cross-talk between HER2 and its family members.

ErbB network Cross-talk

To illustrate the rich cross-talk among members of the ErbB network, and especially the importance of ligand-dependent formation of HER2-based heterodimers, it is of interest to recall lessons learned from the use of tyrosine kinase inhibitors of the EGFR (HER1). In particular, several studies showed that the EGFR tyrosine kinase inhibitor ZD1839 (Iressa) inhibited the growth of HER2 overexpressing breast cancer cells[61, 62 61, 63 45]. An apparently surprising observation that accompanied this cell growth effect was that ZD1839 treatment resulted in the blockade of HER2 phosphorylation and ligand-dependent signaling transduction in intact cells, despite that *in vitro* it does not inhibit HER2 tyrosine kinase activity at the concentrations tested. We know now that this paradox is the result, at least in part, of the rich cross-talk within the ErbB network. This view is supported by experiments showing that the exposure of cells to tyrosine kinase inhibitors of the EGFR results in the formation of an array of inactive ErbB dimers that sequester HER2 and HER3[45]. A complementary observation of these studies was that combined treatments with EGFR inhibitors and trastuzumab resulted in increased anti-tumor activity.

Altogether, these studies support that HER2 as a preferred co-receptor within the family. HER2 has an array of signaling activities that depends on the presence of other ErbB receptors and ligands. A collorary to this is that targeting each mechanism (i.e., trastuzumab targets ligand-independent HER2 homodimers and EGFR inhibitors target ligand-dependent HER2-heterodimers) might be therapeutically advantageous. This concept is of practical interest because biological activity of specific EGFR inhibitors has been proved in patients[27, 64] and anti-tumor responses have been achieved [65]. In fact, clinical studies combining EGFR inhibitors and trastuzumab in breast cancer are underway.

2C4 Disrupts Ligand-dependent HER2 Activation

An alternative approach to prevent HER2 ligand-dependent activation is the use of monoclonal antibodies. Furthermore, as seen with trastuzumab, a potential advantage of monoclonal antibodies is that they may have additional *in vivo* effects beyond the interference with the function the role of HER2 as a co-receptor.

Among the antibodies that targets ligand-activated HER2 (i.e. the role of HER2 as a co-receptor), 2C4 is the one in a more advanced stage of clinical development is called. 2C4 targets the extracellular domain of HER2 and sterically hinders HER2 recruitment into ErbB ligand complexes[2, 11, 66, 67] (Figure 1), hence allowing an effective disruption of HER2 ligand dependent activation (Figure 4).

Since the HER3 receptor contains an inactive tyrosine kinase domain and HER2 is a ligand-less receptor, the formation of dimers of HER2/HER3 following addition of the HER3 ligand heregulin is a prerequisite to activate signalling[68]. Therefore, tumor cells that express both receptors are a good model to study the ability of anti-HER2 antibodies to disrupt heregulin-dependent formation of HER2/HER3 dimers and hence to prevent signalling activation. In experiments addressing this question, 2C4 was much more effective in disrupting ligand dependent HER2/HER3 complexes as compared to trastuzumab[11]. A finding of practical importance was that this effect was seen in both low- and high-HER2-expressing systems. When the ability of the two antibodies was assayed in terms of signalling, 2C4 was very effective in blocking heregulin-mediated HER3/HER2 signaling, while trastuzumab was poorly effective. This was concluded from assays that assessed the phosphorylation of HER2, MAPK, Akt and GSK3 (a downstream marker of Akt kinase activity) following a short exposure to ligand and antibodies[11]. 2C4 also blocked TGF-α mediated MAPK activation, indicanting that also interferes with EGFR-based dimers. The short exposure time to the antibodies in such experiments did not allow for trastuzumab-mediated downmodulation and, in consecuence, the results reflect the ability of the antibodies tested to act on ligand-driven signalling. In another study, 2C4 also inhibited ligand dependent activation of signalling transduction pathways in colorectal cancer cells, except for TGF-α mediated MAPK activation[69].

Collectivey, these studies demonstrate that 2C4 and trastuzumab differ greatly in their ability to target the role of HER2 as a co-receptor, being 2C4 much more efficient in the prevention of HER2-based heterodimers (Figure 4). Another difference between trastuzumab and 2C4 is that the later does not prevent HER2 cleavage while trastuzumab blocks this event[38].

2C4 Inhibits the Growth of Tumors with High or Low HER2 Expression

Several studies have investigated the antitumor activity of 2C4 against breast and prostate tumors that do not have high HER2 expression and, therefore, would be not adequate targets for treatment with trastuzumab[11, 67]. In these studies, it has been shown that the *in vitro* and *in vivo* growth of several breast and prostate tumor models is inhibited by 2C4 treatment. The antitumor activity *in vivo* was seen both in tumor xenografts with low or high HER2 expression. In tumor xenografts overexpressing HER2, the antitumor effects of 2C4 or murine 4D5 (the precursor of trastuzumab) was similar. This observation led the authors to propose that 2C4 shares the inhibitory activity of trastuzumab in tumor systems whose growth is driven by ligand-independent HER2 activation[11]. In prostate cancer models, 2C4 was effective in both androgen-dependent and independent tumors[11, 67], supporting a role for this antibody in the treatment of these malignancies. An additional finding was that, in contrast with the important role for ADCC for trastuzumab *in vivo* activity in animal models, monovalent versions of 2C4 that do not have an intact Fc region retain the antitumor potential of the antibody[11]. In another study, 2C4 was also active against lung tumor xenografts[70].

Prospects

2C4, in addition to its activity as a single agent, has potential for studies combining this antibody with other anti-tumor treatments. The different antitumor activities of 2C4 and trastuzumab raised the interest of combination studies (Figure 4). In experiments using co-treatment with 2C4 and trastuzumab, there was an enhanced antitumor activity against breast cancer xenografts in animals treated with both antibodies[70]. 2C4 has been also tested in combination with small molecule ErbB tyrosine kinase inhibitors. As an example, the EGFR tyrosine kinase inhibitor OSI-779 (Tarceva) augmented the antitumor activity of 2C4 against human breast tumor cells that have an autocrine ErbB loop[71]. These result adds to prior ones supporting combined treatments with drugs that target HER2 and EGFR, showing enhanced inhibition of tumor growth in those tumors that co-express both receptors. Studies combining 2C4 with standard chemotherapeutic agents or with other biological agents are also promising.

Given the good preclinical activity of 2C4 and its potential to target a broad range of human tumors, including those with low HER2 expression, the antibody has been humanised for clinical use. Phase I trials have been undertaken and the results are eagerly awaited.

Refences

1. Yarden Y, Sliwkowski MX. Untangling the ErbB signalling network. Nat Rev Mol Cell Biol 2001; 2:127-37.
2. Fendly BM, Winget M, Hudziak RM, Lipari MT, Napier MA, Ullrich A. Characterization of murine monoclonal antibodies reactive to either the human epidermal growth factor receptor or HER2/neu gene product. Cancer Res 1990; 50:1550-1558.
3. Carter P, Presta L, Gorman CM, et al. Humanization of an anti-p185HER2 antibody for human cancer therapy. Proc.Natl.Acad.Sci.USA 1992; 89:4285-4289.
4. Baselga J, Tripathy D, Mendelsohn J, et al. Phase II study of weekly intravenous recombinant humanized anti-p185[HER2] monoclonal antibody in patients with HER2/neu-overexpressing metastatic breast cancer. J.Clin.Oncol 1996; 14:737-744.
5. Cobleigh MA, Vogel CL, Tripathy D, et al. Multinational study of the eficacy and safety of humanized anti-HER2 monoclonal antibody in women who have HER2-overexpressing metastatic breast cancer that has progressed after chemotherapy for metastatic disease. Journal of Clinical Oncology 2000; 17:2639-48.
6. Slamon D, Leyland-Jones B, Shak S, et al. Addition of Herceptin™ (humanized anti-HER2 antibody) to first line chemotherapy for HER2 overexpressing metastatic breast cancer (HER2+/MBC) markedly increases anticancer activity: a randomized, multinational controlled phase III trial. Proc.Am.Soc.Clin.Oncol. 1998.
7. Salomon D, Brandt R, Ciardiello F, Normanno N. Epidermal growth factor-related peptides and their receptors in human malignancies. Crit Rev Oncol Hematol 1995; 19:183-232.
8. Slamon DJ, Clark GM, Wong SG, Levin WJ, Ullrich A, McGuire WL. Human breast cancer: correlation of relapse and survival with amplification of the HER-2/*neu* oncogene. Science 1987; 235:177-182.
9. Slamon DJ, Godolphin W, Jones LA, et al. Studies of the HER-2/neu Proto-oncogene in Human Breast and Ovarian Cancer. Science 1989; 244:707-712.
10. Albanell J, Bellmunt J, Molina R, et al. Node-negative breast cancers with p53(-)/HER2-neu(-) status may identify women with very good prognosis. Anticancer Res. 1996; 16:1027-1032.
11. Agus D, Akita R, Fox W, et al. Targeting ligand-activated ErbB2 signaling inhibits breast and prostate tumor growth. Cancer Cell 2002; 2:127.

12. Olayioye MA, Neve RM, Lane HA, Hynes NE. The ErbB signaling network: receptor hetero-dimerization in development and cancer. Embo J 2000; 19:3159-67.

13. Lemmon MA, Schlessinger J. Regulation of signal transduction and signal diversity by receptor oligomerization. Trends Biochem Sci 1994; 19:459-463.

14. Thor AD, Liu S, Edgerton S, et al. Activation (tyrosine phosphorylation) of ErbB-2 (HER-2/neu): a study of incidence and correlation with outcome in breast cancer. J Clin Oncol 2000; 18:3230-9.

15. Samanta A, LeVea CM, Dougall WC, Qian X, Greene MI. Ligand and p185c-neu density govern receptor interactions and tyrosine kinase activation. Proc Natl Acad Sci U S A 1994; 91:1711-5.

16. Hudziak RM, Schlessinger J, Ullrich A. Increased expression of the putative growth factor receptor p185HER2 causes transformation and tumorigenesis of NIH3T3 cell. Proc.Natl.Acad.Sci.USA 1987; 84:7159-7163.

17. Katsumata M, Okudaira T, Samanta A, et al. Prevention of breast tumour development in vivo by downregulation of the p185neu receptor. Nat Med 1995; 1:644-8.

18. Tzahar E, Waterman H, Chen X, et al. A hierarchical network of interreceptor interactions determines signal transduction by Neu differentiation factor/neuregulin and epidermal growth factor. Mol Cell Biol 1996; 16:5276-5287.

19. Tzahar E, Pinkas-Kramarski R, Moyer JD, et al. Bivalence of EGF-like ligands drives the ErbB signaling network. EMBO J 1997; 16:4938-4950.

20. Klapper LN, Glathe S, Vaisman N, et al. The ErbB-2/HER2 oncoprotein of human carcinomas may function solely as a shared coreceptor for multiple stroma-derived growth factors. Proc.Natl.Acad.Sci.USA 1999; 96:4995-5000.

21. Graus-Porta D, Beerli RR, Daly JM, Hynes NE. ErbB-2, the preferred heterodimerization partner of all ErbB receptors, is a mediator of lateral signaling. Embo J 1997; 16:1647-55.

22. Pinkas-Kramarski R, Soussan L, Waterman H, et al. Diversification of Neu differentiation factor and epidermal growth factor signaling by combinatorial receptor interactions. EMBO J 1996; 15:2452-2467.

23. Pinkas-Kramarski R, Alroy I, Yarden Y. ErbB receptors and EGF-like ligands: cell lineage determination and oncogenesis through combinatorial signaling. J Mammary Gland Biol Neoplasia 1997; 2:97-107.

24. Lenferink AE, Pinkas-Kramarski R, van de Poll ML, et al. Differential endocytic routing of homo- and hetero-dimeric ErbB tyrosine kinases confers signaling superiority to receptor heterodimers. Embo J 1998; 17:3385-97.

25. Alimandi M, Romano A, Curia MC, et al. Cooperative signaling of ErbB3 and ErbB2 in neoplastic transformation and human mammary carcinomas. Oncogene 1995; 10:1813-21.

26. Gee JM, Robertson JF, Ellis IO, Nicholson RI. Phosphorylation of ERK1/2 mitogen-activated protein kinase is associated with poor response to anti-hormonal therapy and decreased patient survival in clinical breast cancer. Int J Cancer 2001; 95:247-54.

27. Albanell J, Codony-Servat J, Rojo F, et al. Activated extracellular signal-regulated kinases: association with epidermal growth factor receptor/transforming growth factor alpha expression in head and neck squamous carcinoma and inhibition by anti- epidermal growth factor receptor treatments. Cancer Res 2001; 61:6500-6510.

28. Yu D, Jing T, Liu B, et al. Overexpression of ErbB2 blocks taxol-induced apoptosis by upregulation of p21^{cip1}, which inhibits p34^{cdc2} kinase. Molecular Cell 1998; 2:581-591.

29. Lane HA, Beuvink I, Motoyama AB, Daly JM, Neve RM, Hynes NE. ErbB2 potentiates breast tumor proliferation through modulation of p27^{Kip1}/Cdk2 complex formation: receptor overexpression does not determine growth dependency. Molecular Cell Biology 2000; 20:3210-3223.

30. Viglietto G, Motti ML, Bruni P, et al. Cytoplasmic relocalization and inhibition of the cyclin-dependent kinase inhibitor p27Kip1 by PKB/Akt-mediated phosphorylation in breast cancer. Nat Med 2002; 8:1136-44.

31. Liang J, Zubovitz J, Petrocelli T, et al. PKB/Akt phosphorylates p27, impairs nuclear import of p27 and opposes p27-mediated G1 arrest. Nat Med 2002; 8:1153-60.

32. Shin I, Yakes FM, Rojo F, et al. PKB/Akt mediates cell-cycle progression by phosphorylation of p27Kip1 at threonine 157 and modulation of its cellular localization. Nat Med 2002; 8:1145-52.

33. Lewis GD, Figari I, Fendly B, et al. Differential responses of human tumor cell lines to anti-p185HER2 monoclonal antibodies. Cancer Immunol Immunother 1993; 37:255-263.

34. Baselga J, Norton L, Albanell J, Kim YM, Mendelsohn J. Recombinant humanized anti-HER2 antibody (Herceptin) enhances the antitumor activity of paclitaxel and doxorubicin against HER2/neu overexpressing human breast cancer xenografts. Cancer Res. 1998; 58:2825-2831.

35. Sliwkowski MX, Logfren JA, Lewis GD, et al. Nonclinical studies addressing the mechanism of action of Trastuzumab (Herceptin®). Semin.Oncol. 1999; 26 (suppl. 12):60-70.

36. Baselga J, Albanell J, Molina MA, Arribas J. Mechanism of action of trastuzumab and scientific update. Semin.Oncol. 2001; 28:4-11.

37. Baulida J, Kraus MH, Alimandi M, Di Fiore PP, Carpenter G. All ErbB receptors other than the epidermal growth factor receptor are endocytosis impaired. J Biol Chem 1996; 271:5251-7.
38. Molina MA, Codony-Servat J, Albanell J, Rojo F, Arribas J, Baselga J. Trastuzumab (herceptin), a humanized anti-Her2 receptor monoclonal antibody, inhibits basal and activated Her2 ectodomain cleavage in breast cancer cells. Cancer Res. 2001; 61:4744-4749.
39. Lee S, Yang W, Lan KH, et al. Enhanced Sensitization to Taxol-induced Apoptosis by Herceptin Pretreatment in ErbB2-overexpressing Breast Cancer Cells. Cancer Res 2002; 62:5703-10.
40. Yarden Y. Biology of HER2 and its importance in breast cancer. Oncology 2001; 61:1-13.
41. Drebin JA, Link VC, Stern DF, Weinberg RA, Greene MI. Down-modulation of an oncogene protein product and reversion of the transformed phenotype by monoclonal antibodies. Cell 1985; 41:695-706.
42. Klapper LN, Vaisman N, Hurwitz E, Pinkas-Kramarski R, Yarden Y, Sela M. A subclass of tumor-inhibitory monoclonal antibodies to ErbB-2/HER2 blocks crosstalk with growth factor receptors. Oncogene 1997; 14:2099-2109.
43. Klapper LN, Waterman H, Sela M, Yarden Y. Tumor-inhibitory Antibodies to HER-2/ErbB-2 May Act by Recruiting c-Cbl and Enhancing Ubiquitination of HER-2. Cancer Res 2000; 60:3384-3388.
44. Yakes FM, Chinratanalab W, Ritter CA, King W, Seelig S, Arteaga CL. Herceptin-induced inhibition of phosphatidylinositol-3 kinase and Akt Is required for antibody-mediated effects on p27, cyclin D1, and antitumor action. Cancer Res 2002; 62:4132-41.
45. Anido J, Albanell J, Rojo F, Codony-Servat J, Arribas J, Baselga J. Inhibition by ZD1839 (Iressa) of Epidermal Growth Factor (EGF) and heregulin Induced signaling pathways in human breast cancer cells. Proc Am Soc Clin Oncol 2001; 20:1712A.
46. Petit AM, Rak J, Hung MC, et al. Neutralizing antibodies against epidermal growth factor and ErbB-2/neu receptor tyrosine kinases down-regulate vascular endothelial growth factor production by tumor cells in vitro and in vivo: angiogenic implications for signal transduction therapy of solid tumors. Am J Pathol 1997; 151:1523-1530.
47. Izumi Y, Xu L, di Tomaso E, Fukumura D, Jain RK. Tumour biology: herceptin acts as an anti-angiogenic cocktail. Nature 2002; 416:279-80.
48. Codony-Servat J, Albanell J, Lopez-Talavera JC, Arribas J, Baselga J. Cleavage of the HER2 ectodomain is a pervanadate-activable process that is inhibited by the tissue inhibitor of metalloproteases-1 in breast cancer cells. Cancer Res. 1999; 59:1196-1201.
49. Christianson TA, Doherty JK, Lin YJ, et al. NH2-terminally truncated HER-2/neu protein: relationship with shedding of the extracellular domain and with prognostic factors in breast cancer. Cancer Res 1998; 15:5123-5129.
50. Albanell J, Molina MA, Codony-Servat J, et al. The production of cleaved intracellular HER2 fragment is inducible in breast cancer cells and this fragment is phosphorylated in breast tumors. Biological Therapy of Breast Cancer 2001; 2:10-13.
51. Molina MA, Saez R, Ramsey EE, et al. NH(2)-terminal truncated HER-2 protein but not full-length receptor is associated with nodal metastasis in human breast cancer. Clin.Cancer Res. 2002; 8:347-353.
52. Clynes RA, Towers TL, Presta LG, Ravetch JV. Inhibitory Fc receptors modulate in vivo cytotoxicity against tumor targets. Nature Med. 2000; 6:443-446.
53. Pegram MD, Baly D, Wirth C, et al. Antibody dependent cell-mediated cytotoxicity in breast cancer patients in Phase III clinical trials of a humanized anti-HER2 antibody (Meeting abstract). Proc Annu Meet Am Assoc Cancer Res 1997; 38:A4044.
54. Jurianz K, Maslak S, Garcia-Schuler H, Fishelson Z, Kirschfink M. Neutralization of complement regulatory proteins augments lysis of breast carcinoma cells targeted with rhumAb anti-HER2. Immunopharmacology 1999; 42:209-18.
55. Pegram M, Hsu S, Lewis G, et al. Inhibitory effects of combinations of HER-2/neu antibody and chemotherapeutic agents used for the treatment of human breast cancers. Oncogene 1999; 18:2241-2251.
56. Ligibel JA, Winer EP. Trastuzumab/chemotherapy combinations in metastatic breast cancer. Semin Oncol 2002; 29:38-43.
57. Slamon DJ, Leyland-Jones B, Shak S, et al. Use of chemotherapy plus a monoclonal antibody against HER2 for metastatic breast cancer that overexpresses HER2. N Engl J Med 2001; 344:783-792.
58. Albanell J, Baselga J. Unraveling resistance to trastuzumab (Herceptin): insulin-like growth factor-I receptor, a new suspect. J.Natl.Cancer Inst. 2001; 93:1830-1832.
59. Lu Y, Zi X, Zhao Y, Mascarenhas D, Pollak M. Insulin-like growth factor-I receptor signaling and resistance to trastuzumab (Herceptin). J Natl Cancer Inst 2001; 93:1852-7.
60. Dugger D, Hollingshead P, Wong D, Romero M, Erickson S, Schwall R. Acquisition of Herceptin [reg] (Trastuzumab) resistance by HER2 mutation in a HER2-transgenic mouse breast cancer. Proc Am Assoc Cancer Res 2002; 43:LB12 (meeting abstract).

61. Moulder SL, Yakes FM, Muthuswamy SK, Bianco R, Simpson JF, Arteaga CL. Epidermal growth factor receptor (HER1) tyrosine kinase inhibitor ZD1839 (Iressa) inhibits HER2/neu (erbB2)-overexpressing breast cancer cells in vitro and in vivo. Cancer Res. 2001; 61:8887-8895.
62. Moasser MM, Basso A, Averbuch SD, Rosen N. The tyrosine kinase inhibitor ZD1839 ("Iressa") inhibits HER2-driven signaling and suppresses the growth of HER2-overexpressing tumor cells. Cancer Res 2001; 61:7184-8.
63. Ye D, Mendelsohn J, Fan Z. Augmentation of a humanized anti-HER2 mAb 4D5 induced growth inhibition by a human-mouse chimeric anti-EGF receptor mAb C225. Oncogene 1999; 18:731-738.
64. Albanell J, Rojo F, Averbuch S, et al. Pharmacodynamic studies of the epidermal growth factor receptor inhibitor ZD1839 in skin from cancer patients: histopathologic and molecular consequences of receptor inhibition. J.Clin.Oncol. 2002; 20:110-124.
65. Baselga J, Rischin D, Ranson M, et al. Phase I Safety, Pharmacokinetic, and Pharmacodynamic Trial of ZD1839, a Selective Oral Epidermal Growth Factor Receptor Tyrosine Kinase Inhibitor, in Patients With Five Selected Solid Tumor Types. J Clin Oncol 2002; 20:4292-4302.
66. Lee H, Akita RW, Sliwkowski MX, Maihle NJ. A naturally occurring secreted human ErbB3 receptor isoform inhibits heregulin-stimulated activation of ErbB2, ErbB3, and ErbB4. Cancer Res 2001; 61:4467-73.
67. Mendoza N, Phillips GL, Silva J, Schwall R, Wickramasinghe D. Inhibition of Ligand-mediated HER2 Activation in Androgen-independent Prostate Cancer. Cancer Res 2002; 62:5485-8.
68. Sliwkowski MX, Schaefer G, Akita RW, et al. Coexpression of erbB2 and erbB3 proteins reconstitutes a high affinity receptor for heregulin. J Biol Chem 1994; 269:14661-14665.
69. Jackson J, St Clair P, Sliwkowski M, Brattain M. Blockade of ErbB2 activation with the anti-ErbB2 monoclonal antibody 2C4 has divergent downstream signaling and growth effects following stimulation by epidermal growth factor or heregulin. Proc Am Assoc Cancer Res 2002; 43:4123a.
70. Lewis-Phillips G, Totpal K, Kang K, Crocker L, Schwall R, Sliwkowski M. In vitro and in vivo efficacy of a novel HER2 antibody, rhuMAb 2C4, on human breast and lung tumor cells. Proc Am Assoc Cancer Res 2002; 43:3556 (meeting abstract).
71. Totpal K, Lewis G, Balter I, Sliwkowski M. Augmentation of rhuMAb2C4 induced growth inhibition by TARCEVA™ the EGFR tyrosine kinase inhibitor on human breast cancer cell line. Proc Am Assoc Cancer Res 2002; 43:3889 (meeting abstract).

EORTC RESEARCH AND DEVELOPMENT: ACHIEVEMENTS AND FUTURE PERSPECTIVES

Denis Lacombe, Assistant Director New Drug Development Program

Ralph Crott, Coordinator Health Economics Unit

Françoise Meunier, Director General

EORTC, Brussels, Belgium

The European Organisation for Research and Treatment of Cancer (EORTC) is an international association under Belgian law. It was established as a cancer research organisation in 1962 by the eminent Belgian cancer expert Professor Henri Tagnon (formerly head of the Institut Bordet, the cancer center of the Free University of Brussels-Belgium) and other leading European oncologists working in the main cancer research institutes and hospitals. It was initially called 'Groupe Européen de Chimiothérapie Anticancéreuse (GECA) and became the European Organisation for Research and Treatment of Cancer (EORTC) in 1968. The main reason to join forces at that time was the perceived need to conduct large-scale clinical studies which were beyond the capacity of individual centers and even national organisations.

The intention was to firmly establish a unique research organisation in Europe to promote and co-ordinate high-quality laboratory research and clinical trials and also to provide a central facility with scientific expertise and administrative support for this network of scientists and clinical investigators. Ahead of its time and ready for the united Europe, the EORTC promoted multidisciplinary cancer research and collaboration with leading biomedical research settings around the world.

The organisation encompasses all aspects of cancer research, from laboratory research and new drug development to large Phase III clinical trials, including also quality of life, health economics, meta-analysis and outcome research.

The EORTC's unique network comprises more than 2,500 scientists and clinicians, all collaborating on a voluntary basis in about 30 multidisciplinary Groups in 32 countries. These Groups organise laboratory research and clinical trials for almost all types of cancers such as breast, gynecological, lung, gastrointestinal, genito-urinary, hematological cancers and others. Overall, there are more than 6,500 new patients with cancer treated each year in EORTC protocols.

The aims of the European Organisation for Research and Treatment of Cancer (EORTC) are to conduct, develop, co-ordinate, and stimulate research in Europe on the experimental and clinical bases of treatment of cancer and related problems.

The ultimate goal of the EORTC is to improve the standard of cancer treatment in Europe, through the development of new drugs and other innovative approaches or modalities, and to test more effective therapeutic strategies, using agents which are

New Trends in Cancer for the 21st Century, edited by
Llombart-Bosch and Felipo, Kluwer Academic/Plenum Publishers, 2003

269

already commercially available, or surgery and radiotherapy. Via laboratory and clinical research, the EORTC offers an integrated approach to drug development as well as to therapeutic strategy programs. Clinical research is accomplished mainly through the execution of large, prospective, randomised, multi-center, cancer clinical trials. In this way, the EORTC facilitates the passage of experimental discoveries into state-of-the-art treatment and minimises the delay between discovery of new active agents and their therapeutic benefit for patients.

DRUG DEVELOPMENT AT EORTC: A CONSTANTLY EVOLVING FIELD

Since 1976 The EORTC has conducted early clinical development studies through various co-operative groups. These groups dedicated to early drug development have been particularly subject to organisational changes in order to adapt to the rapidly changing regulatory requirements of oncology drug development. This has resulted in the establishment of a solid and dedicated network of medical oncologists with focussed expertise in cancer drug development. Through the EORTC network, this expertise has cross–fertilized with the disease/tumor-oriented groups, and also back to the laboratory research groups. Despite the fact that many aspects of clinical research have been completely revisited at the EORTC, it is strongly believed that this approach to drug development is still valid today. The EORTC continues to build on such a networking approach and cross-fertilisation of scientific know-how.

The life threatening character of cancer and the adverse drug reactions inherent to the molecules traditionally used in oncology, have determined the development of these drugs in cancer patients from phase I to phase III. This approach is directed initially at patients with a range of tumor types (in phase I) and then specific tumors (in phase II and III). More recently, the discovery of new targets and signalling pathways have emphasized the importance of defining specific patient populations in novel ways other than histology or site of origin of a tumor. Therefore, drug development in oncology requires close knowledge of this rapidly evolving field.

The role of the EORTC in drug development in Europe has greatly increased over the last 10 years. The results of EORTC studies have been an important part of the registration dossier for several important agents. This was, for example, the case for docetaxel[1,2,3], CPT11[4,5], topotecan[6], ET743 and Glivec which is currently being considered for soft tissue sarcomas. Nevertheless, cancer drug development nowadays has many new features reflecting a more rational approach and greater insight into the mechanism of action of the drugs. This prompted the EORTC to again completely revisit its drug development pathway and operational structures in parallel.

EORTC DRUG DEVELOPMENT PATHWAY

The laboratory and clinical research groups are now linked by translational studies which allow for a swift continuation of scientific activities from pre-clinical testing to clinical research. Increasingly, clinical research projects incorporate relevant laboratory scientific end-points such as pharmacokinetics and pharmacodynamics in close cooperation with the pre-clinical groups, especially the Pharmacology and Molecular Mechanisms (PAMM) Group. This approach also extends to collaboration with the Functional Imaging Group. At a later stage in drug development, phase III trials may be implemented with additional objectives such as quality of life and health economics that are highly relevant in randomised evaluations of new treatments. The EORTC has implemented and validated mechanisms for performing large phase III in cooperation with other European and/or American groups (intergroup studies). The EORTC has taken compounds through from phase I to phase II, as with E7070 and glufosfamide and into phase III trials with docetaxel. This has ensured continuity in the clinical development of these compounds.

EORTC NOVEL APPROACH FOR EARLY DRUG DEVELOPMENT

The EORTC Drug Development strategy is based on four basic policy principles:
- quality of the clinical work and documentation
- speed of patient accrual
- rapid communication within the group and between the group and partners (pharmaceutical industry)
- striving for prioritising innovative treatment concepts.

This can be best achieved by integrating the clinical networks, the EORTC Data Center New Drug Development Program as well as decisional committees such as the New Drug Advisory Committee and the Translational Research Committee, all coordinated by tight working procedures.

THE EORTC NEW DRUG ADVISORY COMMITTEE AND TRANSLATIONAL RESEARCH COMMITTEE

The EORTC New Drug Advisory Committee (NDAC) supports all new drug initiatives within the EORTC. It is composed of medical oncologists with specific expertise in new drug development, chemistry and laboratory research. The mission of NDAC is multifold.
- Stimulate, organize and prioritize new drug acquisition at the EORTC
- Review all Phase I and early phase II study outlines prior to submission to Protocol Review Committee
- Coordinate advisory boards performed for the pharmaceutical industry
- Facilitate and stimulate intergroups studies between new drug developers and EORTC disease oriented groups
- Support EORTC Data Center New Drug Development Program with methodology issues inherent to innovative agents with new mechanism of action in the approach of phase I and early phase II design

The EORTC Translational Research Advisory Committee supports all EORTC initiatives in order to implement the most relevant translational research projects in clinical trials. It offers therefore unique opportunities to combine a high quality network of investigational sites with a network of European research laboratories covering a large range of various expertise.

The missions of TRAC are as follows:
- To provide expert advice on any Translational Research (TR) Project conducted within EORTC both from scientific and practical perspectives.
- To stimulate TR projects either as Side Studies of EORTC clinical trial protocols or as TR projects not linked to a specific EORTC clinical trial (i.e. EORTC Translational Research Fund Program).
- To ensure optimal flow of information between EORTC Laboratory and Clinical Research Divisions.

Specific process of communication between the laboratories and the clinical groups guarantee rapid exchange of information allowing new agents to reach the clinic.

Conversely clinical trials generate biological material to the laboratories in order to document the insight mechanisms of new agents and promote translational research.

Since 1996, almost 2000 patients have been enrolled in phase I and early phase II studies. Over the last 2 years alone the EORTC New Drug Development Group (NDDG) and the New Drug Development Program (NDDP) have initiated about 25 studies which have accrued close to 600 patients. Phase II trials have so far been conducted in 11 different tumor types. The NDDP based at the EORTC Data Center is now structured to give full support to early drug development activities from Phase I to pivotal phase III; from protocol preparation to final publication. The NDDP has designated staff for GCP compliance and documentation handling and received support from the quality assurance unit for day to day management and auditing procedures. Specific working procedures have been created for phase II and phase III trials to encourage collaboration with the disease-oriented groups as part of the new drug development pathway.

Networking of new drug developers and disease specialists has been established in order to ensure a consistent and straightforward development process of new drugs into the therapeutic strategies The example of cooperation with the EORTC Brain Tumor Group (BTG) can best illustrate the potential of such networks. Specific criteria have been applied to identify medical oncologists who have expertise in drug development and brain tumor specialists with experience of assessing efficacy against these tumors to select a limited number of high quality centers. These centers are capable of managing early drug development in brain tumors with close cooperation on site between medical oncologists and neuro-oncologists supported by dedicated clinical research teams. This resulted in the creation of a network (figure 1) which has successfully conducted a series of 4 phase II studies of remarkable quality over a very short period of time.

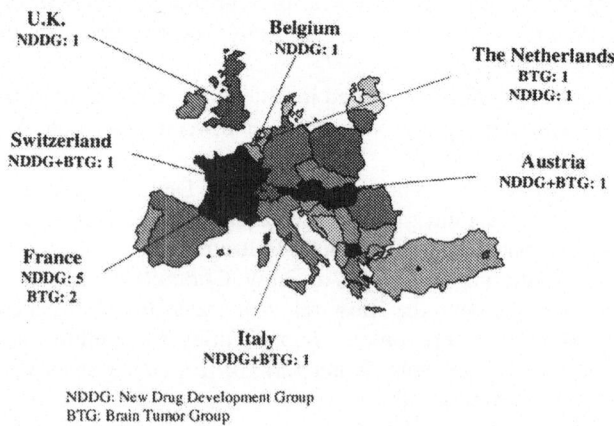

Figure 1. EORTC High Grade Glioma Drug Development Network .

EORTC CLOSELY FOLLOWS THE DEVELOPMENT OF EUROPEAN REGULATORY FRAMEWORK FOR CLINICAL RESEARCH

While cancer research is faced with many potential new drugs to be developed, only a few will reach medical practice after a long and expensive drug development process. This process for conducting clinical trials under current varying national and international requirements has become extremely complex and requires a number of different competencies in a multidisciplinary environment to ensure high quality of science and full compliance to regulatory frameworks.

Therefore drug development and the conduct of clinical trials are more and more expensive and results in high cost for innovative drugs. Cancer is usually treated by agents that may eventually be used in combination with other modalities such as radiotherapy and surgery. Innovative new drugs should be correctly assessed taking into account the full scientific environment and their contribution into the therapeutic arsenal.

Europe urgently needs to be equipped with an optimized network to develop in an objective and independent manner awaited new drugs in life threatening diseases such as cancer. Patients are desperately waiting for better quality of care and improvement in survival and scientists are living a fantastic era where potential new molecules and breakthrough discoveries are more numerous than ever. The challenge consists in investing enormous resources to afford more targeted treatments including for example the recently developed drugs such as Glivec and Herceptin, which threatens health budgets.

In oncology, two types of clinical trials are required: those aiming at bringing new agents from bench into human use, i.e. drug development trials with registration purposes and those aiming at optimizing therapeutic strategies and which include other modalities such as radiotherapy, surgery and others. The context of these two types of trials is completely different and subsequently their conduct raises different concerns. As an example, safety concerns of developing a new agent are not the same as those for optimizing the role of a well-known agent into a therapeutic strategy. Optimal therapeutic strategy addresses major public health issues leading to improvement of standards of care. Regulatory and economically wise, these trials should also be viewed from different angles as they will benefit to patients, scientific community but also to society and health insurance as they lead to optimized use of resources and funds.

A recent article[7] showed that, for 12 new cancer drugs approved in Europe between 1995-2000 by the EMEA, the cost per single cycle taking only into account the drug costs, ranged from twice up to 350 times the cost of the (older) reference drug.

Although drug costs are only part of the total cost of a cancer therapy (typically between 15% and 30%), such high prices for new drugs can have a large impact on the already stretched health care budgets, whether national, regional or at the institutional level.

Furthermore over their life-cycle the use of (new) anticancer drugs (when successful) is generally shifting from late stage and/or second –third line indications towards first line or earlier stage use, thereby exacerbating the financial impact.
A case in point is the current thinking about chemoprevention in early stages for a number of (new) drugs in breast and colorectal cancer.

A major point that is often forgotten is that, within fixed or at least constrained health care budgets, a careful assessment is required on the balance between the clinical benefits of new treatment strategies and their cost for the health care system and patients.

Despite some attempts in a selected number of instances to take economic aspects into consideration, most market authorization decisions are made in an ideal world in which there are no financial limits and where the economic and budgetary impact of those decisions are not forecasted neither assessed ex-post.

The consequence is that often new approved drugs can only be afforded by a (wealthy) minority of patients or that they are allocated in practice according to some (mostly hidden or implicit) rationing scheme (first come-first served, postcode rationing, etc..).

There is therefore a need for an independent and continuous clinical-economic evaluation of new therapies before (usually at the phase III development stage) and after market authorization not only at the national level but also at the local institutional level in daily practice in order to establish their cost-effectiveness.

The EORTC through its Health Economics Unit has been involved since 1996 in assessing the economics of new treatments in parallel with European-wide clinical trials[8].

Public health authorities should also muster up the political will to revise previous reimbursement decisions if the promises (clinical and economic) seen in the trial phase are not supported by observational evidence in real practice by well conducted phase IV studies, so as to weed out less effective therapies.

A major impediment to such an undertaking is the lack in Europe (both at national and at European level) of public health funding organizations that would have the resources to fund such independent studies.

Sponsors are also faced with increased costs for drug development which may be generated by ill-delineated regulatory frameworks, and while sponsors and society need an easier system to select candidate drugs in an independent way, regulations keep being more and more complex, such as the new directive for clinical research in Europe, without guaranty for harmonization of the legal framework throughout Europe. The implementation of the directive by national authorities may create major obstacles to independent pan European evaluations of drugs but may even lead to a split between drug trials and other therapeutic strategies at a time when only multidisciplinary approach of cancer research will lead to therapeutic benefits and change of practice. Such evaluations can only be best performed by recognized independent academic research networks, which should be unique partners to sponsors and society in such decision process from Phase I to marketing authorization.

While academic networks are constantly evolving toward international standards guaranteeing high quality clinical research, their role in this process should be better recognized[9]. It also allows addressing and developing new methodologies as the understanding of the processes of cell division and growth is constantly evolving with the support of molecular research.

This leads to the development of new drugs which may no longer lead to cytotoxicity but to agents which will be integrated in treatment strategies such as cytostatics. Therefore there is a need to revisit appropriate end-points on which decision rules are made to take a potential new drug any further. New study templates, designs and appropriate statistical methodology need to be validated and conducted by highly knowledgeable networks supported by research methodologists to ensure that the appropriate decision is taken.

The EORTC network for brain tumors described above can also be shown as an example of networks of excellence which have developed standard procedures to screen new drugs in an efficient manner independently from the industry. This constitutes a unique European setting which allows to eventually select promising new drugs and evaluate them taking into account the full scientific standards for best positioning.

Time has come for society to revisit its modus operandi for leading effective innovative agents to all patients. At a time when budget constraints and tight regulations are streamlining strategies for drug developments, more effective ways should be explored to evaluate all possible new candidate anti cancer agents that are emerging due to the revolution of molecular biology. This is the challenge to translate cancer research into practice in the coming years.

FUTURE DIRECTIONS

The tremendous increase in our understanding of tumor cell biology coming from molecular research in the laboratory, creates the need to review trial design and analysis as well as study performance.

The traditional approach of defining the maximum tolerated dose (MTD) and dose limiting toxicities (DLT) may not be valid in trials of novel biological or cytostatic agents given on a chronic basis. There is increasing emphasis on "proof of principle" and identifying a biologically active drug dose. New end-points have to be established and validated, on which "stop/go" decision can reliably be based. The NDDP is currently exploring modified versions of the continuous reassessment method. This allows a 3 stage phase I design implementing an efficient dose escalation process at the lower dose levels, a safe approach as the highest dose levels and information on chronic administration. These methodologies are oriented to the clinic as safety observations are fed back into the models, which subsequently determine the next dose level. The role of clinical investigators in assessing the relationship between adverse events and the study drug is, therefore of the highest importance. In parallel, the EORTC has developed software where such algorithms are taken on board to allow rapid but safe assessment of increasing dose levels. In a similar approach, more appropriate designs and end-points are being tested for phase II trials of novel agents. Brain tumors are again a good example where tumor shrinkage is not the only criterion for a drug to be of potential clinical importance. Indeed, in such aggressive tumors, stabilisation of tumor growth is of considerable clinical interest. This emphasizes the need for new approaches that not only challenge the definition of "positive" outcomes in a phase II trial but may allow biological activity to be confirmed as part of initial trials rather than in the sequential phase I/phase II model.

References

1. Dieras V., Chevallier B., Kerbrat P.; et al. A multicenter phase II study of docetaxel 75 mg/m² as first line chemotherapy for patients with advanced breast cancer: report of the Clinical Screening Group of the EORTC. European Organisation for Research and Treatment of Cancer. Br. J. Cancer. 1996 Aug; 74(4): 650-6.
2. Fumoleau P., Chevallier B., Kerbrat P., et al. A multicenter phase II study of the efficacy and safety of docetaxel as first-line treatment of advanced breast cancer: report of the Clinical Screening Group of the EORTC. Ann. Oncol. 1996 Feb;7(2):165-71.
3. Chevallier B., Fumoleau P., Kerbrat P., et al. Docetaxel is a major cytotoxic drug for the treatment of advanced breast cancer: a phase II trial of the Clinical Screening Cooperative Group of the European Organisation for Research and Treatment of Cancer. J; Clin. Oncol. 195 Feb; 13(2)314-22.
4. Lhomme C., Fumoleau P., Fargeot P., et al. Results of a European Organisation for Research and Treatment of Cancer/Early Clinical Studies Group phase II trial of first-line irinotecan in patients with advanced or recurrent squamous cell carcinoma of the cervix. J.Clin. Oncol. 1999 Oct;17(10):310-42.
5. Wagener D.J.Th., Verdonk H.E.R., Dirix L.Y., Catimel G., Siegenthaler P., Buitenhuis M., Mathieu-Boué A. and Verweij J. Phase II trial of CPT-11 in patients with advanced pancreatic cancer, an EORTC Early Clinical Trials Group study. Ann. Oncol. 6: 129-132, 1995.
6. Creemers G.J., Wanders J., Calabresi F., Valentin S., Dirix L.Y., Schöffksi P., Franklin H., McDonald M., and Verweij J. Topotecan in colorectal cancer: a phase II study of the EORTC Early Clinical Trials Group. Ann. Oncol. 6:844-846,1995
7. Garattini S., Bertele V. Efficacy, Safety and Costs of New Cancer drugs, BMJ, vol 325, 3 Aug 2002, 269-271.

8. Crott R., Neymark N. (editors). Economics of Cancer, Special Issue, EJC, Sept 2001, vol 37, No 14.,1729-1804.
9. 40 Years of Excellence in Developing New Standards of Cancer Care, EJC Supplement, March 2002, vol 38, Suppl 1.,S1-178.

For more information on EORTC; website: http://www.eortc.be

CONTRIBUTORS

ALBANELL, J.
ICMHO
Laboratory of Oncology Research
Medical Oncology Service
Hospital Clinic I Provincial
Barcelona
Spain

ANDRE, F.
ERIT-M 02-08 INSERM
Department of Clinical Biology
Institut Gustave Roussy (IGR)
94805 Villejuif,
France

BALBÍN, M.
Departamento de Bioquímica
Instituto Universitario de Oncología
Universidad de Oviedo
33006-Oviedo
Spain

BARBACID, M.
Molecular Oncology Progamme
Centro Nacional de Investigaciones
Oncológicas
Madrid
Spain

BARBERA GUILLEM, E.
1555 Picardae Court
Powell, OH 43065
USA

BECKERM K.
Institut für Pathologie
Technische Univeristät München
GSF-Forschungszentrum für Umwelt
Gesundheit Neuherberg
Germany

CAO, Y.
Microbiology and Tumor Biology Center
Karolinska Institutet
S-171 77 Stockholm
Sweden

CHAPUT, N
ERIT-M 02-08 INSERM
Department of Clinical Biology
Institut Gustave Roussy (IGR)
94805 Villejuif,
France

CODONY, J.
ICMHO
Laboratory of Oncology Research
Medical Oncology Service
Hospital Clínic i Provincial
Barcelona
Spain

CROTT, R.
Coordinator Health Economics Unit
EORTC
Brussels
Belgium

DUBUS, P.
University of Bourdeaux
Bourdeaux
France

ELLIS, M. J.
Duke University Breast Cancer Program
Duke University Medical Center, DUMC
PO Box 3446,
Durham, NC 27710
USA

ESTELLER, M.
Cancer Epigenetics Laboratory
Spanish National Cancer Center (CNIO)
28029 Madrid
Spain

FREIJE, J. M. P.
Departamento de Bioquímica
Instituto Universitario de Oncología
Universidad de Oviedo
33006-Oviedo
Spain

GASCON, P.
ICMHO
Laboratory of Oncology Research
Medical Oncology Service
Hospital Clínic i Provincial
Barcelona
Spain

GEORGE, D.
Dana-Farber Cancer Institute
Boston, MA
USA

GRIFFIN, J. D.
Department of Medical Oncology
Dana-Farber Cancer Institute
Boston, Massachusetts 02115
USA

GRÜNWALD, V.
The Sidney Kimmel Comprehensive
Cancer Center at Johns Hopkins
Baltimore, MD
USA

HANASH, S. M.
Department of Pediatrics
Comprehnsive Cancer Center
University of Michigan
Ann Arbor 48109-0944
USA

HIDALGO, M.
The Sidney Kimmel Comprehensive
Cancer Center at Johns Hopkins
Baltimore, MD
USA

HÖFLER, H.
Institut für Pathologie
Technische Univeristät München
Trogerstrasse 18
D-81675 München
Germany

HUNT, S.L.
Molecular Oncology Progamme
Centro Nacional de Investigaciones
Oncológicas
Madrid
Spain

KOVAR, H.
Children's Cancer Research Institute
St. Anna Kinderspital
Vienna
Austria

LACOMBE, D.
Assistant Director New Drug
Development Program
EORTC
Brussels
Belgium

LI, J. J.
Division of Etiology & Prevention of
Hormonal Cancers
Department of Pharmacology, Toxicology
and Therapeutics
University of Kansas Medical Center
Kansas City, KS 66160-7417
USA

LI, S. A.
Division of Etiology & Prevention of
Hormonal Cancers
Department of Pharmacology, Toxicology
and Therapeutics
University of Kansas Medical Center
Kansas City, KS 66160-7417
USA

LIOTTA, L.
FDA/NCI Clinical Proteomics Program
Laboratory of Pathology
Center for Cancer Research
National Cancer Institute
Bethesda, MD 20892
USA

LOPEZ-OTIN, C.
Departamento de Bioquímica
Instituto Universitario de Oncología
Universidad de Oviedo
33006-Oviedo
Spain

MADOZ-GURPIDE, J.
Department of Pediatrics
Comprehnsive Cancer Center
University of Michigan
Ann Arbor 48109-0944
USA

MALUMBRES, M.
Molecular Oncology Progamme
Centro Nacional de Investigaciones
Oncológicas
Madrid
Spain

MANEGOLD, C.
Thoraxklinik-Heidelberg gGmbH
69126 Heidelberg
Germany

MARTÍN, A.
Molecular Oncology Progamme
Centro Nacional de Investigaciones
Oncológicas
Madrid
Spain

MARTÍN, J.
Molecular Oncology Progamme
Centro Nacional de Investigaciones
Oncológicas
Madrid
Spain

MASFERRER, J. L.
Science Fellow, Pharmacia Corporation
700 Chesterfield parkway
St. Louis MO 63017
USA

MELLADO, B.
ICMHO
Laboratory of Oncology Research
Medical Oncology Service
Hospital Clínic i Provincial
Barcelona
Spain

MEUNIER, F.
Director General
EORTC
Brussels
Belgium

ODAJIMA, J.
Molecular Oncology Progamme
Centro Nacional de Investigaciones
Oncológicas
Madrid
Spain

ORTEGA, S.
Molecular Oncology Progamme
Centro Nacional de Investigaciones
Oncológicas
Madrid
Spain

PAWELETZ, C. P.
FDA/NCI Clinical Proteomics Program
Laboratory of Pathology
Center for Cancer Research
National Cancer Institute
Bethesda, MD 20892
USA

PENDAS, A. M.
Departamento de Bioquímica
Instituto Universitario de Oncología
Universidad de Oviedo
33006-Oviedo
Spain

PETRICOIN III, E. F.
FDA/NCI Clinical Proteomics Program
Center for Biologics Evaluation and
Research
Food and Drug Administration
Bethesda, MD 20892
USA

PUENTE, X. S.
Departamento de Bioquímica
Instituto Universitario de Oncología
Universidad de Oviedo
33006-Oviedo
Spain

ROVIRA, A.
ICMHO
Laboratory of Oncology Research
Medical Oncology Service
Hospital Clínic i Provincial
Barcelona
Spain

SAMPSEL, J. W.
860 W4th st.
Marysville, OH 43040
USA

SANCHEZ, L. M.
Departamento de Bioquímica
Instituto Universitario de Oncología
Universidad de Oviedo
33006-Oviedo
Spain

SATTLER, M.
Professor of Medicine
Harvard Medical School
Department of Adult Oncology
Dana-Farber Cancer Institute
Boston, Massachusetts 02115
USA

SCHARTZ, N.
ERIT-M 02-08 INSERM
Department of Clinical Biology
Institut Gustave Roussy (IGR)
94805 Villejuif,
France

SCHEIJEN, B.
Department of Medical Oncology
Dana-Farber Cancer Institute
Boston, Massachusetts 02115
USA

SCHIRRMACHER, V.
German Cancer Research Center
Division of Cellular Immunology
D-69120 Heidelberg
Germany

SERRANO, M.
Departamento de Inmunología y
Oncología
Centro Nacional de Biotecnología
Campus de Cantoblanco
28049 Madrid

SOTILLO, R.
Molecular Oncology Progamme
Centro Nacional de Investigaciones
Oncológicas
Madrid
Spain

SPECHT, K.
Institut für Pathologie
Technische Univeristät München
GSF-Forschungszentrum für Umwelt
Gesundheit Neuherberg
Germany

STEEG, P. S.
Women's Cancers Section
Laboratory of Pathology
Center for Cancer Research
National Cancer Institute
Bethesda, MD 20892
USA

WEISBERG, E.
Department of Medical Oncology
Dana-Farber Cancer Institute
Boston, Massachusetts 02115
USA

WULFKUHLE, J. D.
FDA/NCI Clinical Proteomics Program
Laboratory of Pathology
Center for Cancer Research
National Cancer Institute
Bethesda, MD 20892
USA

ZITVOGEL, L.
ERIT-M 02-08 INSERM
Department of Clinical Biology
Institut Gustave Roussy (IGR)
94805 Villejuif,
France